Essentials of Clinical Surgery

Pocket Essentials

Series Editors

Professor Parveen Kumar

Professor of Clinical Medical Education, Barts and the London, Queen Mary's School of Medicine and Dentistry, University of London, and Honorary Consultant Physician and Gastroenterologist, Barts and the London Hospitals NHS Trust and Homerton University Hospital NHS Foundation Trust, London, UK

and

Dr Michael Clark

Honorary Senior Lecturer, Barts and the London, Queen Mary's School of Medicine and Dentistry, University of London, UK

For Elsevier
Commissioning Editor: **Pauline Graham**
Development Editor: **Ailsa Laing**
Project Manager: **Sruthi Viswam**
Designer: **Miles Hitchen**
Illustration Manager: **Jennifer Rose**
Illustrators: **Paul Banville, Gillian Lee and Barking Dog**

Essentials of Clinical Surgery

Second Edition

IAN J. FRANKLIN
MS FRCS(GenSurg)
Consultant Surgeon, Imperial College Healthcare NHS Trust,
London, Honorary Consultant Surgeon, West Middlesex
University Hospital, London and Honorary Clinical Senior Lecturer,
Faculty of Medicine, Imperial College, London

PETER M. DAWSON
MS FRCS
Consultant Surgeon, Imperial College Healthcare NHS Trust,
London, Honorary Consultant Surgeon, West Middlesex
University Hospital, London and Honorary Clinical Senior Lecturer,
Faculty of Medicine, Imperial College, London

ALEXANDER D. RODWAY
MD FRCS(GenSurg)
Senior Specialist Registrar, Imperial College Healthcare
NHS Trust, London

SERIES EDITORS

PARVEEN KUMAR and MICHAEL CLARK

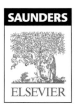

Edinburgh   London   New York   Oxford
Philadelphia   St Louis   Sydney   Toronto   2012

SAUNDERS
ELSEVIER

© 2012 Elsevier Ltd. All rights reserved.

No part of this publication may be reproduced or transmitted in any form or by any means, electronic or mechanical, including photocopying, recording, or any information storage and retrieval system, without permission in writing from the publisher. Details on how to seek permission, further information about the Publisher's permissions policies and our arrangements with organizations such as the Copyright Clearance Center and the Copyright Licensing Agency, can be found at our website: www.elsevier.com/permissions.

This book and the individual contributions contained in it are protected under copyright by the Publisher (other than as may be noted herein).

First edition 2008
Second edition 2012
ISBN 9780702043628

British Library Cataloguing in Publication Data
A catalogue record for this book is available from the British Library

Library of Congress Cataloging in Publication Data
A catalog record for this book is available from the Library of Congress

Notices
Knowledge and best practice in this field are constantly changing. As new research and experience broaden our understanding, changes in research methods, professional practices, or medical treatment may become necessary.

Practitioners and researchers must always rely on their own experience and knowledge in evaluating and using any information, methods, compounds, or experiments described herein. In using such information or methods they should be mindful of their own safety and the safety of others, including parties for whom they have a professional responsibility.

With respect to any drug or pharmaceutical products identified, readers are advised to check the most current information provided (i) on procedures featured or (ii) by the manufacturer of each product to be administered, to verify the recommended dose or formula, the method and duration of administration, and contraindications. It is the responsibility of practitioners, relying on their own experience and knowledge of their patients, to make diagnoses, to determine dosages and the best treatment for each individual patient, and to take all appropriate safety precautions.

To the fullest extent of the law, neither the Publisher nor the authors, contributors, or editors, assume any liability for any injury and/or damage to persons or property as a matter of products liability, negligence or otherwise, or from any use or operation of any methods, products, instructions, or ideas contained in the material herein.

Printed in China

Series Preface

Medical students and doctors in training are expected to travel to different hospitals and community health centres as part of their education. Many books are too large to carry around, but the information they contain is often vital for the basic understanding of disease processes.

The *Pocket Essentials* series is designed to provide portable, pocket-sized companions for larger texts like our own *Kumar & Clark's Clinical Medicine*. They are most useful for clinical practice, whether in hospital or the community, and for exam revision.

All the books in the series have the same helpful features:
- succinct text
- simple line drawings
- emergency and other boxes
- tables that summarise causes and clinical features of disease
- examination questions and answers.

They contain core material for quick revision, easy reference and practical management. The modern format makes them easy to read, providing an indispensable 'pocket essential'.

Parveen Kumar and Michael Clark
Series Editors

Acknowledgements

The authors acknowledge with thanks the many figures and tables in this book which are drawn from Henry and Thompson's *Clinical Surgery*, 2nd edn (Saunders 2005, ISBN: 0-7020-2719-7, ISBN 13: 978-0-7020-2719-2). Intended as a companion to that text, our own is considerably enriched by the inclusion of these materials.

Preface

This book is written primarily as a practical reference/aide-mémoire for medical students, foundation doctors and surgical trainees that can be carried in the pocket or on a PDA file while they are 'on the job' treating surgical patients. The emphasis of the book is on the general surgical take for those on call, providing a knowledge base for conditions that occur frequently in the emergency setting. The principles of the common general surgical operations are given along with practical procedures used in everyday surgical practice. The second edition has been revised and updated using the same principles as the first. The chapter on critical care has been rewritten by Alex Rodway in line with modern trauma management principles. Senior students may find the book useful as an overview of surgery in general, fulfilling most of the requirements of membership of the Royal College of Surgeons. The book is intended to be used as a companion to Henry and Thompson's *Clinical Surgery* which provides a more detailed background to the topics.

We have not attempted to explain operative techniques in detail but rather the principles that a trainee can expect to see and understand while assisting senior colleagues at common operations in each specialty. To give the book unity, we have adopted, as far as possible, standard headings for each of the conditions described with box format headings where lists of differential diagnoses or symptoms are necessary.

We are indebted to all those who assisted at various stages in the preparation of the text, in particular the series editors Parveen Kumar and Mike Clark, whose feedback, experience and insights were invaluable. We are also grateful to the contributing authors of *Clinical Surgery* and to Mrs Isabella Karat for additional contributions to the text. Finally, we thank the staff of Elsevier for their expertise in transforming the manuscript into a beautifully produced volume.

Feedback from readers is greatly appreciated.

We hope you enjoy this book, use it frequently, make notes on it and find it a helpful and friendly companion for your surgical studies and practice.

IJF
PMD
ADR
London

Contents

SECTION 4: Practical skills in surgery

SECTION 5: Self-assessment

Abbreviations

AAA	abdominal aortic aneurysm
ABG	arterial blood gas
ABPI	ankle–brachial pressure index
AC	acromioclavicular
ACL	anterior cruciate ligament
ACTH	adrenocorticotrophic hormone
ADH	antidiuretic hormone
A&E	accident and emergency
AFP	alpha-fetoprotein
ALP	alkaline phosphatase
ALS	advanced life support
AMD	age-related macular degeneration
APTR	activated prothrombin time ratio
APUD	amine precursor uptake and decarboxylation
ARDS	acute respiratory distress syndrome
ARF	acute renal failure
ARMD	age-related macular degeneration
ASA	American Society of Anesthesiologists
ATLS	advanced trauma life support
AXR	abdominal X-ray
BLS	basic life support
BMI	body mass index
BP	blood pressure
2,3-BPG	2,3-biphosphoglycerate
BPH	benign prostatic hyperplasia
CA125	carcinoma antigen 125
CABG	coronary artery bypass grafting
CAD	coronary artery disease
CCK	cholecystokinin
CEA	carcinoembryonic antigen
CJD	Creutzfeldt–Jakob disease
CLI	critical limb ischaemia
CMV	cytomegalovirus
CNS	central nervous system
COPD	chronic obstructive pulmonary disease
CRF	chronic renal failure
CRP	C-reactive protein

CSF	cerebrospinal fluid
CT	computed tomography
CTA	CT angiography
CTU	CT urogram
CVP	central venous pressure
CXR	chest X-ray
DCIS	ductal carcinoma in situ
DDH	developmental dysplasia of the hip
DIC	disseminated intravascular coagulation
DNA	deoxyribonucleic acid
DPL	diagnostic peritoneal lavage
DSA	digital subtraction angiography
DU	duodenal ulcer
DVT	deep vein thrombosis
DXT	radiotherapy
EBV	Epstein–Barr virus
ECG	electrocardiogram
EMR	endo-mucosal resection
ENT	ear, nose and throat
ER	(o)estrogen receptor
ERCP	endoscopic retrograde cholangiopancreatography
ESR	erythrocyte sedimentation rate
EUA	examination under anaesthesia
EVAR	endovascular aneurysm repair
FAST	focused assessment with sonography for trauma
FB	foreign body
FBC	full blood count
FEV_1	forced expiratory volume in the first second
FFP	fresh frozen plasma
FiO_2	fractional concentration of oxygen in inspired gas
FNA	fine-needle aspiration
FNAC	fine-needle aspiration cytology
FSH	follicle-stimulating hormone
FVC	forced vital capacity
GA	general anaesthetic
GI	gastrointestinal
GRH	gonadotrophin-releasing hormone
GORD	gastro-oesophageal reflux disease
G&S	group and save serum
GTN	glyceryl trinitrate
GU	(1) genitourinary; (2) gastric ulcer
Hb	haemoglobin
HBV	hepatitis B virus
HCG	human chorionic gonadotrophin
HCL	hydrochloric acid

HCV	hepatitis C virus
HDU	high-dependency unit
HER2	human epidermal growth factor receptor 2
HIV	human immunodeficiency virus
HLA	human leucocyte antigen
HNPCC	hereditary non-polyposis colorectal cancer
HRS	hepatorenal syndrome
HRT	hormone replacement therapy
IC	intermittent claudication
ICP	intracranial pressure
INR	international normalised ratio
IHD	ischaemic heart disease
IL	interleukin
ITU	intensive therapy unit
IUCD	intrauterine contraceptive device
IV	intravenous
IVI	intravenous infusion
IVU	intravenous urogram
JVP	jugular venous pressure
LA	local anaesthetic
LATS	long-acting thyroid stimulators
LCIS	lobular carcinoma in situ
LFT	liver function test
LH	luteinising hormone
LHRH	luteinising hormone-releasing hormone
LIF	left iliac fossa
LMWH	low-molecular-weight heparin
LSV	long saphenous vein
LUTS	lower urinary tract symptoms
MAP	mean arterial pressure
MC&S	microscopy, culture and sensitivity
MDT	multidisciplinary team
MEN	multiple endocrine neoplasia
MHC	major histocompatibility complex
MI	myocardial infarction
MRA	magnetic resonance angiography
MRI	magnetic resonance imaging
MRSA	methicillin-resistant *Staphylococcus aureus*
MSU	midstream urine
NAI	non-accidental injury
NICE	National Institute for Health and Clinical Excellence
NSAID	non-steroidal anti-inflammatory drug
NSAP	non-specific abdominal pain
NSTEMI	non-ST elevation MI
OA	osteoarthritis

OGD	oesophago-gastro-duodenoscopy
OPSI	overwhelming post-splenectomy infection
PaCO$_2$	partial pressure of carbon dioxide in arterial blood
PaO$_2$	partial pressure of oxygen in arterial blood
PCA	patient-controlled analgesia
PCL	posterior cruciate ligament
PCO$_2$	partial pressure of carbon dioxide
PE	pulmonary embolism
PEEP	positive end-expiratory pressure
PEG	percutaneous endoscopic gastrostomy
PET	positron emission tomography
PID	pelvic inflammatory disease
PO$_2$	partial pressure of oxygen
PPI	proton pump inhibitor
PR	per rectum, progesterone receptor
PSA	prostate specific antigen
PTA	percutaneous transluminal angioplasty
PTC	percutaneous transhepatic cholangiography
PTCA	percutaneous transluminal coronary angioplasty
PTH	parathyroid hormone
PTS	post-thrombotic syndrome
PUJ	pelviureteric junction
RA	rheumatoid arthritis
RCC	renal-cell carcinoma
Rh	rhesus
RIF	right iliac fossa
RLN	recurrent laryngeal nerve
RNA	ribonucleic acid
RRT	renal replacement therapy
RTA	road traffic accident
SCID	severe combined immune deficiency
SIADH	syndrome of inappropriate secretion of ADH
SIRS	systemic inflammatory response syndrome
SNS	sacral nerve stimulation
SUFE	slipped upper femoral epiphysis
SVR	systemic vascular resistance
T$_3$	triiodothyronine
T$_4$	thyroxine
TAAA	thoracoabdominal aortic aneurysm
TAVI	transcatheter aortic valve implantation
TB	tuberculosis
TCC	transitional cell carcinoma
TEMS	trans-anal endoscopic microsurgery
TEVAR	thoracic endovascular aortic repair
TFT	thyroid function test

THD	transanal haemorrhoid dearterialisation
TIA	transient ischaemic attack
TNF	tumour necrosis factor
TNM	tumour, node, metastasis
TPN	total parenteral nutrition
TSH	thyroid-stimulating hormone
TUR	transurethral resection
TURP	transurethral resection of prostate
TURBT	transurethral resection of bladder tumour
U&E	urea and electrolytes
UGIH	upper GI haemorrhage
UICC	International Union Against Cancer
USS	ultrasound scanning
UTI	urinary tract infection
VEGF	vascular endothelial growth factor
VIP	vasoactive intestinal peptide
VMA	vanillylmandelic acid
WBC	white blood cell count

Section 1

Introduction

Surgery is not just about the operation and technical expertise. It includes expert skills in communication and the delivery of informed consent. Surgeons today need to base their practice on evidence-based material, conduct regular audit and be aware of their accountability in every aspect of their care of the patient. This chapter explores evidence-based practice, audit, accountability, informed consent, avoidance of legal action, and communication skills including breaking bad news.

EVIDENCE-BASED PRACTICE

Evidence-based medicine is the conscientious, explicit and judicious use of current best evidence in making decisions about the care of individual patients. Good surgeons use both individual clinical expertise and the best available external evidence, as neither alone is enough. Without the current best evidence, surgical practice risks becoming rapidly out-of-date to the detriment of patients.

Evidence-based surgery is not restricted to randomised trials and meta-analyses but involves tracking down the best external evidence available to answer clinical questions or problems (see Box 1.1). For example, to find out about the accuracy of a diagnostic test, we need to find proper, cross-sectional studies of patients clinically suspected of harbouring the relevant problem and not a randomised trial. Proper follow-up studies of patients inform about prognosis. Systematic review of several randomised trials (meta-analysis) is much more likely to inform about therapy and whether it does more good than harm.

Evidence-based medicine is a relatively young discipline whose positive impacts are just beginning to be validated, and it will continue to evolve. These days, several undergraduate and postgraduate continuing medical education programmes adopt it and adapt it to their learners' needs, providing further information and understanding about what evidence-based medicine is and what it is not.

CLINICAL GOVERNANCE AND AUDIT

Clinical governance

A widely used definition of clinical governance is:

'A framework through which … organisations are accountable for continually improving the quality of their services and safeguarding high standards of care by creating an environment in which excellence in clinical care will flourish.'

(Scally G & Donaldson L J (1998) Clinical governance and the drive for quality improvement in the new NHS in England. *BMJ* 4 July: 61–65.)

Box 1.1 Examples of classification systems for levels of evidence

The GRADE Working Group, 2004

High = Further research is very unlikely to change our confidence in the estimate of effect.

Moderate = Further research is likely to have an important impact on our confidence in the estimate of effect and may change the estimate.

Low = Further research is very likely to have an important impact on our confidence in the estimate of effect and is likely to change the estimate.

Very low = Any estimate of effect is very uncertain.

United States Preventive Services Task Force, 1989

Level I: Evidence obtained from at least one properly designed randomised controlled trial

Level II-1: Evidence obtained from well-designed controlled trials without randomisation

Level II-2: Evidence obtained from well-designed cohort or case-control analytic studies, preferably from more than one centre or research group

Level II-3: Evidence obtained from multiple time series with or without the intervention. Dramatic results in uncontrolled trials might also be regarded as this type of evidence

Level III: Opinions of respected authorities, based on clinical experience, descriptive studies, or reports of expert committees

National Health Service

Level A: Consistent randomised controlled clinical trial, cohort study, all or none, clinical decision rule validated in different populations

Level B: Consistent retrospective cohort, exploratory cohort, ecological study, outcomes research, case-control study; or extrapolations from level A studies

Level C: Case-series study or extrapolations from level B studies

Level D: Expert opinion without explicit critical appraisal, or based on physiology, bench research or first principles

---

The purpose of clinical governance is to ensure that patients receive the highest quality of care. Clinical governance applies to all treatments and services. The three most recognisable components of clinical governance and those which involve the surgeon in quality improvement are:

- clinical effectiveness activities including audit and redesign
- risk management including patient safety
- patient focus and public involvement.

Healthcare organisations should achieve good clinical governance by:

- having clear, robust national and local systems and structures that help identify, implement and report on quality improvement
- involving health care staff, patients and the public
- establishing a supportive, inclusive learning culture.

Effective clinical governance ensures the continuous improvement of patient services and care, a patient-centred approach to care, a commitment to quality and the prevention of clinical errors.

Clinical audit

An accepted definition of clinical audit is:

> 'A quality improvement process that seeks to improve patient care and outcomes through systematic review of care against explicit criteria and the implementation of change.'

Principles for Best Practice in Clinical Audit (2002) NICE

The National Institute for Health and Clinical Excellence (NICE)

This is an NHS organisation set up in 1999 to ensure everyone has equal access to medical treatments and high quality care from the NHS. It is responsible for providing national guidance for promotion of good health and for the prevention and treatment of ill health. These are often referred to as 'NICE guidelines'; these are easily accessible via www.guidance.nice.org.uk.

Patient safety: the WHO surgical safety checklist

This simple yet effective tool has been introduced around the world by the World Health Organisation and is thought to have already saved many lives (Fig. 1.1).

Peer review

This is a system whereby hospitals or units are scrutinised by independent peers who assess systems and processes against a set of bench marks for diagnosis and treatment, e.g. for cancer.

The reasons for audit include time utilisation/cost-effectiveness, mortality/morbidity assessment, ensuring quality of diagnostic services, monitoring performance, assessment of newer technologies, knowledge of patient satisfaction, exploration of legal implications and research. Research asks, 'Are we doing the right operation?' Audit research asks, 'Are we doing the operation right?'

For audit to be meaningful, it should satisfy the following criteria:
- includes open debate and self-evaluation
- confidentiality of surgeon and patient maintained
- demonstration of change resulting in improvement of patient care
- resources spent are kept to a minimum
- standards set and reviewed periodically
- priority topics audited
- interesting and informative.

The audit cycle involves observation of existing practice, the setting of standards, comparison between observed and set standards, implementation of change, and re-audit of clinical practice (Fig. 1.2).

Audit techniques available include morbidity and mortality, incident review (critical incident reporting), clinical record review, adverse occurrence screening, focused audit studies, global audit (comparison between units), and national studies, for example the National Confidential Enquiry into Patient Outcome and Death (NCEPOD).

Kumar and Clark's Handbook of Medical Management

Kumar and Clark's Handbook of Medical Management

Before induction of anaesthesia

(with at least nurse and anaesthetist)

Has the patient confirmed his/her identity, site, procedure, and consent?
☐ Yes

Is the site marked?
☐ Yes
☐ Not applicable

Is the anaesthesia machine and medication check complete?
☐ Yes

Is the pulse oximeter on the patient and functioning?
☐ Yes

Does the patient have a:

Known allergy?
☐ No
☐ Yes

Difficult airway or aspiration risk?
☐ No
☐ Yes, and equipment/assistance available

Risk of >500ml blood loss (7ml/kg in children)?
☐ No
☐ Yes, and two IVs/central access and fluids planned

Before skin incision

(with nurse, anaesthetist and surgeon)

☐ **Confirm all team members have introduced themselves by name and role.**

☐ **Confirm the patient's name, procedure, and where the incision will be made.**

Has antibiotic prophylaxis been given within the last 60 minutes?
☐ Yes
☐ Not applicable

Anticipated Critical Events

To Surgeon:
☐ What are the critical or non-routine steps?
☐ How long will the case take?
☐ What is the anticipated blood loss?

To Anaesthetist:
☐ Are there any patient-specific concerns?

To Nursing Team:
☐ Has sterility (including indicator results) been confirmed?
☐ Are there equipment issues or any concerns?

Is essential imaging displayed?
☐ Yes
☐ Not applicable

Before patient leaves operating room

(with nurse, anaesthetist and surgeon)

Nurse Verbally Confirms:
☐ The name of the procedure
☐ Completion of instrument, sponge and needle counts
☐ Specimen labelling (read specimen labels aloud, including patient name)
☐ Whether there are any equipment problems to be addressed

To Surgeon, Anaesthetist and Nurse:
☐ What are the key concerns for recovery and management of this patient?

Figure 1.1 The WHO Surgical Safety Checklist (from *The WHO Surgical Safety Checklist*, World Health Organisation 2009, with permission.)

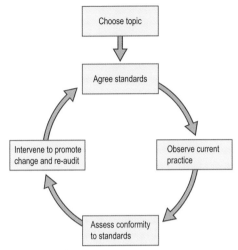

Figure 1.2 The audit cycle.

The essential features of audit include high-quality data collection, relevant and valid measures of outcome, appropriate and valid measures of case mix, a representative population and appropriate statistical analysis.

ACCOUNTABILITY

As surgeons, we are accountable to our patients to inform them about their conditions, educate them about the risks and benefits of their choices, and suggest to them what we would do for ourselves. We then respect their decisions about their own care. It is an essence of our professional life and the basis for our relationship with patients.

At every level of healthcare, the system should be accountable to patients. This demands that patients have access to the information, education and support they need to manage their own healthcare. It also places demands upon patients, holding them responsible for at least a portion of their healthcare decisions and requiring them to be responsible for the consequences of personal decisions that place them at higher risk for illness and disability, e.g. cigarette smoking, alcohol consumption, and obesity (diet).

INFORMED CONSENT

Informed consent is the process by which fully informed patients can participate in choices about their healthcare. It originates from the legal and ethical right the patient has to direct what happens to his or her body and the ethical duty of the surgeon to involve the patient in his or her healthcare.

Complete informed consent includes a discussion of the following:
- nature of the decision/procedure
- reasonable alternatives to the proposed intervention

Kumar and Clark's Handbook of Medical Management

- the risks, benefits and uncertainties related to each alternative
- an assessment of patient understanding
- the acceptance of the intervention by the patient.

In order for the patient's consent to be valid, he or she must be considered competent to make the decision at hand and consent must be voluntary. To encourage the 'voluntariness', the surgeon can emphasise that the patient is participating in a decision, not just signing a form. Comprehension on the part of the patient is as important as the information given. Consequently, the discussion should be carried out in lay person's terms and the patient's understanding should be assessed along the way. This should be done by a surgeon who is competent to do the surgery, within the clinic or ward environment prior to any move toward theatre. Consent taken within a few minutes of surgery is not valid.

Information considered adequate

The law in this area suggests one of three approaches:

- Reasonable physician standard – what would a typical physician say about this intervention?
- Reasonable patient standard – what would the average patient need to know in order to be an informed participant in the decision?
- Subjective standard – what would the patient need to know and understand in order to make an informed decision?

Most interventions now require informed consent. This includes all aspects of general anaesthetic surgery, interventional and invasive procedures, diagnostic procedures (e.g. OGD, colonoscopy) and local anaesthetic procedures.

When it is not clear that a patient is competent to make his or her own decision about consent, (for example during severe illness which causes stress, anxiety, fear and depression) the surgeon's duty is to ensure that the patient does have a capacity to make a good decision, by assessing his or her ability to understand the situation, the risks associated with the decision and to communicate a decision based on that understanding. It should be remembered that competent patients have a right to refuse treatment.

If a patient cannot give informed consent, usually the next of kin becomes the appropriate decision-maker. If no appropriate decision-maker is available, surgeons can be allowed to act in the best interests of the patient, for example in an emergency situation, until an appropriate decision-maker is found. In the above setting, the patient's consent should only be presumed rather than obtained. Care must be taken to assume that consent is implied by the patient's presence in the hospital ward, clinic or intensive care unit.

LEGAL ASPECTS OF SURGICAL PRACTICE

Every surgeon must expect to be the subject of complaint or legal claim from time to time, and be prepared to justify why they have managed the patient in the way that they have. Good surgical practice is defensible practice. This depends on staying within the limits of your expertise, keeping up to date and conducting audit (see above), ensuring effective administration and communicating effectively with patients, their carers and colleagues and ensuring that medical records recall all salient facts relating to the patient. If things go wrong be honest, investigate the facts, explain the situation fully to the patient and do not be afraid to apologise.

While clinical standards continue to improve, complete eradication of error is not possible and there is no foolproof way that surgeons can avoid being litigated against.

Clinical negligence

Claimants have to demonstrate that they were owed a duty of care by their surgeon. This is established as soon as any surgical advice is proffered. Secondly, claimants have to demonstrate that there was a breach of that duty, which requires demonstration that the care provided fell below acceptable standards. In England and Wales this is judged by the Bolam test, which states that care must be provided in accordance with accepted medical practice as determined by experts in the field. Thirdly, claimants must demonstrate that they have suffered harm as a result of substandard care or that harm would have been avoided if adequate care had been provided.

In many hospitals, there are now standard protocols or guidelines for dealing with particular conditions. Surgeons who do not follow unit guidelines must be prepared to justify their management by reference to a responsible body of surgical opinion. If guidelines are not followed, surgeons are making themselves vulnerable to claims of negligence.

Clinical negligence cases are won on evidence, not facts. Inadequate notes, lost records and failing or confused memories may lead to an inability to defend the case. Consequently, some cases which should be defensible are sometimes lost for want of evidence.

It should be remembered that the competence issue extends to the delegation of tasks to others and the delegating surgeon should always check that an individual is competent to a reasonable standard. Equally, delegated duties should not be accepted unless you are confident of completing them to a reasonable standard.

Keeping up to date is important (see above). The use of outdated techniques inevitably makes surgeons vulnerable to criticism. Audit, as defined above, is an integral part of surgical practice which must be demonstrated in these situations.

ADMINISTRATION

The surgeon has a responsibility to ensure that basic systems are in place to deal with patient referral, follow-up, completion of clinical records, correspondence, review of test results and appropriate action taken on discovery of abnormalities. He or she should not rely on administrators for this purpose. Communication skills have been mentioned in terms of informed consent, but it is also vital to ensure good communication between teams and, in particular, between primary and secondary care.

Medical record-keeping is vital and it is essential that each patient contact is adequately recorded so that all clinical developments are noted, together with investigations and actions on results, and that notes for future management, referral and follow-up are recorded. Notes should include a history, examination of the patient, diagnosis, information conveyed to the patient, consent obtained, treatment, follow-up and progress – in a legible form – so that the patient's care can be picked up by other colleagues.

When things go wrong, the surgeon must readily provide a prompt, open, constructive and honest response to any complaint about the patient's care. Where appropriate, an apology should be given. You must co-operate with any further enquiry into the treatment of the patient. You must give (to those who are entitled to ask for it) any relevant information in connection with an investigation into your own or another healthcare professional's conduct, performance or health. Surgeons who prevaricate, appear evasive or refuse to acknowledge fault are far more likely to push their patients towards litigation than those who explain exactly what happened, and apologise for any shortcomings on their part. Patients who are entitled to compensation should receive this swiftly and fairly. It is the surgeon's responsibility to make sure he is adequately insured against the possibility of litigation. Although in the UK a surgeon's NHS practise is indemnified, the terms are limited; 'good Samaritan' acts are not covered for instance.

BREAKING BAD NEWS

Breaking bad news to patients is a common part of surgical life, particularly for those surgeons involved in cancer medicine. The following framework is suggested and many courses are now available to clinicians to practise this skill.

Preparation

An appointment should be made as soon as possible and sufficient uninterrupted time for the consultation made available. Use a comfortable, familiar environment and invite the patient's partner, family member or a friend, as appropriate. Be adequately prepared with the patient's records and background. Be prepared to put aside your personal feelings wherever possible.

Beginning the session

Summarise the situation to date and check this with the patient to find out if anything has happened since the last consultation. Try to gauge how the patient is thinking or feeling and suggest an agenda for the session.

Sharing the information

- Assess the patient's understanding and what they already know.
- Assess how much the patient wishes to know.
- Give a warning that difficult information is coming.
- Basic information should be given simply and honestly.
- Repeat important points if necessary.
- Do not give too much information too early.
- Give information in small chunks.
- Check repeatedly for understanding and the patient's feelings as you proceed.
- Use language carefully with regard to the patient's intelligence, reactions and emotions.
- Avoid technical jargon.

Being sensitive to the patient

- Assess non-verbal clues, for example face or body language, silences or tears.

- Allow the patient time and space, particularly when you feel they might have stopped listening.
- Give adequate breaks for the patient to ask questions.
- Assess if the patient needs further information and listen to their wishes – patients vary greatly in their need for this.
- Try to encourage expression of feelings, 'giving permission' for them to be expressed.
- Respond to these feelings with acceptance, empathy and concern.
- Try to elicit all the patient's concerns.
- Be aware of unshared feelings, i.e. what cancer means for the patient compared with what it means for the surgeon.
- Do not be afraid to show emotion or distress yourself.

Supporting the patient

- Offer to help break down overwhelming feelings into manageable concerns, prioritising and distinguishing the fixable from the unfixable.
- Identify a plan for what is to happen next within a broad time-frame.
- Give hope tempered with realism.
- Ally yourself with the patient and be their advocate.
- Emphasise quality of life where appropriate.

Closing the consultation

- Begin with a summary.
- Check with the patient that they understand what has been said.
- Do not rush the patient into treatment.
- Fix a further appointment if necessary.
- Identify support systems, which may involve relatives and friends.
- Offer to see or tell the spouse or others that whom the patient may wish you to communicate with.
- Provide written materials.

Remember that you yourself will not be invulnerable to anxiety or emotional responses when giving patients bad news. Be aware of your own coping mechanisms and limitations that may be picked up by the patient.

CONTINUING PROFESSIONAL DEVELOPMENT AND REVALIDATION

It is essential to keep up to date with current practice; the most obvious example of which is the 'MDT' or multi-disciplinary meeting, an integral part of the management of cancer cases.

There has always been an expectation that the surgeon should actively keep abreast of developments in his or her field, and refresh skills/ knowledge – a process known as continuing professional development (CPD). There are a multitude of courses available, although funding is always an issue.

A more formal process known as 'revalidation' (the process by which licensed doctors will, in future, regularly demonstrate to the General Medical Council in the UK that they are up to date and fit to practise) is expected to begin in late 2012. It is proposed that each doctor will need to maintain a dossier of 'supporting information' (e.g. CPD course details) which will form the basis of their annual appraisal, with a 'responsible officer' such as a medical director making a recommendation of fitness to practise every five years.

This chapter reviews conditions and generic problems common to all surgical specialties.

WOUND HEALING AND MANAGEMENT

Understanding the principles of wound healing and management is essential in all forms of surgery. Careful wound management reduces complications such as wound breakdown, infection and poor cosmetic result. Oxygen is the crucial ingredient for wound healing. Adequate oxygen delivery depends on heart and lung function, haemoglobin level and blood supply to the wounded tissue. Box 2.1 highlights local and systemic factors affecting wound healing. These same factors apply whether the healing wound is of skin, bone or any other tissue, e.g. a bowel anastomosis.

First intention

Rapid wound healing occurs by the approximation of wound edges soon after injury. This results in a narrow scar formation with superior cosmetic result. Most surgical skin incisions are closed, to heal by first intention.

There are three phases of wound healing:

Inflammatory phase

Acute inflammatory processes cascade in response to cellular injury. Clot formation, tissue oedema, and increased vascular permeability occur, with fibrin formed in the wound helping to hold the edges together. Clean, healthy surgical incisions are typically approximated with sutures, adhesive strips or glues. There is no inherent strength of the wound during this phase, which lasts up to 3 days.

Reparative phase

There is formation of new capillaries and collagen is deposited by fibroblasts during this phase. Collagen, fibroblasts and capillaries together are known as 'granulation tissue'. The wound becomes stronger as collagen aligns and then contracts. Epithelialisation occurs. This phase usually lasts 3 weeks.

Consolidative phase

The scar matures and becomes paler as vascularity decreases. Abnormal collagen deposition can result in hypertrophic or keloid scar formation. Eighty per cent of original tissue tensile strength is regained at 6 months. This phase is completed after 1 year.

Second intention

Contaminated wounds can be left open to heal by secondary intention. They may require debridement of debris and dead tissue first. The wound heals from the base upward with granulation tissue, and re-epithelialisation occurs from the skin edges.

Box 2.1 Factors which impair wound healing

Local
Infection
Contamination or foreign bodies
Poor blood supply
Previous radiotherapy at the same site
Mechanical factors (excessive movement of wound, poor suture technique, wound tension)

Systemic
Poor cardiac/respiratory function
Anaemia
Age
Malnutrition (all causes)
Diabetes
Chronic renal failure
Jaundice
Corticosteroids, immunosuppression, cytotoxic therapy

Delayed primary closure

This is suitable for wounds where bacterial contamination is high and wound breakdown likely if closed immediately, e.g. anal surgery for fistula-in-ano. Healthy-looking wounds are closed after irrigation, debridement and a period of observation have occurred.

Skin grafting

This may be suitable for large, non-infected, healthy granulating wounds. Indications include burns, traumatic skin loss, ulcers, and wounds following excision of large skin tumours.

Classification of surgical wounds

Clean (low risk of postoperative infection)

Incisions are made under aseptic conditions where the gastrointestinal (GI), biliary and genitourinary (GU) tracts and respiratory organs are not cut open. Antibiotic prophylaxis is not usually needed except in operations where prosthetic materials are required, e.g. joint replacement, hernia repair, abdominal aortic aneurysm (AAA) repair.

Clean/contaminated (medium risk of postoperative infection)

Operations involve incisions into the GI, biliary, GU or respiratory tracts. A low level of contamination is expected, e.g. small bowel resection, gallbladder removal. Prophylactic antibiotics are usually indicated.

Contaminated (high risk of postoperative infection)

A high bacterial load is encountered during surgery, e.g. perforated peptic ulcer, perforated appendicitis. Antibiotics are always needed pre- and post-surgery. Broad-spectrum antibiotics are usually given, e.g. cefuroxime 750 mg to 1.5 g three times a day IV and metronidazole 500 mg three times a day IV. Seek regular advice from a microbiologist where severe infection is anticipated. All hospitals in the UK have their own anti-microbial policy for reference in these situations.

Management of bleeding (haemostasis)

The optimal environment for wound healing is a dry wound with minimal ooze. Inadequate control of bleeding:

- prevents apposition of wound edges, leading to increased fibrous tissue deposition and delayed healing
- may lead to a haematoma which has to be released before the wound edges can be opposed
- increases the risk of postoperative infection – bacteria thrive in a haematoma.

The main techniques used to stop bleeding are:

- compression
- ligation/clipping of vessels
- diathermy coagulation.

Wound closure

Wound closure can be achieved in a number of ways:

- suturing
- adhesive tape
- staples/glue
- plastic surgery procedures to close defects which cannot be treated with the above methods, e.g. skin grafting, flap transfer.

Details of these techniques are given in Chapter 23.

Contaminated wounds require adequate debridement, often in the operating theatre. These result from road traffic accidents, farming accidents or bomb injuries in civilian life. Gravel must be removed and all foreign bodies (FBs) extracted along with bits of clothing etc. X-rays to exclude deeper FBs are mandatory. Bites, human or animal, should be thoroughly cleaned and disinfected. Clean wounds may be primarily sutured but others should be left to granulate.

Blood products

The components of blood, e.g. red cells, platelets, fresh frozen plasma (FFP), are prepared from single donors whilst plasma derivatives, coagulation factor concentrates etc. are made from many donors.

- **Whole blood** is rarely used, as blood is a very scarce commodity. Specific use of the required component is a more effective use of these products. Packed red cells are used for acute haemorrhage in combination with colloid or crystalloid solutions and correction of anaemia after the diagnosis has been established. Platelets may be given to prevent bleeding, whilst FFP is given often in severe coagulopathy states, e.g. leaking aortic aneurysm surgery.
- **Cryoprecipitate** contains fibrinogen, factor VIIIc and von Willebrand factor. Its use is confined in surgery to patients with severe coagulopathy, e.g. severe sepsis.
- **Albumin** may be used for correction of hypoalbuminaemic states.
- **Immunoglobulins** are used to prevent infection in patients with idiopathic thrombocytopenic purpura and specific immunoglobulins may be used for patients who have contracted infections, e.g. antihepatitis B immunoglobulin. Consultation with a haematologist is mandatory in

Kumar and Clark's Handbook of Medical Management

> **Box 2.2** Blood transfusion checking procedure
>
> **Blood must be checked by two nurses, one of whom is a registered nurse, before transfusion**
>
> **Check the blood bag is not leaking or wet and has a compatibility label attached**
>
> **Check the patient's surname, first names, sex, date of birth, hospital number on**
> Patient's name band which the patient must be wearing
> Blood transfusion request form
> Compatibility label
> Medical case notes
> Intravenous fluid prescription chart
>
> **Check the expiry date of the unit of blood on**
> Compatibility label
> Blood bag
>
> **Check the blood group and unit number on**
> Blood transfusion request form
> Compatibility label
>
> **Record the unit number of the blood on**
> Intravenous fluid prescription chart
>
> **Date and time and signature of both nurses on**
> Blood transfusion request form
> Compatibility label
> Intravenous fluid prescription chart
>
> *(from Ballinger & Patchett 2003 Pocket Essentials of Clinical Medicine, 3rd edn, Saunders, Edinburgh, with permission)*

situations where these products are needed. Protocols for massive transfusion exist in all UK hospitals.

Blood groups

Blood groups are determined by antigens on the red cell surface. There are over 400 different types, the most important being the ABO and rhesus (Rh) systems. Incompatibility transfusion reactions involving other blood groups can occur, resulting in haemolytic anaemia. Compatibility testing is always done by the transfusion service; donor blood of the same ABO and Rh group as the recipient is chosen. The patient's serum is also screened for antibodies against other red cell antigens.

Most hospitals now have strict guidelines for the use and ordering of blood for operations and with new technology blood can be available within 20–30 minutes of a request even if the blood is not 'grouped and saved'. The blood transfusion checking procedure is shown in Box 2.2.

BLOOD TRANSFUSION

Blood transfusion is not without risk. Other therapies must always be considered before prescribing a blood transfusion, e.g. plasma substitutes

---

Box 2.3 Complications of blood transfusion

Early
Fluid overload
Hyperkalemia
Disordered coagulation
Incompatibility reactions
Thrombophlebitis

Late
Transmission of infection (rare with modern screening)
  Viruses (HBV, HCV, HIV, CMV, EBV)
  Parasites (malaria, toxoplasma)
  Bacteria
  Prions (variant CJD)
Haemochromatosis (seen in repeated transfusions for
  haemoglobinopathies)

---

or iron therapy. The introduction of screening programmes for hepatitis B and C and HIV have now made transfusion safer. For the first 48 hours after transfusion, donated blood does not have the same oxygen-carrying capacity as normal blood due to red blood cell depletion of 2,3-biphosphoglycerate (2,3-BPG), which shifts the oxygen-haemoglobin dissociation curve to the left. Blood transfusion also deranges fluid balance, electrolytes and coagulation (Box 2.3). For this reason, when required, preoperative blood transfusions should wherever possible be given at least 48 hours preoperatively. It is now possible for patients to store their own blood prior to big operations.

Complications of blood transfusion

Early

- **Volume overload** Patients with limited cardiac and renal reserve are prone to pulmonary oedema if transfused too quickly; 20 mg furosemide administered IV with every second unit is a common precaution for these patients. This does NOT apply in the emergency situation with a shocked patient.
- **Hyperkalaemia** Transfused red cells are tired and leaky and allow potassium to diffuse out. This increases the serum potassium concentration. Patients with normal kidneys will clear this without difficulty but those with renal impairment may develop dangerously high potassium levels. In such patients, the urea and electrolytes should be checked before starting transfusion and after every 2–4 units.
- **Coagulation problems** Transfused blood consists of packed red cells only, so transfusion dilutes the patient's own platelets and coagulation factors. Transfused blood contains citrate, which is an anticoagulant, to prevent the blood clotting during storage. Blood is stored at 4°C and it is easy inadvertently to cause hypothermia by a large blood transfusion (ameliorated by blood warming devices). For these reasons it is important to monitor a patient's clotting after every 4 units and correct impaired coagulation by administering clotting factors in the form of FFP.

- **Incompatibility reactions** Transfusion reactions vary from anaphylaxis to a mild rash/headache/temperature. The former is usually the result of administering the wrong blood to the wrong patient, leading to a major ABO mismatch. The latter are due to lesser antibodies, which are not included in the cross-match.
- **Impaired oxygen-carrying capacity** Due to 2,3-BPG depletion, transfused red cells take 48 h before they deliver oxygen to the tissues.

Because of these potential early complications of blood transfusion, if an anaemic patient requires a transfusion preoperatively, it is most unwise to do it the day before. Allow at least 48 hours for the volume, potassium, coagulation and 2,3-BPG to equilibrate.

Late

- **Transfer of infection** The viruses hepatitis C and HIV are the most important infections caused by transfusion of infected blood. Malaria (a protozoan) can also be transmitted by transfusion and there is a risk of spreading diseases caused by prions, e.g. CJD.
- **Depression of cell-mediated immunity** There is some evidence that wound infections and metastases are commoner in patients who receive blood transfusions at the time of cancer surgery.
- **Haemochromatosis** Patients with haemoglobinopathies who need multiple transfusions over many years may suffer from the effects of iron overload. This is seldom seen in the surgical setting.

Alternatives to blood transfusion

Concerns about blood transfusion safety have resulted in alternative strategies for its use. Artificial haemoglobin solutions are being developed along with autologous blood transfusion and intraoperative blood salvage (e.g. the cell saver system).

FLUID BALANCE

Water

The basic principle behind fluid balance is that what goes out must come in. Water losses occurring through the skin, the lungs as water vapour, kidneys as urine and GI tract as faeces approximate to 2500 mL/day (Table 2.1).

These losses can be much greater due to pyrexia, vomiting and diarrhoea, bowel preparation, or intestinal obstruction. On average, 3 litres of fluid per day will be adequate for normal losses, but much greater volumes are required when there is a deficit to be made up.

Electrolytes

The main electrolytes are Na^+ and K^+. Sodium is lost mainly in the urine at 100 mmol/day with an additional 40 mmol lost in sweat. Potassium (also lost in urine) loss is 80 mmol/day. These amounts should be added to water replacement. A typical regime in a surgical patient might be 1 L 0.9% saline plus 20 mmol KCl in 8 hours followed by 1 L dextrose 5% plus 20 mmol KCl in 8 hours followed by another litre of dextrose 5% plus 20 mmol KCl in the final 8 hours of a 24-hour period. This gives 150 mmol Na^+ and 60 mmol K^+; this regime would of course only replace losses in a healthy patient, as these totals are the normal daily requirement.

Table 2.1 24-hour intake and output of water and electrolytes in health

Substance	Intake	Excretion and route
Water	2000–2500 mL (plus 500 mL of water of oxidation – needs consideration if renal excretion is limited)	Kidney (1500 mL) and insensible loss (respiratory and sweating, 1000 mL)
Sodium	100 mmol	Kidney (but sweat also up to 120 mmol/L)
Potassium	Up to 100 mmol	Kidney; restricted input not followed by fall in excretion

Alternating sodium-rich fluid with dextrose solution may be required if sodium-rich fluid is lost pre- or perioperatively.

In addition to losses suffered during an operation, surgical patients can also 'lose' fluids in the postoperative phase, e.g. during paralytic ileus into interstitial spaces (third space losses). These fluids will return to the normal spaces upon recovery, often seen in the diuretic phase after intestinal surgery or recovery from shock.

Specific electrolyte problems

- **Hyponatraemia** This is usually due to water overload with inappropriate administration of dextrose 5%. If mild, fluid restriction is all that is required with furosemide diuresis, but if severe with symptoms (convulsions, confusion, and coma), hypertonic saline may have to be given with full support.
- **Hypernatraemia** This occurs with dehydration in the postoperative surgical patient or when too much saline is given when aldosterone secretion is high. It may be a complication of Conn's syndrome (see Ch. 11). In the former case, rehydration is needed, and in the latter case, sodium restriction. Electrolytes need to be checked twice daily in these situations.
- **Hypokalaemia** Hypokalaemia may be a preoperative problem secondary to the disease state (e.g. villous adenoma of the rectum or pyloric stenosis) or as a result of diuretic therapy, but inadequate replacement postoperatively is the most common cause. Muscle weakness and ECG changes (T-wave flattening) are seen and corrected by potassium replacement. Care should be taken with rate of administration to prevent cardiac arrhythmia.
- **Hyperkalaemia** Hyperkalaemia may be caused by crush syndrome, massive blood transfusion or chronic renal failure preoperatively. Postoperatively excessive administration is the usual cause, often asymptomatic. Treatment by intravenous insulin and glucose should be given with calcium gluconate if ECG changes are present. A level of >7 mmol/L is dangerously high and is considered an emergency. Calcium resonium orally and rectally may also be given to further reduce the levels on the subsequent days.

Kumar and Clark's Handbook of Medical Management

ACID–BALANCE BALANCE

The pH of body fluids is slightly alkaline maintained between 7.36 and 7.44. If it moves outside this range, body metabolism is deranged. A pH <7 or >7.8 is usually fatal. The constant production of CO_2 in the body forms carbonic acid in solution (H_2CO_3), which together with the bicarbonate ion of the sodium salt ($NaHCO_3$) forms the most important buffer system in the body. Carbonic acid dissociates to H^+ and HCO_3^-, the mixture being in equilibrium ($H_2CO_3 = H^+ + HCO_3^-$). The addition of hydrogen ions causes a shift to the left and withdrawal a shift to the right. The equilibrium keeps the hydrogen ion concentration constant.

Because there is a constant production of H_2CO_3 and therefore hydrogen ions these must be eliminated. The major routes excreting CO_2 are the lungs (fast) and the kidney (slowly). Dehydration reduces the efficacy of the buffering system, promoting acidosis. Haemoglobin is an additional important base buffer after oxygen has been removed.

Metabolic acidosis

This is commonly seen in surgery where there is a failure of oxygen transport and excess acid production due to anaerobic metabolism (lactic acidosis). Fluid loss, bleeding or sepsis may cause peripheral circulatory failure (see Ch. 3). Initial compensation occurs in the lungs but when, for example, sepsis is prolonged, ventilatory failure also occurs. Mechanical ventilation often restores the balance whilst additional compensation is provided by the kidneys. If acidosis is persistent despite the above measures, intravenous administration of sodium bicarbonate may correct the situation.

Respiratory acidosis

Chronic lung disease is the commonest cause of this condition. The renal system compensates by excreting acid urine. Patients should have intensive pre- and postoperative physiotherapy to maximise their lung function or alternative methods of anaesthesia should be considered (e.g. epidural, local block). Patients often require prolonged weaning from ventilators due to a metabolic alkalosis induced by ventilation itself (high HCO_3^-), the renal system taking a long time to excrete the HCO_3^-.

Metabolic alkalosis

Gastric outlet obstruction is a cause of this situation due to prolonged vomiting and loss of HCl. Sodium and potassium loss compound the problem due to their preferential retention by the kidneys instead of H^+. There is paradoxically acid urine in the presence of a metabolic alkalosis. Treatment consists of fluid and electrolyte correction allowing the kidneys to redress the alkalosis.

Respiratory alkalosis

Apart from the ventilatory problems described above, respiratory alkalosis may be seen in patients who hyperventilate (hysteria, panic attacks). Breathing into a paper bag to increase the level of inspired CO_2 usually stabilises the H_2CO_3 levels in the blood.

Measurement of acid–base balance

The pH, PO_2, PCO_2, standard bicarbonate, corrected bicarbonate and base excess/deficit can be easily measured on an arterial sample in a blood gas

---

Box 2.4 Factors predisposing to infection

Malnutrition	Age
Malignancy	Obesity
Jaundice	Diabetes

---

analysis machine. The base deficit figure may be used to calculate the amount of bicarbonate required to correct a metabolic acidosis, given by the equation: sodium bicarbonate infusion (mmol) = base deficit multiplied by weight (kg) divided by 3.

INFECTIONS AND ANTIBIOTICS

The propensity for an infection to develop depends on the size of the inoculum, the pathogenicity of the organism and ability of the patient to resist the infection. Steroid therapy, diabetes, malnutrition, lower resistance, alcoholism, AIDS and immunosuppression from any cause (Box 2.4) all promote infection, while locally the main factors are necrotic tissue, blood clot, foreign bodies and ischaemia.

Infection control and prevention

The patient and healthcare worker both need protection. Risks emanate from both the environment and the patient's own flora. Frequent handwashing and a mixture of (a) disinfectants that kill most pathogens but not spores or slow viruses, (b) antiseptics that can be used on living tissues and (c) sterilisation will prevent infection.

The patient is protected by knowledge of the risk factors that are associated with an increased risk of infection, namely (a) operations lasting more than 2 hours, (b) abdominal procedures, (c) endogenous or exogenous contamination and (d) more than three diagnoses for the patient. Aseptic surgical technique, preparation of the skin and bowel, and antibiotic prophylaxis reduce the risks substantially.

Antibiotic prophylaxis

Patients at high risk should be given antibiotic prophylaxis. The choice of antibiotic depends on the type of operation, the most likely organisms to be encountered, the likelihood of the development of resistance, and financial costs involved (risk management) (Table 2.2). Cephalosporins are widely used in general and orthopaedic surgery and given at the time of induction. Two further doses over 24 hours are sufficient thereafter. Antibiotics may be administered orally, rectally, intravenously or topically. Long-term prophylaxis, for example in post-splenectomy patients, is given to prevent overwhelming infections.

Principles of antibiotic usage

Intravenous administration of antibiotics is the route of choice in seriously ill patients, ensuring high serum levels. Oral therapy requires a functioning bowel and ability to tolerate by mouth. Topical antibiotics should be avoided as they lead to colonisation, resistance and sensitivity reactions.

Table 2.2 Examples of antibiotic prophylaxis*

Operation	Infection site	Likely organisms	Prophylactic antibiotics
Colectomy	Wound	*E. coli* Anaerobes *Bacteroides*	Cefuroxime Metronidazole
Hip replacement	Prosthesis	*Staph. aureus*	Cefuroxime
Bladder instrumentation	Urinary tract	*E. coli* *Klebsiella spp.*	Gentamicin
ERCP	Biliary tract	*E. coli*	Ciprofloxacin
Vascular graft	Graft	*Staph. aureus* *Staph. albus*	Cefuroxime

ERCP, endoscopic retrograde cholangiopancreatography.
*Check with the hospital's local policy.

The dose of antibiotic varies with the patient's weight and age. Most paediatric doses are calculated to this formula, but adults tend to have a fixed dose despite their weight and their serum levels may therefore fluctuate to suboptimal levels. Aminoglycoside antibiotics need careful monitoring to achieve the therapeutic level required. The length of a prescribed course is debatable. Prophylactic prescriptions need only one dose, which must be given before the operation starts. The length of the course is based on the patient's general condition. A 5–7 day course is the norm.

The choice of agent is often directed by microbiological advice. The more expensive drugs are not necessarily the best. A suggested list of antimicrobial chemotherapy is shown in Table 2.3.

Infections acquired in hospital

Common sites include an operative site, in relation to a prosthesis, respiratory or GI tract translocation, urinary tract from catheters, infections from intravenous lines and cross-infection from any site (MRSA – see below).

Specific infections

Septicaemia

In septicaemia, bacteria are not just present in the blood (bacteraemia), but are using it as a culture medium. Fever, tachycardia, hypotension, acute respiratory distress syndrome (ARDS) and multiple organ failure may ensue (see Chapter 3). In some instances with shock, it is not the organisms that are found but circulating endotoxins (Gram-negative). Symptoms may be severe with malaise or related to the focus of infection. Repeated blood cultures may be negative. Leucocytosis is common. 'Best-guess' antibiotics are given immediately, usually of broad-spectrum activity.

Systemic inflammatory response (SIRS)

SIRS is the name given to a physiological state of septic collapse (see Chapter 3). The mechanism appears to be activation of macrophages and release of tumour necrosis factor (TNF). The situation is worsened by cell injury leading to deficient uptake of oxygen, tissue hypoxia and lactic

Table 2.3 Common antibiotics and their uses

Antibiotic	Common uses	Notes
Penicillin	All cocci: strepto-, staphylo-, pneumo-	85% of staphylococci resistant due to beta-lactamase production Allergies common: simple rash to fatal anaphylaxis
Flucloxacillin	Anti-staphylococci; included in treatment of cutaneous infections	
Co-amoxiclav	Broad-spectrum: soft tissue infections, pneumonia, UTI and antibiotic prophylaxis	Combination of amoxicillin (amoxycillin) and clavulanic acid; latter prevents action of beta-lactamases
Amoxicillin	Active against Gram-negative and -positive organisms: urinary tract and respiratory infections	An amino group added to the basic penicillin molecule gives increased antimicrobial activity
Piperacillin	For severe infections in combination with gentamicin (for Gram-negative, resistant organisms)	Later-generation penicillin that has activity against *Pseudomonas*

Table 2.3 Common antibiotics and their uses *(Continued)*

Antibiotic	Common uses	Notes
Ticarcillin + clavulanic acid	Same uses as piperacillin	
Cefuroxime	Broad-spectrum: prophylaxis bowel and biliary operations; treatment of GI conditions – cholecystitis, appendix mass, diverticulitis	Second-generation cephalosporin In common use in GI surgery often in combination with metronidazole 10% of those allergic to penicillin similarly affected by cephalosporins
Cefotaxime or ceftazidime	Second-line treatment for sepsis insensitive to cefuroxime	Third-generation cephalosporin Some improvement in activity against Gram-negative organisms but slightly poorer against staphylococci
Imipenem	Broad-spectrum – for use in ICU	A carbapenem–thienamycin beta-lactam best combined with cilastatin – an enzyme inhibitor of its metabolism by the kidney
Tetracycline	Pelvic inflammatory disease; other sexually transmitted diseases	Bacteriostatic rather than bactericidal, but active against *Chlamydia*
Gentamicin	Severe sepsis (in combination with penicillin or metronidazole)	Aminoglycoside active against Gram-negative organisms and *Pseudomonas*; inactive against anaerobes and streptococci

Table 2.3 Common antibiotics and their uses (*Continued*)

Antibiotic	Common uses	Notes
	Prophylaxis during urinary tract instrumentation	Potentially nephrotoxic; serum levels must be regularly checked
Erythromycin	Soft tissue and chest infections	Active against staphylococci and *H. influenzae* Useful in those allergic to penicillin
Clarithromycin	Similar to erythromycin	Used for *Helicobacter pylori* infections of the upper GI tract
Vancomycin	Gram-positive infections resistant to penicillins and cephalosporins (MRSA and pseudomembranous colitis)	
Teicoplanin	Similar uses to vancomycin	Requires administration by intramuscular or intravenous route
Trimethoprim	Urinary tract infections	
Co-trimoxazole	*Pneumocystis carinii* pneumonia	
Metronidazole	Anaerobic abdominal infections (including prophylaxis and usually in combination) Gas gangrene Amoebic infections Pseudomembranous colitis	
Ciprofloxacin	Gram-negative infections – *Salmonella, Shigella, Campylobacter*	4-Quinolone – the traveller's antibiotic

Table 2.3 Common antibiotics and their uses *(Continued)*

Antibiotic	Common uses	Notes
Examples of typical antibiotic choices for particular clinical infections		
Infection	First choice	Alternatives
Chest infection	Penicillin + erythromycin	Co-amoxiclav
Wound Infection (cellulitis)	Penicillin + flucloxacillin	Co-amoxiclav
Intra-abdominal infection (endogenous organisms likely)	Cefuroxime + metronidazole	Cefotaxime Gentamicin
Cholecystitis-cholangitis	Cefuroxime + metronidazole	Piperacillin
Urinary tract infection	Trimethoprim	Gentamicin Co-amoxiclav
Pelvic inflammatory disease	Tetracyclines + cefuroxime + metronidazole	
Severe sepsis	Gentamicin + metronidazole + penicillin	Imipenem Ticarcillin
MRSA	Vancomycin	Teicoplanin
Pseudomembranous colitis	Metronidazole	Vancomycin
Gas gangrene	Penicillin + metronidazole	Metronidazole

acidosis. Clinically this leads to fever, oliguria, respiratory and multi-organ failure.

Abscess

An abscess is a localised collection of pus. Symptoms include *rubor* (redness), *dolor* (pain), *calor* (warmth) and *functio laesa* (loss of function) if the pus is in an enclosed space, along with a swinging pyrexia and general malaise. After drainage it is essential to ensure that continued drainage is allowed. Deep abscesses will require drains, whilst superficial abscesses need deroofing to allow healing by secondary intention. Antibiotics are not required unless there is surrounding cellulitis.

Deep-seated abscesses may be primary (e.g. pyogenic liver abscess) or secondary, e.g. after surgery for peritonitis. The latter patients may be difficult to diagnose and require repeated imaging to find the source of the sepsis. Investigations most usually used are ultrasound, CT scan and white cell scan (autologous leucocytes labelled with ^{111}In). Increasingly, percutaneous drainage under ultrasound- or CT-guided control is being used instead of open surgical approaches.

Cellulitis

This is inflammation of the tissues without suppuration. It is commonly seen in the lower limb but may occur deep in the retroperitoneum. There may be associated lymphangitis. The organisms most usually found are *Streptococcus* or *Staphylococcus*. A combination of flucloxacillin and penicillin intravenously should be given until appropriate cultures and sensitivities have been found. Adequate analgesia, bed rest and exclusion of diabetes are essential.

Streptococcal and staphylococcal infection

Streptococcal infections are sensitive to penicillins and these are the first-line choice for cellulitis (see above). Staphylococcal infections are an increasingly common problem in hospitals and the community, especially if they are methicillin-resistant. Hand-washing policies are now in force throughout hospitals in the UK and with political backing hygiene measures are strictly enforced to reduce this problem. Hospital policies include isolation, barrier nursing, topical mupirocin (similar to vancomycin), regular screening to determine if the infection has been eradicated, with IV vancomycin for serious infections. New agents active against MRSA (e.g. linezolid), which may be administered orally, are now available.

Clostridial infections

Clostridial infections are anaerobic Gram-positive bacilli which produce a variety of serious exotoxins causing tetanus (*C. tetani*), gas gangrene (*C. perfringens*) (see 'Necrotising infections', below), pseudomembranous colitis (*C. difficile*) and botulism (*C. botulinum*).

Tetanus is caused by *C. tetani*. There is muscle spasm caused by the exotoxin tetanospasmin. The main cause is through dirty wounds due to agricultural injuries and war wounds. There is a variable incubation period. Symptoms include jaw stiffness progressing to spasm *(risus sardonicu)* and back-arching spasms with impaired ventilation. There is a high risk of cardiopulmonary arrest with brain damage and death.

Management consists of human tetanus immunoglobulin (5000–10 000 units), adequate wound toilet and penicillin antibiotics. Spasms are controlled by medical means from diazepam to full ventilatory support.

Prevention is better than cure and routine tetanus toxoid immunisation was introduced to the UK in 1961. All babies are immunised from 2 months of age, with a course of four further booster doses into adulthood.

Gangrene

Gangrene is black necrotic tissue. Two types are recognised.

- **Dry gangrene** The tissue (usually the toes) is dry and does not smell. It is colonised by bacteria but not actively infected with proliferating organisms. Provided the blood supply is adequate the tissue will autoamputate.
- **Wet gangrene** The tissue is wet and offensive, actively infected with bacteria. The condition spreads to threaten the limb and life of the patient. Amputation of the affected limb is necessary.

Necrotising infections

There are a number of rapidly spreading soft tissue infections which cause tissue necrosis. These conditions are sometimes classified according to the infecting organism but in practice this is unhelpful since the organisms are not identified until after the patient is on the mend or has died.

Fournier's gangrene is a mixed streptococcal and staphylococcal infection which starts in the perineum and rapidly spreads to the surrounding tissues. Gas gangrene is another example of necrotising infection caused by *C. perfringens*.

Necrotising fasciitis is the general term given to these conditions. Despite their disastrous progression and outcome, the early stages may be quite difficult to diagnose. The skin wound, if any, may be trivial and the skin necrosis does not develop until later. The diagnosis should be considered in a systemically unwell patient with signs of a soft tissue infection. Drug users, the immunocompromised, diabetics and cancer patients are all more susceptible, as are so-called battle field wounds that are contaminated with clostridia. The skin may be discoloured (purple or brown) before black necrosis occurs. There is severe pain. If there is gas in the tissues, crepitus will be felt.

The white blood cell count and C-reactive protein are raised but this is not specific for necrotising infections. The creatine kinase level is helpful since it is very elevated. Plain X-rays may show gas in the tissues. Ultrasound, CT and MRI may all help confirm the diagnosis.

Treatment requires resuscitation, high-dose IV antibiotics and wide surgical debridement of the infected tissue. Mortality is high, and survivors face extensive reconstructive plastic surgery.

Candida

This is an omnipresent fungus that causes opportunistic infection in patients who are ill for other reasons or who are on antibiotics. The commonest sites are oral and oesophageal, perianal and vaginal, especially in the elderly, young or immunosuppressed. IV drug users are prone to endocardial infection. Characteristic white plaques are seen on mucous membranes or as a discharge. Diagnosis is confirmed on culture. Topical ointments (nystatin) are used commonly. Severe cases of systemic disease warrant intravenous anti-fungal agents such as amphotericin or caspofungin, and correction of pre-existing disease.

Human immunodeficiency virus

Surgeons are presented with HIV patients usually as a complication of their disease. The risk of infection is small provided precautions are taken.

Early stage disease may present with conditions linked to lifestyle, e.g. anal warts, perianal abscess and carcinoma or complications associated with injections (venous thrombosis, false aneurysm, injection site abscess).

Later stages of disease may require surgical assistance for central venous lines, Hickman lines or percutaneous gastrostomy. Interventions may be needed for Kaposi's sarcoma in the intestine, lymph node biopsy or splenectomy for thrombocytopenia.

DEEP VEIN THROMBOSIS

Deep vein thrombosis (DVT) and pulmonary embolus (PE) are an important cause of morbidity and mortality in surgical patients, since they often have one or more of Virchow's triad (Box 2.5).

The main risk factors for DVT in surgical patients are:
- age over 40
- obesity
- operation for cancer
- previous DVT/PE
- contraceptive pill/HRT.

Other risk factors are summarised in Box 2.6.

The commonest site for DVT to start is in the veins of the calf. Small thrombi may lyse spontaneously but some will propagate to form large

---

Box 2.5 Virchow's triad: factors which lead to thrombosis

Stasis (i.e. sluggish blood flow)
Increased blood viscosity
Endothelial trauma

Box 2.6 Risk factors for thromboembolic disease in surgical patients

Age >40
Obesity
Immobility
Coma
Lower limb amputation
Pelvic/lower limb surgery (e.g. hysterectomy or hip replacement)
Long distance travel
Malignancy
Oestrogen therapy
Previous DVT/PE
Polycythaemia (high haemoglobin)
Thrombocytosis (high platelets)
Thrombophilia (e.g. protein C or S deficiency, antithrombin III deficiency)
Smoking

> **Box 2.7** Enhanced recovery
>
> Enhanced recovery is an innovative approach to elective surgery incorporating evidence-based steps to ensure patients are in optimal condition for surgery, and receive the best evidence-based care during and after their operation to optimise surgery. Other terms used are accelerated- or rapid-recovery. The underlying principle is to enable patients to recover from surgery and leave hospital sooner by minimising the stress-response of the body during surgery.

ileofemoral DVTs which carry a high risk of pulmonary embolism and post-thrombotic symptoms (limb swelling, skin pigmentation and ulceration, pain and swelling).

Clinical features

Many DVTs are asymptomatic; indeed a patient may drop dead of pulmonary embolism with no previous symptoms at all. Typical DVT symptoms are lower limb swelling and calf pain. Signs include calf tenderness, ankle oedema, distension of superficial veins, superficial thrombophlebitis and limb discoloration. The differential diagnosis includes ruptured popliteal cyst, torn muscle fibres and local trauma (all rare in the post-operative patient).

Management (see Box 2.7)

The diagnosis is best confirmed by duplex scanning. Venography is not required for acute diagnosis.

Immediate treatment requires anticoagulation with low molecular weight heparin to prevent extension of the thrombus. Surgical or endovascular methods to lyse and remove the thrombus are unproven but may reduce the long-term incidence of post-phlebitic problems.

Assuming there are no contraindications, anticoagulation with warfarin for at least 6 months is recommended to prevent recurrence.

If a clear precipitating factor for the DVT is not identified, it is necessary to exclude an underlying thrombophilia or occult malignancy. Clinical examination, blood tests (thrombophilia screen) and CT scanning (of chest, abdomen and pelvis) are required.

Anti-DVT prophylaxis

Anti-DVT prophylaxis is critical to prevent unnecessary deaths after surgery. The key steps in prophylaxis are:

- low molecular weight heparin given subcutaneously
- graduated compression stockings
- early mobilisation after surgery.

The exact choice of heparin is less crucial than ensuring patients do not slip through the net and receive no prophylaxis at all (a monotonously common occurrence).

Contraindications to anti-DVT prophylaxis are few, but patients with peripheral vascular disease should not be prescribed compression stockings and heparin may be inadvisable in some patients with bleeding problems.

Pulmonary embolism

The mortality of untreated PE is 30%. Symptoms include pleuritic chest pain, dyspnoea, haemoptysis, and collapse/loss of consciousness. There may be hypotension, raised jugular venous pressure, tachycardia and arrhythmias. Examination may elucidate a pleural rub, signs of consolidation and pyrexia. The most common clinical finding, however, is of sinus tachycardia alone.

Chest X-ray is normal or with a wedge of consolidation. CT pulmonary angiography is the quickest way to confirm the diagnosis. Radio-isotope scan (ventilation perfusion or V/Q scan) using technetium-99-labelled albumin demonstrates areas of underperfusion, but this is less frequently used. ECG changes include tall peaked P waves, right bundle-branch block and axis deviation and T-wave inversion. Blood gas analysis shows relative or absolute hypoxia, dependent on the percentage of inhaled oxygen given to the patient. Differential diagnosis includes myocardial infarction, severe fluid overload, sepsis, tension pneumothorax, cardiac tamponade and aortic dissection.

Treatment entails resuscitation and anticoagulation; thrombolysis is employed by some for massive PE but a significant risk of bleeding remains a major issue.

NUTRITION

The average daily energy requirement for a middle-aged woman is 8100 kJ (1940 kcal) and for a man 10 600 kJ (2550 kcal). Nutritional requirements increase during periods of growth, pregnancy, lactation and sepsis. A balanced diet is made up of 50% carbohydrate, 35% fat and 15% protein. A balance of energy intake and output determines body weight. Weight gain is the product of excess intake over expenditure. Weight loss due to chronic disease or cancer is due to a reduction in intake nearly always due to appetite suppression.

Adequate diet also requires vitamins and minerals. These may be deficient in patients in underdeveloped countries, patients with hepatobiliary disease (fat-soluble vitamins A, D, E and K) and patients with enteropathies. Some drugs can interfere with pyridoxal phosphate, causing vitamin B_6 deficiency (e.g. isoniazid). Vitamin B_{12} and D deficiencies are discussed elsewhere.

Patients should be assessed for nutritional status on admission to hospital. Dietary history is necessary, and weight and height must be recorded to ascertain body mass index (BMI, normal range male 20–25 kg/m², female 19–24 kg/m²). Poor nutrition results in postoperative morbidity and mortality due to poor wound healing and decreased resistance to infection.

Major causes of malnutrition (severe = BMI ≤ 15) include increased catabolism (sepsis, major surgery), increased losses (liver disease, enteropathy), decreased intake (vomiting, dysphagia), decreased absorption (fistulae, short bowel), other (trauma, chemotherapy, radiotherapy).

Nutritional support
Enteral nutrition
Enteral nutrition is cheaper, more physiological and has fewer complications than parenteral nutrition. It should be used if the GI tract is working normally. Dietary feeding regimes can be calculated by the dietician

> **Box 2.8** Complications of total parenteral nutrition
>
> Catheter related: sepsis, thrombosis, embolism and pneumothorax
> Metabolic, e.g. hyperglycaemia, hypercalcaemia
> Electrolyte disturbances
> Liver dysfunction
>
> *(from Ballinger 2011* Pocket Essentials of Clinical Medicine, *5th edn, Saunders, Edinburgh, with permission)*

(under the guidance of a multidisciplinary nutrition support team) and delivered either by mouth, fine-bore feeding tube, percutaneous endoscopic gastrostomy (PEG), or percutaneous jejunostomy (often inserted at laparotomy when nutritional problems are foreseen).

Total parenteral nutrition

Total parenteral nutrition (TPN) is given via a feeding catheter placed into the subclavian vein or superior vena cava. This can be placed percutaneously under radiological guidance. The risk of infection is high and strict aseptic conditions must be observed during placement and after care. The complications are shown in Box 2.8.

Patients should be monitored closely (weight twice a week, regular review for catheter complications, strict fluid and electrolyte balance). In addition, liver function, glucose and serum magnesium, calcium, zinc and nitrogen should be monitored. The aim of any regime is to achieve positive nitrogen balance (12 g per 24 hours), with catabolic patients requiring more (15 g per 24 hours).

Postoperative pyrexia

The cause of fever in a postoperative patient is not always apparent. Non-infective causes, e.g. DVT, haematoma and malignancy, should be borne in mind whilst new conditions (e.g. cholecystitis, pancreatitis, viral infections) may also be a possibility.

The most likely causes will, however, be:

- chest infection
- wound/surgical site infection
- anastomotic leakage
- subphrenic/pelvic abscess
- urinary tract (catheter)
- infection of intravenous lines.

ANAESTHESIA

The purpose of anaesthesia is to allow the patient to undergo surgery in a safe and pain-free way. A number of different techniques and agents are used to achieve this. In the main there are two types, general (with the patient unconscious) and local/regional anaesthesia. Pre-operative preparation of the patient is crucial for the safe delivery of anaesthetic. Mostly this is straightforward but for complex procedures patients may need to be in hospital for investigations and optimisation of their underlying medical health several days before surgery. Validated scoring systems are

---

Box 2.9 Parameters used to calculate APACHE II score

Temperature – core	Arterial pH
Mean arterial pressure	Serum sodium
Heart rate	Serum potassium
Respiratory rate – ventilated	Serum creatinine
or non-ventilated	Haematocrit
Oxygenation	White blood cell count
FiO$_2$ >0.5 record A-aDO$_2$	Glasgow coma score
FiO$_2$ <0.5 record PaO$_2$	

(Knaus WA et al. APACHE II: A severity of disease classification system. Critical Care Medicine. 1985; 13(App)pp828-829)

---

increasingly being used for estimating the likely risks of surgery and can also be used to compare outcome data of different hospitals/surgeons (allows a correction for case-mix). POSSUM (physiological and operative severity score for the enumeration of morbidity and mortality) and APACHE (acute physiology and chronic health evaluation) score are two of the most widely used tools (see Box 2.9).

Pre-assessment

Pre-assessment of patients for elective cases often occurs in an outpatient setting. A full history is taken of pre-existing co-morbidity, drugs and previous hospital admissions and reactions/problems with anaesthetics. Further investigations may be required to assess cardiac or respiratory status. Blood pressure medication may need to be reviewed and diabetes stabilised. The opportunity for fully informed consent can also be taken. A list of indications for preoperative investigations is shown in Table 2.4. An overall preoperative grading, using the American Society of Anesthesiologists (ASA) system, is decided (Box 2.10).

Airway examination is mandatory to assess mouth opening, jaw protrusion, neck movement, dental condition and a view of the posterior pharyngeal structures. Increasingly, pre-medication is not a necessity, particularly with day-case surgery. The commoner complications of anaesthesia are shown in Box 2.11.

Local and regional anaesthesia

Many procedures can now be performed without a general anaesthetic. Local anaesthetic agents block the generation and propagation of nerve impulses at several sites, e.g. the spinal cord, spinal nerve roots, peripheral nerves and local nerves at the site of the procedure. Factors affecting the choice of regional anaesthesia are shown in Table 2.5. Overdose can occur and the maximum safe doses of commonly used agents are shown in Box 2.12. Local anaesthetic can be administered topically, subcutaneously, by Bier's block (intravenous regional anaesthesia, see Box 2.13), nerve block or epidural/spinal routes. The anatomy of the latter is shown in Figure 2.1. Complications of spinal and epidural anaesthesia can be very serious, ranging from prolonged headache, prolonged hypotension and nerve root damage to epidural haematoma or abscess (which can result in paraplegia).

Table 2.4 Indications for preoperative investigations

Investigation	Indication
Full blood count	History of bleeding, major surgery, cardiorespiratory disease, premenopausal women
Electrolytes	History of vomiting, diarrhoea, renal disease, cardiac disease, diabetes, diuretics, ACE inhibitors, anti-arrhythmics, steroids, hypoglycaemics
Glucose	History of diabetes, abscesses, steroids
Liver function tests	History of liver disease, alcoholism, bleeding, pyrexia of unknown origin
Clotting studies	History of liver disease, bleeding
Sickle cell test	Afro-Caribbeans if sickle cell status unknown
Electrocardiogram	History of hypertension, cardiorespiratory disease, age >55 years
Chest X-ray	History of cardiorespiratory disease, heavy smoker, potential metastases, recent immigrants from area where TB is endemic
Pulmonary function tests	Respiratory disease, thoracic surgery
Arterial blood gases	Respiratory disease, thoracic surgery
Cervical spine X-ray	Rheumatoid arthritis, trauma

Box 2.10 Preoperative grading system of the American Society of Anesthesiologists (ASA)

ASA I	Healthy patient
ASA II	Mild systemic disease, no functional disability
ASA III	Moderate systemic disease, functional disability
ASA IV	Severe systemic disease, constantly life-threatening
ASA V	Moribund patient, unlikely to survive 24 hours with or without an operation

Monitoring and charting the anaesthetised patient

Apart from clinical observation, standard monitoring is directed to the cardiovascular and respiratory systems (Box 2.14). Continuous ECG and automated blood pressure measurement are mandatory. Pulse oximetry provides continuous oxygenation information. Measurement of exhaled

Table 2.5 Factors to consider in choosing regional anaesthesia

Advantages	Disadvantages
Avoids complications of general anaesthetic	Toxic effects of local anaesthetics
Contributes to postoperative analgesia	Patient unhappy to be awake
Less postoperative nausea and vomiting	Inadequate anaesthesia
Patient satisfaction (e.g. caesarean section)	Possible nerve damage
Reduces incidence of DVT	Can be slow onset

Box 2.11 Complications of anaesthesia

Hypoxia
Hypercapnia
Hypotension
Arrhythmias
Pulmonary embolism
Allergic reactions
Hypothermia

Awareness
Minor trauma, e.g. sore throat
Headache
Malignant hyperpyrexia
Nausea and vomiting

Box 2.12 Maximum safe doses of local anaesthetics

Lidocaine 4 mg/kg
Bupivacaine 2 mg/kg
Prilocaine 5 mg/kg

NB: 1% solution of drug = 10 mg/mL.

Box 2.13 History of spinal anaesthesia

The first planned spinal anaesthesia for surgery in man was administered by August Bier (1861–1949), a German surgeon, on 16 August 1898, in Kiel, Germany.

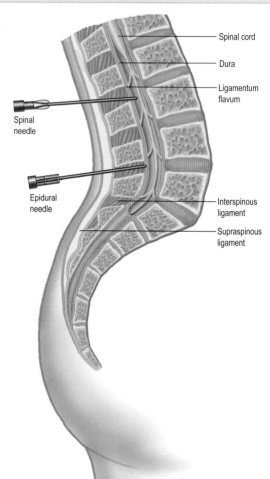

Spinal cord

Dura

Ligamentum flavum

Spinal needle

Epidural needle

Interspinous ligament

Supraspinous ligament

Figure 2.1 The anatomy of spinal and epidural anaesthesia.

gases also occurs, indicating if ventilation is adequate. Complex cases often utilise further monitoring, e.g. intra-arterial lines, central venous pressure measurement, cardiac output devices (e.g. oesophageal Doppler) and urine output. All these methods carry a small measure of morbidity and complication rate. However, it is increasingly recognised that optimal fluid management using these devices optimises outcome and shortens in-patient hospital stay.

Box 2.14 Standard monitoring

ECG	Temperature
Non-invasive blood pressure	Degree of muscle relaxation
Pulse oximetry	Inspired oxygen
End-tidal carbon dioxide levels	concentration

Box 2.15 Standard criteria for discharge from the recovery unit

Awake and cooperative	Surgical site uncomplicated
Cardiovascularly stable	Postoperative fluids and
Well oxygenated	drugs charted
Pain controlled	

The anaesthetic machine also needs monitoring. This is achieved by a variety of devices, namely: flow meters, vaporisers, and the ventilator, all of which have alarm systems in place to detect malfunction.

The agents used during the procedure may be classified into:

(a) induction agents (e.g. thiopentone or propofol)
(b) inhalational maintenance agents (halothane, sevoflurane, isoflurane, nitrous oxide)
(c) neuromuscular blocking agents (suxamethonium, vecuronium)
(d) analgesics (opioids, simple analgesics and NSAIDs).

The criteria for discharge from the recovery unit are shown in Box 2.15. Specific signs that may be important in the early postoperative phase are shown in Table 2.6.

Pain and its relief

Tissue damage (surgical intervention) causes release of pain mediators (e.g. histamine, bradykinins) at the site of injury. Nerve fibres are stimulated to transmit the sensation of pain via the spinal cord to the brain. Anti-inflammatory agents can inhibit release of pain mediators, whilst local blocks prevent impulses reaching the brain. Opiate analgesics exert a central effect.

Post-operative pain is inevitable for most patients. It can have serious physiological and psychological consequences (Table 2.7). Intensity of pain is influenced by cultural and family background, personality, past experience and motivation. Pre-operative literature can inform and allay anxiety while a calming, reassuring attitude from the medical and nursing staff will contribute to pain reduction. Pain management has become a subspecialty in its own right and principles only will be discussed here.

Therapy

All agents are better given on a regular basis. Mild pain may be treated with NSAIDs and paracetamol. Moderate pain responds well to mixtures

Table 2.6 Specific signs that may be important in the early postoperative period

Sign	Possible meanings
Respiratory distress: tachypnoea, cyanosis	Hypoxia
CNS signs:	
CNS depression	Oversedation
Agitation	Carbon dioxide retention Blood loss Hypoxia Pain
Disorientation	Inappropriate sedation Hypoxia
Severe inappropriate pain	Local complication at site of operation – bleeding, leakage of secretions, ischaemia
Wound:	
Bleeding	Uncontrolled blood vessel
Soft tissue haematoma	Clotting disorder
Irregular pulse	Unrecognised cardiac disorder Hypoxia
Skin pallor, empty veins, hypotension, tachycardia	Hypovolaemia

Table 2.7 Effects of postoperative pain

Effect	Outcome
Decreased respiratory excursion	Hypoventilation Pulmonary collapse/consolidation
Gastrointestinal atony	Ileus, nausea and vomiting
Bladder atony	Urinary retention
Catecholamine release	Vasoconstriction; increased blood viscosity, clotting activity and platelet aggregation; raised cardiac work

of codeine and paracetamol. Narcotic analgesics (e.g. morphine) are widely used for severe pain and are delivered in a variety of regimens (orally, subcutaneous infusion, intramuscularly and intravenously, more often controlled by the patient – PCA) (Table 2.8). A combination of these drugs usually produces the best results. Pre-emptive analgesia before the operation has been started is also useful (e.g. infiltrating the skin prior to incision).

Table 2.8 Standard postoperative analgesia regimens (fit, adult, male, 70 kg)

Grade of surgery	Example	Postoperative analgesia
Minor	Lipoma removal	Paracetamol, 1 g, 6-hourly
Intermediate	Arthroscopy Hernia repair	Co-dydramol, 2 tablets, 6-hourly + diclofenac, 50 mg orally, 8-hourly
Major	Laparotomy Hip replacement	Morphine PCA, 1 mg bolus, 5 min lock-out + diclofenac, 50 mg orally, 8-hourly

PCA, patient-controlled analgesia.

The management of chronic pain is a complex subject managed by anaesthetists with an interest in this area. The skills of a number of other specialists are enlisted including psychologists, physiotherapists and relaxation therapists. Antidepressants are increasingly used in this field.

The general surgical take

Care of the critically ill surgical patient 3

INTRODUCTION

The term 'critical illness' describes the condition of a patient who has a likely, imminent or established requirement for organ support; in simple terms where death is possible without timely and appropriate intervention. Some patients are at greater risk of developing critical illness than others (Box 3.1). Also certain conditions bring a likelihood of severe physiological stress (Box 3.2). It is unfortunately commonplace for the junior surgeon to be faced with a critically ill surgical patient, in various situations-from the peritonitic teenager admitted to A&E to the elderly postoperative hip replacement on HDU. It is crucial that a systematic approach is taken to assessment and treatment.

While it is more challenging to manage the patient with multiple organ failure it is rarely rewarding; rescuing the elderly post-laparotomy patient from cardiac failure brought about by fast atrial fibrillation is far harder than anticipating the hypokalaemia (causing the cardiac irritability) associated with ileus: *prediction and prevention is essential*. Prediction can begin with pre-operative assessment (such as identifying chronic airways disease or poor nutritional state) but continues through knowledge of the common problems associated with the condition/operation (such as the risk of chest infection after laparotomy). Prevention encompasses specific steps such as adequate replacement of fluid and electrolytes, adequate analgesia, chest physiotherapy and thromboprophylaxis, but the role of regular review (e.g. ward rounds) cannot be overstated.

Conversely a failure to assess patients regularly, to identify and act upon abnormal findings, to check whether one's interventions have been carried out and whether they have been effective/sufficient, will make successful management less likely.

Finally, communication has become ever more important. The maxim *'if it's not in the notes it didn't happen'* is not only for the benefit of the medical defence unions but reminds us that colleagues rely heavily on written information, not only if the case is complex but especially if the author is not available to discuss the case in person. The junior surgeon will often be working shifts and be responsible for many patients, in different clinical areas and will also have to leave the hospital at the end of his/her shift. Continuity of care relies entirely on this written 'handover' information. A schematic is suggested in Box 3.3.

IMMEDIATE MANAGEMENT

There are two broad clinical scenarios facing the surgeon in critical care management: those patients who are 'unstable' (newly arrived or recently deteriorated on the ward) and those who are more 'stable' (typically on HDU/ITU with organ support established). Even in such a place of relative

---

Box 3.1 Risk factors for developing critical illness

Being very young or elderly
Co-morbidity
Recent (non-critical) illness
Recent operation
Prior complication
Delay in presentation
Delay in diagnosis

Delay in intervention
Multiple interventions
Complex surgery
Prolonged surgery
Massive transfusion
Emergency presentation

Box 3.2 Conditions likely to result in critical illness

Perforated viscus (including anastomotic leak)
Pancreatitis
Intestinal obstruction
Major GI haemorrhage
Ischaemic bowel
Undrained sepsis (pyelonephritis, cholangitis, intra-abdominal
 abscess, empyema)
Major non-GI haemorrhage (ruptured AAA, spleen, postoperative
 bleeding)

Box 3.3 Information required in notes after assessing a critically ill
surgical patient

Who and when
Date, time, name, grade, specialty, bleep number

Assessment
Summary of events, clinical features, response to treatments
already given by others

Differential diagnosis
Compile a list of active problems

Treatment given
What ABCDE measures have been taken, investigations
performed, medications given, responses to the treatment?

Communication
Who has been informed (nurses, seniors, relatives, ITU)

Plan of action
What is planned (investigations, definitive treatment, when should
next review occur)?

safety, 'stable' patients can become destabilised; the approach, even on the HDU/ITU ward round, should be structured as for the 'unstable' patient. This also assists the creation of an ordered management plan for the rest of the shift.

Unfortunately the junior surgeon is faced more often, as the attending doctor, with an unstable patient and there is a need to identify *what is going on* at the *same time* as institution of resuscitative measures (see Table 3.1). The mnemonic ABCDE is used as an *aide-memoire* for this systematic approach to the initial phase of critical care management, 'immediate assessment and treatment'. By the end of this phase some common steps should have occurred:

● Oxygen therapy to saturation above 94%
● Intravenous access and fluid administration
● Moving of patient to appropriate level of care bed and institution of intensive monitoring (cardiac monitor, pulse oximeter, catheter)
● Involving senior colleague
● Involving intensivist colleague
● Baseline investigations (see Box 3.4).

It is essential to reassess the patient regularly to ensure that some measure of improvement has occurred and that time has been bought for a more thorough 'full assessment'.

FULL ASSESSMENT

This will depend upon the clinical scenario – the longer the patient has been in hospital the greater the amount of available information. Relative/ carer history is of paramount importance in the newly-admitted patient whereas identification of trends (from charts, clinical notes and/or blood results) is often rewarding in identifying *what is going on* in a previously 'stable' ward patient.

Knowledge of the patients' pre-existing conditions and functional performance is essential to guide treatment. There may be poor cardiac/ respiratory and/or renal reserve; not only are those patients more likely to become critically ill from a lesser degree of severity of illness, therapeutic measures (and even the investigations) may also place the patient at further danger. Large fluid boluses may overload the failing heart and intravenous contrast can provoke renal failure.

DEFINITIVE TREATMENT

When all information is collated, and the clinical situation reassessed, the patient may have returned to stability (a 'hiccup') and enhanced monitoring can form part of the routine daily plan. This conclusion should be reached with caution. It is more likely that there remains a degree of instability and/or uncertainty as to exactly what has happened. Specialist opinions and investigations should occur while resuscitative measures in a 'place of safety' (usually HDU or ITU) continue. The aim is to identify pathology and establish definitive treatment as soon as possible. Definitive treatments may be medical or surgical and may need to be tailored to severity or response – the best example is the bleeding duodenal ulcer: a proportion of patients with this condition will stop bleeding spontaneously (and thus require supportive care such as blood transfusion), others will require injection sclerotherapy at oesophago-gastroduodenoscopy and some will require laparotomy and oversew of the ulcer. What is crucial

Table 3.1 The ABCDE approach to the ill patient

Observe	Examine	Treat
Airway		
Look for: oral FB, cyanosis, 'seesaw', abdominal respiration. Listen for: stridor, hoarseness, grunting	Feel for airflow	Chin-lift, suction, oral vomit, denture, airway, bag & mask, anaesthetic support
Breathing		
Look for: respiration rate, accessory muscle use equal expansion, sweating, JVP. Listen for: full-sentences	Trachea central. Surgical emphysema, percussion note, auscultate	High flow O_2. Treat as per cause, e.g. chest drain for pneumothorax
Circulation		
Look for: external haemorrhage, BP, heart rate, pallor, sources of fluid loss, charts	Cool/warm peripheries. Pulse rate/rhythm/ volume	IV fluid control external haemorrhage
Dysfunction		
Alert/verbal stimulus. Pain response/unresponsive. Glasgow Coma Score. Pupils reactive/equal		Exclude hypoxia/hypercapnia, sedatives, hypoglycaemia
Expose		
As required to aid diagnosis (while respecting patient dignity)		Allowing access for therapeutic intervention

Box 3.4 Baseline investigations (and look up/acquire any older tests for comparison/trends)

ECG
Rhythm, ischaemic changes

Blood monitoring
Bedside glucose

CXR
Acute lung pathology (atelectasis, pneumonia, pleural effusion), chronic lung pathology, cardiac overload, perforated viscus (pneumoperitoneum)

Bloods
Full blood count, urea & electrolytes, clotting, LFTs, amylase, CRP

ABG
Oxygenation level, CO_2 level, acid-base balance

Micro
Cultures (sputum, urine, blood)

is that, by regular systematic assessment, confirmation is obtained that a strategy is working, and if not that a new strategy is pursued post haste.

COMMON CRITICAL CARE PROBLEMS

Although they may overlap in the severely ill surgical patient, there are common clinical scenarios that may occur. While it is worth considering these separately, by adopting a systematic approach, the assessment and management of the patient (along with a sound understanding of physiology) in most situations is straightforward.

Respiratory failure

This is the commonest cause of admission to an intensive care unit. Respiratory failure may be indicated by (ABCDE):
- Tachypnoea
- Cyanosis
- Use of accessory muscles
- Saturations <95%
- Distress
- Confusion.

Immediate management (assuming patent airway) is to sit the patient upright and to institute high-flow oxygen therapy, exclude easily-reversible causes of respiratory distress (eg tension pneumothorax) and complete the ABCDE.

Alongside baseline investigations, the full patient assessment will reveal what is the likely cause of the respiratory impairment (Table 3.2). The severity of impairment can be estimated by arterial blood gas measurement; alongside the CXR this is the most important investigation.

Technically a patient is regarded as suffering respiratory failure if the arterial partial pressure of oxygen (PO_2) is <8 kPa; a higher level of oxygen

Kumar and Clark's Handbook of Medical Management

Table 3.2 Management of respiratory failure

	Management steps
Generic steps	Humidified O_2, sit-up, IV access, monitoring in a place of safety, ABG, ECG, CXR, bloods, senior help especially if likely to need respiratory support (CPAP, BIPAP) or definitive airway
Airway obstruction	Relieve obstruction, adjunctive airway measures
Pulmonary oedema (including iatrogenic overload)	Diuretics
Atelectasis	Physiotherapy
Bronchial obstruction (acute/chronic)	Nebulised bronchodilators
Pneumonia	Antibiotics
Pulmonary embolus*	Maintain high preload, anti-coagulate
Myocardial infarction	Analgesia, ACS protocol
Pleural effusion	Consider aspiration
ARDS	Treat underlying cause**
Pneumothorax	Chest drain (needle thoracocentesis if tension)
Anaemia	Transfuse to 10 g/dL
Neurological dysfunction (e.g. sedation)	Give antidote if available, e.g. naloxone for opiate overdose, 'bag & mask' if poor ventilation

*See Box 3.5.
**See Box 3.6.

obtained on blood gas may still be seen if the patient has already been receiving supplementary oxygen. Respiratory failure is further divided into type 1 and type 2. The failure to oxygenate, despite adequate ventilation (with normal or even low CO_2 levels), is termed type 1 respiratory failure; the failure to oxygenate because of inadequate ventilation (with high CO_2 levels) is type 2.

In general terms, hypoxia improves with increases in the inhaled oxygen concentration. Predicting/identifying impaired ventilation is the next most crucial step; in hypercapnia measures must be taken to improve ventilation. There may be a significant pre-existing respiratory problem and there may be limits as to what can be achieved with standard ward care. In type 2 respiratory failure, merely increasing the inhaled oxygen concentration will improve arterial oxygenation (and buy time) but may paradoxically worsen the ventilatory drive (and lead to worsening CO_2 levels, respiratory acidosis and confusion). Unless a readily-reversible

Box 3.5 Pulmonary embolism

The migration of thrombus from typically a deep leg or pelvic vein, lodging in the pulmonary vasculature, is an all-too-common complication of surgical care (immobility, hyperviscosity, trauma to veins).

Classic presentation
Day 7–10 postoperative
Dyspnoea
Pleuritic chest pain
Haemoptysis
More often, sinus tachycardia and shortness of breath

Management
ABCDE
O_2
ECG, CXR (as much for a differential)
ABG (PaO_2 is usually low, CO_2 normal or low)
Anticoagulate (IV heparin if may need to stop quickly, low
    molecular-weight heparin more convenient)
IV fluid (increase preload)
Supportive care as necessary (HDU/ITU)

Diagnosis
CT pulmonary angiogram (rarely V/Q scan)
Venous duplex legs to identify source

Occasionally
Catheter-directed thrombolysis
Caval filter (especially if cannot anticoagulate)

Box 3.6 Acute respiratory distress syndrome (ARDS)

A diffuse inflammatory condition of the lungs (often part of a wider systemic inflammatory response syndrome) where there is leak of inflammatory fluid into the alveoli and progressively impaired oxygenation and ventilation (stiffening of lung tissue). Can occur rapidly and CXR signs may occur late therefore suspicion, recognition and escalation (typically to ITU) is key.

Causes
Any shock state
Severe infection
Pancreatitis
Trauma
Major surgery

Kumar and Clark's Handbook of Medical Management

factor is identified, the patient will require respiratory support (and often intubation) which usually necessitates asking for senior help.

Shock/circulatory failure

Shock is defined as the failure of the circulation to maintain adequate tissue perfusion. In immediate management (ABCDE), it is usually (but not always) associated with low systolic blood pressure (<100 mmHg) and tachycardia (HR >100); other signs vary according to the underlying cause. 'Hard' signs of reduced tissue perfusion include oliguria and metabolic acidosis. Immediate management may involve definitive treatment (e.g. control of external haemorrhage or the need to follow the advanced life support pathway) but the common generic steps are:

Immediate management

- Oxygen
- Large bore intravenous access
- *Initial* volume expansion (almost all forms of shock respond to fluid bolus)
- Baseline investigations (ECG, bloods, ABG)
- Senior help.

Full assessment

Clinical assessment (and data gathered from charts and the notes) will usually point to a typical cause (Box 3.7), but should begin by a targeted examination to establish the likely form of shock. Warm peripheries will point to a 'distributive' shock; that is to say where there is a failure of peripheral resistance (BP= (HR × CO) × TPR). This usually indicates systemic inflammatory response ± sepsis, but may occur in anaphylaxis or 'neurogenic shock' (such as spinal cord transection). Cool peripheries with signs of reduced circulating volume (low JVP, signs of dehydration, obvious fluid losses) may point to hypovolaemic shock. Cool peripheries and high JVP suggest a 'pump failure' – this may be intrinsic 'cardiogenic shock' if there has been a cardiac event (MI, arrhythmia) but can also occur secondarily to extrinsic compromise ('obstructive shock'), tension pneumothorax, cardiac tamponade or pulmonary embolism (Table 3.3).

Further definitive management depends on the exact cause and any easily reversible causes should take priority. The movement of the patient to a critical care area and the institution of invasive monitoring is invariably required, as established shock is not often rapidly reversible. Hypovolaemic states require expansion of circulating volume (to replace losses; see Chapter 4); low peripheral resistance states also require fluid replacement (as the circulating volume requirement increases) but often require inotropic support to increase arteriolar tone (see SIRS/sepsis below). Pump failure situations may require a combination of careful pre- and after-load management and in the case of cardiogenic shock, management is very difficult requiring expert cardiological input. For management of anaphylaxis see Box 3.8.

Sepsis and multi-organ failure

The body's response to threat of injury or infection is complex, involving multiple mediators (e.g. TNF, IL-1) to co-ordinate the inflammatory response. There is clearly a balance struck between pro- and anti-inflammatory mediators, and if the inflammatory response is excessive the process may ultimately harm the patient, with the development of a shock

Box 3.7 Causes of cardiac compromise in surgical patients

Hypovolaemia (most common in surgical patients)
Bleeding (revealed or concealed)
Burns
GI losses (vomit, diarrhoea, fistula, stoma)
Renal losses (post-obstructive diuresis, diuretics)
Inflammatory 'third space' losses (ileus, pancreatitis)
Iatrogenic (fasting preoperatively, bowel preparation)

Cardiogenic
Myocardial infarction
Cardiac failure (often iatrogenic fluid overload)
Arrhythmia (fast atrial fibrillation)

Systemic
Severe sepsis

Inflammation
Sepsis-syndrome
Septic shock

Obstructive
Pulmonary embolism
Tension pneumothorax
Cardiac tamponade

Anaphylaxis
Drugs
Transfusion reactions

Neurogenic
Spinal injury
Brainstem injury
Overly successful epidural anaesthesia

state and progressing to multi-organ failure. A continuum exists between the mild derangement of SIRS through to septic shock (Box 3.9). Certain conditions seem to predispose to an inflammatory response (Box 3.10) but there are probably other factors that determine outcome – including the severity of the insult, the delay to treatment and the underlying patient substrate (pre-existing cardiac, respiratory or renal impairment). *Early recognition, immediate resuscitation* and *identification and treatment of any underlying cause* are the key steps in management. If an infective source is suspected, *prompt antibiotic administration* is crucial pending more definitive treatment (e.g. drainage of abscess).

Immediate management
● ABCDE
● O₂
● Intravenous access and fluid bolus
● Intensive, invasive monitoring
● Baseline tests
● Senior help (inotropic and/or respiratory support may be required).

Kumar and Clark's Handbook of Medical Management

Table 3.3 Differentiating shock states (usually with ↓ BP)

Type	Heart rate	CVP	Peripheries	Other pointers
Hypovolaemic	↑	↓	Cool	Signs of haemorrhage, obvious fluid losses
Distributive	↑*	↓	Warm	Rigors (sepsis), urticaria, facial oedema, bronchospasm (anaphylaxis)
Obstructive	↑	↑	Cool	Chest signs (tension pneumothorax), predominant dyspnoea (PE), Kussmauls sign (↑ CVP with inspiration – tamponade)
Cardiogenic	↑, ↓ or →	↑	'Clammy'	Ischaemic ECG, chest pain

*Normo-/bradycardic (neurogenic).

Box 3.8   Management of anaphylaxis

Remove any obvious precipitating cause (e.g. drug infusion)
Give 0.5 mg epinephrine intra*muscularly*
Establish IV access:
    10 mg chlorpheniramine intra*venously*
    200 mg hydrocortisone intravenously
Fluid: initial 1 L bolus colloid
Admit to intensive monitoring area
Seek senior advice

Box 3.9   Definitions in sepsis

Systemic inflammatory response syndrome if any two of the
    following:
    Pyrexia >38°C or hypothermia <36°C
    Tachycardia >90 bpm
    Tachypnoea >20/min
    White cell count >12 or <4
Sepsis = SIRS + documented source of infection
Sepsis syndrome (SIRS +) organ malperfusion: or
Severe sepsis (sepsis +) organ malperfusion:
    Lactate >1.2 mmol/L
    SVR <800 dyne/s/cm^3
    PaO_2/FiO_2 <30
    PaO_2 <9.3 kPa
    Urine <120 mL/4h
    GCS <15 (no sedation or neurological event)
Septic shock = severe sepsis + refractory hypotension in presence
    of infection

Box 3.10   Some causes of an exaggerated inflammatory response

Infective

Central venous catheters   Abscess
Perforated viscus   Prosthetic tissue
Pyelonephritis   Necrotic tissue
Cholangitis

Non-infective

Pancreatitis   Major trauma
Reperfusion injury   Major surgery
Major haemorrhage

Kumar and Clark's Handbook of Medical Management

Full assessment

- History and examination
- Review of all charts
- Specialised tests, e.g. CT.

Definitive management

- Medical (antibiotics, removal of infected catheters)
- Interventional (percutaneous drainage, ERCP in biliary sepsis, nephrostomy in obstructive pyonephrosis)
- Surgical (abscess drainage, bowel resection, amputation).

Renal failure (Box 3.11)

Low urine output is one of the commonest reasons a doctor is called to review a surgical patient. Unfortunately one of the body's natural responses to stress is to reduce urine output, and working out when a patient is appropriately concentrating his urine rather than sliding into acute renal failure can present a challenge.

Renal dysfunction is however a common complication in the critically ill, and a major reason for admission to the ICU. The patients' baseline renal (dys)function is a major risk factor. A baseline creatinine of >140 mmol/L, although in numerical terms 15% above normal (range usually 125 mmol/L or less) represents as much as 80% loss of renal function. These patients should be carefully monitored as there is a much greater chance that the chronically-impaired kidney will fail in critical illness.

The key management steps when asked to see a patient with low urine output (<0.5 mL/kg/hr) are as follows:

- ABCs – is the patient stable? If the renal deterioration is secondary to another factor (such as hypotension due to post-operative bleeding) this must be addressed first. Assess as for all critically-ill patients (ABCDE) and resuscitate:
  - O_2 (adequate oxygenation)
  - IV access, fluid running (fluid challenge appropriate for the frailty of the patient)

> ### Box 3.11 Definitions in renal failure
>
> Acute renal failure (ARF) is defined as the sudden (and potentially recoverable) impairment of the kidneys' ability to excrete the body's nitrogenous waste.
>
> Chronic renal failure (CRF) is the irreversible chronic loss of functioning nephrons, of variable severity. In the critically ill surgical patient the patient may have suffered ARF before presentation due to the pathology, or may suffer ARF post-operatively.
>
> Both situations are made more likely if there is any degree of CRF. The kidney's function is very dependent upon adequate perfusion and oxygenation, and nephrons are extremely sensitive to sepsis and toxins (such as NSAIDS and aminoglycoside antibiotics); *prediction and prevention* in the stable patient is crucial.

Table 3.4 Complications of acute renal failure (and indications for dialysis)

Complication	Manifestation
Hyperkalaemia	Cardiac arrhythmia
Fluid overload	Pulmonary oedema, respiratory failure
Metabolic acidosis	Coma, arrhythmias, cardiac failure
Uraemia	Encephalopathy, pericarditis, gastrointestinal bleeding

Emergent treatment of hyperkalaemia (>6.5 mmol/L and/or ECG changes).
Calcium gluconate (10 mL of 10%), repeat if ECG changes unchanged at 5 min.
Insulin 10 U with 50 mL 50% dextrose over 15–30 min.
(If acidotic) sodium bicarbonate solution *get expert advice*.
Salbutamol 5 mg nebulised.

Box 3.12 Cardiac complications

A wide range of cardiac problems can occur in the critically ill surgical patient.

If presented with a cardiac arrhythmia the reader is referred to the ALS protocol (see www.resus.org.uk/pages/als.pdf

Ischaemic heart disease is widespread among older surgical patients, especially diabetics and in peripheral artery disease. The stress of the critical illness, and particularly combined with a major surgical insult, can precipitate a myocardial infarction (MI) and/or cardiac dysfunction. While the diagnosis is sometimes obvious (anterior chest pain, ischaemic changes on ECG) often the presentation is more obscure. A primary cardiac problem should be suspected in any case where there is a low cardiac output state, failing to respond to fluid resuscitation (obstructive causes, e.g. pneumothorax (tamponade excluded)).

Early advice from a cardiologist is essential but early management steps are:

ABCs: ensure no easily-reversible factors
Oxygen: keep SaO$_2$ >95%
Analgesia: IV diamorphine (for pain relief if symptomatic, distress-relief if severely dyspnoeic)
Anti-platelet agent: aspirin 300 mg if cannot exclude acute infarction
Vasodilator: nitrates (sublingually initially then intravenously; improve coronary blood flow and reduce cardiac workload)
Diuretic: IV furosemide if failure clinically.

Kumar and Clark's Handbook of Medical Management

- Aim BP MAP>70 mmHg (adequate perfusion)
- Bloods
- ECG
- ABG
- Catheter: Insert/hourly urometer/flush/replace.

Although it is crucial to watch out for the complications of established renal failure (and know how to treat – see Table 3.4) these usually take a little time to develop. Fluid overload, hyperkalaemia and metabolic acidosis are easily identified by these initial steps.

What do you think the volaemic status (intravascular, i.e. hydration state) of the patient is? Clinical exam, charts, likely losses and knowledge of pre-existing conditions will all aid an educated guess. If any doubt that the patient is euvolaemic (i.e. adequately hydrated) continue fluid rehydration.

Can you be certain that there is no obstruction? Total anuria is an obstructed urinary system until proven otherwise. Request KUB ultrasound if any doubt.

Take a history – what has happened to the patient recently?

Standard courses of treatment are as follows. Sepsis – treat source as above. Jaundice (the danger of liver and kidney failure 'the hepatorenal syndrome') – relieve any obstructive cause. Nephrotoxic drugs (stop if possible). Rhabdomyolysis (muscle breakdown in trauma or limb ischaemia – myoglobin is nephrotoxic) – aggressive hydration and alkalinize urine.

If renal deterioration is not quickly reversed and it becomes likely that renal replacement therapy will be necessary, get specialist help (renal team, intensive care physician).

For cardiac complications, see Box 3.12.

Trauma remains the leading cause of death in the first four decades of life. Deaths following trauma occur in a trimodal distribution. The first peak is caused by deaths occurring within seconds to minutes of the injury, usually due to non-salvageable conditions such as brain lacerations, major aortic and other vascular injuries. The only way of reducing these deaths is prevention. The second peak occurs within minutes to hours of the injury. The third peak is a broad shape and accounts for deaths occurring weeks to months after the trauma as a result of complications of the injuries and treatment. The advanced trauma life support (ATLS) method of trauma care, developed in Nebraska in the 1970s, is now widely accepted as the optimum approach to treating injured patients.

ATLS protocols focus on reducing the second peak, and optimum care in the so-called 'golden hour' undoubtedly reduces late deaths from complications.

INITIAL ASSESSMENT

Primary survey

Table 4.1 outlines the priorities for the first few minutes of treating an injured patient. Each of the 'ABCDE' priorities is paired with an equally important task. The usual sequence of history, examination, investigation and treatment seen in non-emergency situations is abandoned. Treatment of immediately life-threatening conditions is instigated simultaneously with ongoing assessment.

Airway

The quickest way to establish whether an airway is patent is to get the patient to talk. A patient who is shouting may be distressed but clearly has an adequate airway, whereas an unconscious patient may be assumed to have a compromised airway until proved otherwise.

An airway problem may be suspected in the presence of:

- cyanosis
- tachypnoea/agitation/use of accessory muscles of respiration
- noisy breathing
- foreign body/vomit/blood in the mouth
- facial and neck injuries
- facial burns
- unconsciousness.

Manoeuvres that may help establish a patent airway include:

- chin lift and jaw thrust
- Guedel (oropharyngeal) airway
- endotracheal intubation (oral or nasal)
- cricothyroidotomy
- tracheostomy.

Table 4.1 Sequence and priorities for primary survey

Airway	Cervical spine control
Breathing	100% oxygen
Circulation: assess heart rate and blood pressure, establish IV access	Control of external haemorrhage
Disability (neurological state)	Pupils
Exposure: undress patient	Temperature control

Throughout all these manipulations the cervical spine must be maintained in a stable midline position, by an assistant's hands if necessary. Once the airway is established the cervical spine should be stabilised using a hard cervical collar and taping the head to sandbags on either side of the patient's head.

Breathing

As soon as the airway is established, give 100% oxygen then examine the chest. Even with a patent airway, ventilation is often inadequate. Look for:

- asymmetric chest movements
- open chest wounds
- tracheal deviation (suggesting pneumo- or haemothorax pushing the mediastinum away from the side of the problem)
- abnormal percussion note (hyper-resonant in pneumothorax, dull in haemothorax)
- breath sounds (absent over pneumo- and haemothorax).

Pulse oximetry is a useful indicator of oxygenation and adequacy of ventilation but it is unreliable where the peripheral perfusion is poor.

Circulation

Note the heart rate and blood pressure. Pass two wide-bore cannulae in the antecubital fossae and commence infusion of 2000 mL of warm Hartmann's solution. Subsequent management depends on the patient's response to this initial fluid bolus (see 'Shock', Ch3 p50). Blood should be sent for full blood count, coagulation, cross-match, urea and electrolytes (U&E), glucose and amylase. Alcohol and other drugs may also be measured if indicated.

External haemorrhage should be controlled by direct pressure over the open wound.

If peripheral venous access cannot be established in the arm, surgical cut-down on to the long saphenous vein at the ankle or groin is required. Alternatively central venous access via the internal jugular or femoral veins may be used.

Disability (neurological status)

The simplest assessment of consciousness is the AVPU scale:

A: Alert
V: Responds to verbal stimuli
P: Responds to pain
U: Unresponsive.

If time permits, the more formal Glasgow Coma Score should be determined (see Table 4.5). Observe the pupils for dilatation and reactivity. A fixed, dilated pupil suggests an expanding intracranial haematoma or

> **Box 4.1** Conditions that are either detected or excluded at the end of a primary survey – 'ATOM Football Club'
>
> **A**irway obstruction   **M**assive haemothorax
> **T**ension pneumothorax   **F**lail chest
> **O**pen pneumothorax   **C**ardiac tamponade

cerebral oedema (the third nerve becomes compressed along the edge of the tentorium cerebelli as the brain herniates downward, allowing unopposed sympathetic pupillary dilatation).

Exposure

The patient must be undressed fully but hypothermia prevented by adequate covers or warming devices.

Box 4.1 outlines conditions that must be detected or excluded by the end of the primary survey. The mnemonic 'ATOM Football Club' may help.

Adjuncts to primary survey

Monitoring

ECG monitoring and continuous pulse oximetry are vital.

X-rays

X-rays of the chest, pelvis and lateral cervical spine are required for all seriously injured patients, in addition to other studies that may be indicated. The chest film is the most useful as haemo/pneumothoraces are often identified that were not obvious on clinical examination but which require chest drainage. Note that a normal lateral cervical spine film alone does NOT exclude a neck injury, especially in an unconscious patient.

Nasogastric tube

This reduces the likelihood of aspiration of gastric contents. If a facial or basal skull fracture is suspected, the oral route should be used; a tube passed nasally may end up in the cranium.

Urinary catheter

Urine output is a useful indication of renal perfusion and blood volume and is required in all severely injured patients. Transurethral catheterisation is contraindicated if there is evidence of urethral trauma, in which case a retrograde urethrogram is required. Signs suggestive of urethral damage include:
● blood at the urethral meatus
● scrotal/perineal bruising/haematoma
● high riding prostate on rectal examination
● pelvic fracture.

Log roll

The log roll is a manoeuvre where the patient is rolled onto one side without rotating any part of the spine. It allows full exposure and inspection of the back of the patient's body without exacerbating any undiagnosed spinal injury. The precise timing in the resuscitation sequence is not fixed. Four trained personnel are required.

Kumar and Clark's Handbook of Medical Management

Secondary survey

The secondary survey comprises a complete history and examination and does not take place until the primary survey is complete.

History

The nature of the accident gives useful clues about the injuries that may be expected. Ambulance personnel, paramedics, police and witnesses may all provide useful information. The AMPLE mnemonic may help:

A: Allergies
M: Medication
P: Past medical history/Pregnancy
L: Last meal
E: Events leading to injury.

Examination

A complete head-to-toe examination is required: 'fingers and tubes in every orifice'.

Further specialised investigations may be performed as adjuncts to the secondary survey, e.g. CT scanning or additional plain X-rays. Once the full extent of the injuries has been determined, definitive care may commence.

SHOCK

Shock is defined as acute circulatory collapse causing inadequate perfusion and resultant tissue hypoxia and is extremely common in trauma. Haemorrhagic shock is the most common cause in trauma. Other causes of shock and their clinical features are outlined in Table 3.3 (see pages 50-52) .

Haemorrhagic shock

Severe haemorrhagic shock, characterised by tachycardia, hypotension, cold peripheries and oliguria, is straightforward to recognise, but the early stages may be less obvious, especially in a young and fit patient who can maintain a normal systolic pressure surprisingly well until further bleeding precipitates sudden collapse. Any trauma patient who is tachycardic and has cool peripheries must be assumed to be shocked until proven otherwise.

Haemorrhage is classified into four levels (Table 4.2), which are useful when estimating likely blood loss but are rarely clearly defined in practice. In true emergency situations patients are considered as *responders, transient responders* and *non-responders,* depending on the change in circulatory status following infusion of the initial bolus of 2000 mL warm crystalloid solution. Rapid responders who remain stable after the initial bolus do not need transfusion. Transient and non-responders need urgent blood transfusion and surgical intervention to identify and stem ongoing bleeding. When tracking down major haemorrhage in a hurry it is helpful to remember blood loss can only be in four places (and how to identify each in parentheses):

● chest (CXR, CT, in the chest drain)
● abdomen/pelvis (FAST ultrasound scan, X-ray of the pelvis, CT, DPL)
● surrounding long bone fractures (plain X-ray)
● on the floor (on the floor, witness accounts).

Blood in the chest, long bone fractures and major external haemorrhage are fairly easy to detect; most major occult blood loss is into the abdomen (see 'Abdominal trauma', p. 65).

Table 4.2 The four classes of haemorrhagic shock

	I	II	III	IV
Blood loss	750 mL	750–1500 mL	1500–2000 mL	>2000 mL
Percentage blood loss (think of tennis)	15	30	40	>40
Heart rate	<100	>100	>120	>140
Systolic pressure	Normal	Normal	Low	Low/unrecordable
Pulse pressure	Normal	Narrowed	Narrowed	Unrecordable
Level of consciousness	Normal	Anxious	Confused	Unconscious
Respiratory rate	Normal	20–30	30–40	>30–40
Urine output (mL/h)	>30	Oliguric	Oliguric	Anuric

It is important to realise that the early stages of haemorrhagic shock may not be obvious, and if unrecognised may suddenly progress to collapse which may be too late to reverse. This is especially true in the elderly and athletes, and in hypothermia and pregnancy. Beware beta-blockers and pacemakers, which may prevent the patient mounting a tachycardia.

Arterial blood gas estimation is very useful in assessing whether a patient is adequately resuscitated, since shock causes inadequate perfusion and the tissues become hypoxic, shifting to anaerobic respiration leading to acidosis. Urine output is also a useful guide.

Fluid resuscitation

When using crystalloid fluid for resuscitation, each unit volume of lost blood must be replaced by three times the volume of the crystalloid solution. Fully cross-matched blood is best for transfusion but takes time to prepare. Type-specific (ABO) blood is available much more quickly. Group O rhesus-negative blood is reserved for catastrophic exsanguinating haemorrhage (but see Box 4.2).

Routes of administration of fluids

- Peripheral intravenous infusion – the most effective route for fast infusion of fluids is a wide-bore IV cannula in each antecubital fossa.
- Central line – percutaneous catheterisation of the femoral or internal jugular or subclavian veins allows central venous access. The long length of these catheters restricts the rate at which fluid may be given. Short, wide-bore peripheral lines are better.
- Venous cut-down – the long saphenous vein is easy to find just anterior to the medial malleolus or medial to the femoral pulse in the groin. It is quickly exposed through a small incision that permits catheterisation under direct vision. This technique is especially useful when all peripheral veins are collapsed and difficult to cannulate percutaneously.
- Intra-osseous needle (proximal tibia) – used for emergency resuscitation of children under 6 years of age, where no other access is available.

Kumar and Clark's Handbook of Medical Management

> **Box 4.2** Permissive hypotension/hypotensive haemostasis 'The only way to stop the bleeding is to stop the bleeding'
>
> There are several factors in haemorrhagic shock that challenge standard ATLS fluid-resuscitation:
>
> Hypotension in haemorrhage is a natural protective mechanism
> Hypotension facilitates in vivo coagulation
> Hypotension secondary to haemorrhage can be tolerated for some time with moderately-well preserved cerebral and renal perfusion
> Animal models have demonstrated that clot formed at the vessel bleeding point can be 'pushed out' at systolic pressures >80 mmHg
> Aggressive fluid resuscitation with crystalloid has the following additional consequences:
> dilution coagulopathy
> hypothermia and sequelae
> metabolic acidosis
> acute respiratory distress syndrome.
>
> The change in approach to major haemorrhage management is most clearly demonstrated with respect to the management of the ruptured abdominal aortic aneurysm (AAA). The patient has suffered a tear in the wall of a very large artery but often with a combination of clot, tamponade in the retroperitoneal space and hypotension (hypovolaemia plus autoregulation), the bleeding temporarily stops. Trying to bring the blood pressure up to normal levels results in reactivation of the haemorrhage, and unless treatment is imminent the patient will expire.
>
> However there are limitations to the concept of permissive hypotension: in general, prolonged organ ischaemia is bad. Traumatic brain injury outcomes are inversely proportional to duration of hypotension for example. Patients with critical stenosis in coronary, carotid or renal vessels may be prone to occlusion of the vessel and/or infarction in the end-organ.
>
> It is ultimately a question of balance with the emphasis on prevention of continuing haemorrhage; *if surgical control is likely to be necessary* then permissive hypotension is a logical management strategy.

CHEST TRAUMA

Most chest injuries, whether penetrating or blunt, can be managed with a combination of chest drainage and assisted ventilation. Thoracotomy is not needed very often; the priority is to provide the simple measures promptly and to be alert to more serious injuries that might need further treatment.

Initial management follows the ABCDE protocol of the primary survey. Immediately life-threatening chest injuries that should be detected during the course of the primary survey are listed in Box 4.1 (p. 59).

Tension pneumothorax: needle thoracocentesis

A tension pneumothorax occurs when the pleura is breached, allowing air to escape into the pleural cavity. Trapped air accumulates in the pleural cavity under increasing pressure, squashing the remainder of the chest contents. This causes hypoxia, agitation ('I can't breathe'), tachycardia, tachypnoea, cyanosis, distended neck veins, tracheal deviation away from the affected side, hyper-resonant percussion note and absent breath sounds. It is a clinical diagnosis and requires immediate treatment: the patient will die if you wait for a chest X-ray.

Decompress the tension immediately passing a large-bore IV cannula into the pleural cavity through the midclavicular line in the second inter-costal space. An immediate 'hiss' will be heard as the high pressure air escapes. This converts a tension pneumothorax into an open pneumothorax and buys enough time to insert a formal chest drain.

Open pneumothorax

An open chest wound allows air to be sucked into the pleural cavity on inspiration and forced out on expiration (hence the term 'sucking chest wound'). If the hole in the chest is wider than the diameter of the trachea, air is sucked in and out of this opening in preference to moving air in and out of the lungs via the airway. The patient rapidly becomes exhausted and hypoxic trying to breathe with the futile effort of forcing air in and out of the open wound.

Immediate management is to close the defect with an occlusive dressing taped down on three sides. This allows air out of the pleural cavity on expiration but on inspiration the dressing is sucked against the chest wall preventing re-entry of air. This improves the situation long enough for a formal chest drain to be inserted at a site away from the wound.

Massive haemothorax

The accumulation of over 1500 mL of blood in the chest causes hypoxia by restricting lung expansion and shock due to class III/IV (i.e. major) blood loss. The chest is dull to percussion over the haemothorax and breath sounds are absent.

Management requires immediate fluid resuscitation and simultaneous decompression of the pleural cavity with a chest drain.

If available, auto-transfusion equipment allows large volumes of blood collected via the chest tube to be transfused immediately.

A patient who drains more than 1500 mL blood on initial insertion of the chest drain, or who continues to drain more than 200 mL per hour for 2–4 hours, is likely to need a thoracotomy. These volumes are guidelines; the indication for surgery depends more on the patient's general state, and the diagnostic and surgical facilities available.

Flail chest

A flail chest (or flail segment) occurs when one or more ribs are fractured in more than one place. This results in a segment of the rib cage losing bony continuity with the rest of the chest wall. Flail segments usually result from severe blunt trauma and the underlying lung is often severely contused, exacerbating the respiratory difficulty. The work of breathing is inefficient (as the flail segment is sucked in as the chest is expanded, and vice versa – this is known as 'paradoxical respiration') and painful.

Crepitus of fractured ribs may be palpable but the presence and extent of a flail chest is best shown by a chest X-ray. The patient may cope for some hours but most patients with flail segment injuries develop respiratory failure (evidenced by deteriorating oxygen saturations and arterial blood gases) and the majority will require a period of assisted ventilation while the underlying lung recovers. In less severe cases, an intercostal nerve block may ease the pain of breathing sufficiently to avoid artificial ventilation.

Cardiac tamponade

Cardiac tamponade is a similar phenomenon to tension pneumothorax in that blood collects in the pericardial cavity following cardiac injury and has nowhere to escape to. The blood accumulates and compresses the heart, preventing venous return and limiting cardiac output. The signs are tachycardia, with hypotension, distended neck veins and muffled heart sounds (Beck's triad). Immediate pericardial aspiration is required.

Cardiac tamponade may be difficult to diagnose. Additional clues are increased pulsus paradoxus (decrease in systolic pressure on inspiration) and Kussmaul's sign (increase in venous pressure on inspiration) but these signs are difficult to elicit with confidence in the emergency setting.

Pulseless electrical activity in the absence of hypovolaemia or pulmonary embolism is suggestive of cardiac tamponade. Echocardiography, if available, may confirm the diagnosis.

Other chest injuries

While the 'ATOM-FC' (Box 4.1) injuries must be detected early, there are other thoracic problems that may not be obvious initially but which can be lethal if missed.

Simple pneumo/haemothorax

Small pneumo- and haemothoraces may not be detected on clinical examination but will be diagnosed on the chest film. Most require insertion of a chest drain, especially if the patient is to have a general anaesthetic (as a simple pneumothorax may become a tension pneumothorax once the patient is ventilated under anaesthetic).

Pulmonary contusion

Often associated with rib fractures, lung contusions may lead to gradual onset of respiratory failure over 2–3 days following the injury. Careful monitoring with regular clinical reassessment, chest radiography, pulse oximetry and arterial blood gas analysis is required.

Mediastinal injuries

Injuries to the trachea and bronchi, aortic disruption, blunt and penetrating cardiac trauma, oesophageal and diaphragmatic injuries all have a high mortality and require expert assessment and treatment.

The chest X-ray in trauma

A systematic approach helps to detect all the useful information that a CXR provides for injured patients (Table 4.3). Rib fractures and pneumothoraces are more easily spotted if the film is rotated 90°.

CT scanning and aortography may help confirm or exclude abnormalities suspected on the chest film.

Table 4.3 Systematic approach to the chest X-ray in trauma

Lungs, pleural cavities, trachea and bronchi	Look for pneumothorax, haemothorax, pulmonary contusions, tracheal and bronchial disruptions. Since the patient is usually supine, even quite large haemothoraces may manifest only as a vague whitening of the lung field
Mediastinum	Widening of the mediastinum suggests aortic disruption. Air in the mediastinum may indicate oesophageal perforation
Diaphragm	Diaphragmatic rupture (usually on the left) Free gas under the diaphragm
Bones	Rib fractures, flail segments, scapular, sternum, clavicle and shoulder injuries. Fractures of the first rib and scapula are associated with high-velocity injuries and usually with serious organ damage. Lower left rib fractures raise the probability of splenic rupture
Soft tissues	Surgical emphysema is often seen with pneumothoraces
Tubes and lines	The positions of endotracheal, chest and nasogastric tubes and central venous line may all be checked on the CXR

Insertion of a chest drain

Chest drains are required for the relief of a large pneumothorax (after release of a tension pneumothorax), surgical emphysema, haemothorax and pleural effusion/empyema – see Chapter 24.

ABDOMINAL TRAUMA

In contrast to the chest, the abdomen in the trauma patient is difficult to examine, problematic to image and more likely to require surgery for haemorrhage. The main difficulty is determining whether or not there is significant abdominal bleeding. It is helpful to recall that the hypovolaemic patient may have lost blood into only four places: the chest, the abdomen, at the site of long bone fractures and on the floor (i.e. external haemorrhage). The abdomen is the only site that is difficult to account for. The availability of CT scanning has reduced the number of exploratory laparotomies, and many injuries that in the past would have led to surgery may now be managed conservatively.

History

Any penetrating trauma to the trunk, or high impact injury (high speed car crash or fall from height) is likely to cause intra-abdominal damage.

Examination

The abdominal examination of the traumatised patient is surprisingly unhelpful, even in experienced hands. Coexisting pain in other parts of the body, alcohol, depressed level of consciousness, shivering and superficial trunk injuries all confound the assessment of the abdomen. Surprising amounts of blood may be lost into an apparently painless and soft abdomen. Equally, broken ribs and muscular bruising may cause extreme pain and guarding while palpating an otherwise unharmed torso. Thus even a careful inspection/palpation/percussion/auscultation examination may neither confirm nor exclude underlying injury.

The examination must include inspection of the back and perineum and a rectal examination, best done at the time of the log roll.

There are four things to check during the rectal examination:

- sphincter tone
- high riding prostate (suggesting urethral disruption)
- bony fragments (a pelvic fracture penetrating the rectum constitutes an open pelvic fracture with a >50% mortality)
- blood in the lumen.

Urethral trauma is suggested by blood at the meatus, perineal/scrotal bruising, a high riding prostate or a pelvic fracture.

Some signs are helpful pointers. The imprint of a steering wheel, seat belt or tyre mark on the trunk suggests serious damage. A fractured pelvis is often associated with abdominal (usually extraperitoneal venous) bleeding. A penetrating wound which when probed reveals bile or bowel content (use a culture swab; the gentle cotton tip is ideal) obviously needs laparotomy, but around a third of stab wounds do not penetrate the peritoneum, and not all those that do require surgery.

Investigation

Table 4.4 outlines the advantages and disadvantages of ultrasound, diagnostic peritoneal lavage (DPL) and CT scanning for abdominal trauma. For all but very unstable patients, CT scanning is by far the superior modality.

Blood tests

The blood tests performed when blood is taken during the primary survey must include a serum amylase (retroperitoneal trauma can be difficult to diagnose – the first indication may be a raised serum amylase).

Plain films

Broken ribs on the CXR or a fractured pelvis raise the likelihood of abdominal trauma.

CT scanning

Unless the patient is very unstable, CT scanning is the best way to diagnose (or exclude) intra-abdominal injury.

Diagnostic peritoneal lavage

Popular at one time, but now largely superseded by CT scanning.

Ultrasound

Quick and accurate in skilled hands but limited information about retroperitoneal structures and not sufficient to exclude splenic rupture.

Contrast studies

Intravenous urography and retrograde urethrography may help define urological trauma. Contrast studies are occasionally indicated for gastrointestinal trauma.

Table 4.4 Comparison of ultrasound, diagnostic peritoneal lavage and CT scanning for abdominal trauma

	Advantages	Disadvantages
Ultrasound	Quick Non-invasive Cheap	Needs skilled operator Unreliable for retroperitoneal and bowel damage Does not exclude splenic rupture Detail inadequate to quantify complex injuries
Diagnostic peritoneal lavage	Quick Sensitive for bleeding	Needs skilled operator Non-specific and over-sensitive Prejudices subsequent imaging Difficult in obese or scarred abdomens No information on retroperitoneum
CT scanning	Highly accurate, sensitive and specific Detailed information on all compartments of the abdomen including retroperitoneum Distinguishes intraperitoneal from retroperitoneal and pelvic bleeding Allows accurate diagnosis and monitoring of injuries and avoids the need for many laparotomies	Takes time Expensive Requires IV contrast for best results

Laparoscopy

Popular in some trauma centres; laparoscopy is particularly accurate in confirming/excluding diaphragmatic trauma in upper abdominal/lower chest stabbings.

Treatment

Laparotomy

Indications for laparotomy include:

- persistent hypotension despite resuscitation where the blood loss is suspected to be abdominal; in these patients there is no time for complex investigations, they must be taken straight to theatre
- peritonitis
- penetrating or gunshot wounds which obviously enter the peritoneal cavity
- radiological evidence of perforated viscus or severe organ damage.

Since a traumatised retroperitoneum is not easy to assess at laparotomy, patients who have clear clinical indications for exploratory laparotomy may still benefit from prior CT scanning if they are sufficiently stable.

Non-operative management

Accurate CT diagnosis of certain injuries, for example contained splenic haematoma or blunt renal trauma, may allow conservative treatment of conditions which would in the past have required surgery. Such patients need close monitoring ('active re-observation') and serial imaging with CT or ultrasound. See also Box 4.3.

Pelvic fractures

Unstable pelvic fractures cause massive haemorrhage, usually from large pelvic veins. This will not stop until the pelvis is stabilised using an external fixator. Laparotomy for suspected bleeding should never be performed until after the pelvis has been stabilised, and indeed may become unnecessary once the fracture is controlled, allowing the bleeding to tamponade.

HEAD INJURIES

Primary brain damage occurs at the time of the injury due to direct impact. This ranges from mild concussion (transient reversible diffuse brain injury) to massive brain contusions and lacerations.

Secondary brain damage results from cerebral oedema and intracranial haemorrhage. The cranium is a rigid cavity of fixed volume. As an injured brain swells or an intracranial haematoma expands, cerebrospinal fluid and venous blood is squeezed out of the skull, allowing the intracranial pressure to remain constant until a point of decompensation is reached and the intracranial pressure rises sharply. This decreases cerebral blood flow with resultant brain hypoxia. The problem is even more acute in the hypotensive, shocked patient with other injuries.

Box 4.3 Interventional radiology extends the role of non-operative management

In many cases of trauma the surgical treatment required to arrest bleeding is difficult and potentially carries risk of major morbidity. Transcatheter embolisation is a technique available to the specialised radiologist wherein occlusion of a vessel is achieved by deposition of thrombogenic materials directly into the vessel via an angiographic catheter.

This is particularly desirable when:
Rapid occlusion is desired
Surgical access is difficult
Patient is a poor anaesthetic risk
Surgery would likely result in the loss of a greater amount of tissue by ligation.

Typically metallic coils are used, although cyanoacrylates and fibrin sealant have also been used in trauma.

Patients with rising intracranial pressure collapse into deepening coma, and develop bradycardia and hypertension (the Cushing reflex). A fixed dilated pupil (due to third nerve compression as the cerebrum herniates through the tentorium cerebelli) is a late sign.

Minor head injuries

This category includes patients who arrive at hospital having been knocked out, but who are essentially back to normal (i.e. no neurological signs) when examined. In general, those with only a short period of loss of consciousness, no amnesia, no skull fracture and who have reliable, sensible relatives may be discharged with instructions to return should problems develop (all A&E units have 'head injury instructions' for carers).

Those who were unconscious for longer periods, who have been drinking alcohol or have a skull fracture should be admitted for a minimum of 24 hours for neurological observation. Patients who have a clinical indication for admission (e.g. no carer at home) do not necessarily require skull X-rays; they simply require observation, with immediate CT scanning if they deteriorate (Fig. 4.1). CT has become the first-line investigation in head injury assessment.

Major head injuries

The Glasgow Coma Score (Table 4.5) is a reproducible way of quantifying depression of consciousness and should be assessed in all significant head injuries.

Types of brain injury

Extradural haematoma (Fig. 4.2a)

The classic history is of a boxer knocked out in the ring who returns to normal (the *lucid interval*) then subsequently collapses unconscious. The extradural haematoma is usually the result of damage to the middle meningeal artery.

Subdural haematoma (Fig. 4.2b)

This typically presents with gradually deteriorating consciousness some time after an apparently innocuous injury in an elderly person. Clotting is often abnormal (beware antiplatelet or warfarin therapy).

Contusions, intracerebral haematomas and diffuse axonal injury

These patients often remain unconscious for a long time and require prolonged intensive care support.

Treatment

Assume all head-injured patients have a cervical spine injury until proved otherwise. The priority is to prevent secondary brain injury by providing maximum perfusion and oxygen delivery to the brain while the type of injury is determined by CT scan. Intubation, ventilation with 100% oxygen and resuscitation of the shocked patient is paramount. Isolated head injuries never cause hypotension, therefore search for other causes of shock in hypotensive patients. For isolated head injuries, some neurosurgical units advise mannitol and hydrocortisone to reduce cerebral oedema.

Kumar and Clark's Handbook of Medical Management

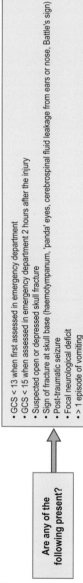

Are any of the following present?

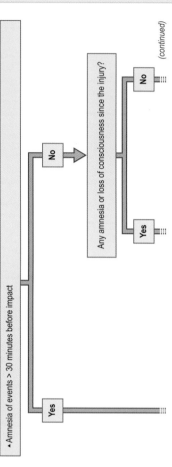

- GCS < 13 when first assessed in emergency department
- GCS < 15 when assessed in emergency department 2 hours after the injury
- Suspected open or depressed skull fracture
- Sign of fracture at skull base (haemotympanum, 'panda' eyes, cerebrospinal fluid leakage from ears or nose, Battle's sign)
- Post-traumatic seizure
- Focal neurological deficit
- > 1 episode of vomiting

▲ Amnesia of events > 30 minutes before impact

Yes

No

Any amnesia or loss of consciousness since the injury?

Yes

No

(continued)

a

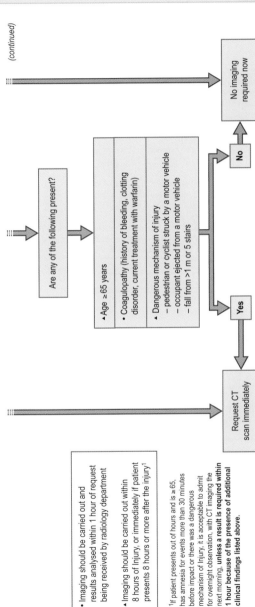

(continued)

Are any of the following present?

- Age ≥65 years
- Coagulopathy (history of bleeding, clotting disorder, current treatment with warfarin)
- Dangerous mechanism of injury
  - pedestrian or cyclist struck by a motor vehicle
  - occupant ejected from a motor vehicle
  - fall from >1 m or 5 stairs

Yes → Request CT scan immediately

No → No imaging required now

- Imaging should be carried out and results analysed within 1 hour of request being received by radiology department
- Imaging should be carried out within 8 hours of injury, or immediately if patient presents 8 hours or more after the injury†

†If patient presents out of hours and is ≥65, has amnesia for events more than 30 minutes before impact or there was a dangerous mechanism of injury, it is acceptable to admit for overnight observation, with CT imaging the next morning, **unless a result is required within 1 hour because of the presence of additional clinical findings listed above.**

a (continued)

Figure 4.1 NICE guidelines for investigating clinically important brain injury. Selection of a) adults and b) children for CT (from Head injury: Triage, assessment, investigation and early management of head injury in infants, children and adults. Clinical Guideline 56. NICE 2007, with permission)

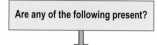

Are any of the following present?

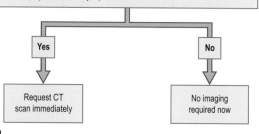

- Witnessed loss of consciousness lasting > 5 minutes
- Amnesia (antegrade or retrograde) lasting > 5 minutes
- Abnormal drowsiness
- 3 or more discrete episodes of vomiting
- Clinical suspicion of non-accidental injury
- Post-traumatic seizure but no history of epilepsy
- Age > 1 year: GCS < 14 on assessment in the emergency department
- Age < 1 year: GCS (paediatric) < 15 on assessment in the emergency department
- Suspicion of open or depressed skull injury or tense fontanelle
- Any sign of basal skull fracture (haemotympanum, 'panda' eyes, cerebrospinal fluid leakage from ears or nose, Battle's sign)
- Focal neurological deficit
- Age < 1 year: presence of bruise, swelling or laceration > 5 cm on the head
- Dangerous mechanism of injury (high-speed road traffic accident either as pedestrian, cyclist or vehicle occupant, fall from > 3 m, high-speed injury from a projectile or an object)

Yes

No

Request CT scan immediately

No imaging required now

b

Figure 4.1 cont'd

Intracranial haematomas need neurosurgical consultation with a view to evacuation. Intracranial pressure measurement may be helpful to monitor progress.

Prognosis

See Table 4.6. Hypotension is thought to have particular relevance: intracranial perfusion pressure = MAP–ICP.

SPINAL INJURIES

Types of spinal injury

Spinal cord injury may occur without bony injury (SCIWORA; spinal cord injury without radiological abnormality), and *vice versa,* but they usually coexist.

Like the brain, injury may be primary due to damage on impact, or secondary resulting from hypoxia, hypoperfusion, haematoma or

Table 4.5 The Glasgow Coma Score

A normal individual scores 15, whilst a corpse still scores 3.

Anyone with a score under 8 is by definition in coma and requires intubation and urgent CT scan

	Score
Best motor response	
Obeys commands	6
Localises pain	5
Withdraws to pain	4
Flexes to pain	3
Extends to pain	2
None	1
Speech	
Normal	5
Confused	4
Inappropriate	3
Incomprehensible sounds (grunts etc.)	2
None	1
Eyes	
Open spontaneously	4
Open to command	3
Open to pain	2
None	1

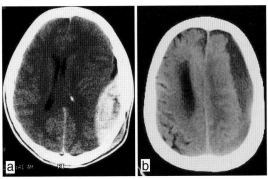

Figure 4.2 CT scans. (a) Left extradural haematoma obliterating the ventricle and shifting the midline to the right. (b) Left chronic subdural haematoma.

Kumar and Clark's Handbook of Medical Management

Table 4.6 Outcome in head injury with coma on admission

Status	Percentage of patients
Complete recovery	30
Some disablement but able to look after themselves	20
Severe disablement: vegetative state or unable to care for themselves	10
Death	40

movement of an unstable spinal fracture. Cord function below the lesion is lost.

Damage below the cervical spine spares the arms (see Fig. 4.3); lesions above C3 paralyse the diaphragm and are lethal without immediate ventilation (e.g. the 'hangman's fracture'; fracture dislocation of C2 on C3).

Stable and unstable fractures

Vertebral column injuries may be stable or unstable. Expert interpretation of imaging is required to determine this, and the injury must be assumed to be unstable until proved otherwise. This requires all movement of the patient to be undertaken with the spine immobilised in a neutral position.

Complete and incomplete cord injuries

Spinal cord injuries may be complete or incomplete. Function below a complete transection is lost and no recovery is expected. Partial injuries have a much better outcome.

- **Central cord syndrome** Motor power is lost in the arms but the legs are spared. This is seen in elderly patients with pre-existing osteoarthritis of the cervical spine after a hyperextension injury to the neck. There may be no fracture but the blood supply to the central cervical cord is compromised.
- **Posterior cord syndrome** Sensation is lost but motor function is preserved.
- **Anterior cord syndrome** Power is lost but sensation is preserved.
- **Brown–Séquard syndrome** The classic hemi-section of the spinal cord is rare. It results in ipsilateral power and proprioceptive loss below the lesion with contralateral loss of pain and temperature sensation.

Spinal and neurogenic shock

Spinal shock

Immediately after a cord trauma there is flaccid paralysis and loss of reflexes below the lesion. This may occur after incomplete injuries and recovery is possible. This is a neurological, not a cardiovascular, phenomenon.

Neurogenic shock

Sympathetic vasomotor tone is lost distal to a cord transection. This allows the peripheral microcirculation to vasodilate, and if the lesion is high, unopposed parasympathetic activity to the heart causes bradycardia. Patients with neurogenic shock are therefore hypotensive with warm extremities, with a normal or low heart rate even in the presence of hypovolaemia.

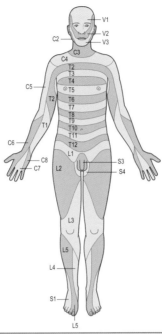

UPPER LIMB	
Reflexes	Predominant roots
Biceps	C5, C6
Triceps	T2
Supinator	C6
Major motor groups	Predominant roots
Trapezius	C3, C4
Shoulder abduction	C5
Elbow flexion	C5, C6
Elbow extension	C7
Finger flexion/extension	C8
Intrinsic muscles of hand	T1

Figure 4.3 Dermatomes of the body.

Management

Follow the ATLS primary and secondary survey protocols, maintaining oxygenation and perfusion. Establish whether the cord injury is partial or complete (largely a clinical decision) and whether the vertebral fracture is stable or unstable (requires plain X-rays or CT scanning).

Specialised spinal injury care must be provided as soon as possible; with high quality rehabilitation some useful recovery may be achieved.

BURNS

History

Establish the type of burn: flame, scald, direct contact, chemical, electrical, radiation. The history will give an idea of the likelihood of inhalational injury and associated carbon monoxide poisoning.

Examination

Site

Burns round the face and neck are more dangerous than elsewhere since the probability of inhalational damage is high. Such patients may walk into the casualty department conscious but collapse shortly afterwards with airway obstruction due to laryngeal oedema.

Circumferential burns of limbs constrict blood supply as the burn contracts. Burns of the face, hands, feet and genitals require special care, since the scarring is highly disabling.

Area

The 'rule of nines' is most convenient (Fig. 4.4). Alternatively the palm of an individual accounts for 1% of their surface area. For infants a Lund–Browder chart is used.

Depth

- **First-degree burns** There is erythema only without blisters, equivalent to sunburn. They are painful but heal rapidly.
- **Second-degree or partial thickness burns** These involve the epidermis and parts of the dermis, and are sometimes subclassified into sub-dermal and deep dermal burns. They are very painful, blistered with a mottled appearance. Healing is from the surviving dermal remnants which regenerate.
- **Third-degree or full thickness burns** The full thickness of epidermis and dermis is destroyed and the surface is painless and of variable colour. Without skin grafting, healing is by scarring, not skin regeneration.

Treatment

Initial treatment is following ABCDE primary and secondary survey protocols. Burns patients are prone to massive fluid loss. The Parkland formula helps guide initial fluid resuscitation:

Volume required (mL of Hartmann's solution) in 24 h = 4 times body weight (in kg) × the percentage of the total body surface burnt.

Half this volume should be given during the first 8 h after the injury. This formula is merely a guide and fluid replacement must be guided by monitoring of cardiovascular status, urine output and U&Es.

Large burns should be covered with clingfilm to reduce fluid loss. Flamazine may ease discomfort and additional analgesia may be needed. A tetanus booster should be given for non-immune patients. Antibiotics

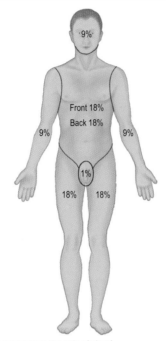

Figure 4.4 Burn assessment, the 'rule of nines'.

are of no benefit at this stage. Subsequent treatment involving surgical debridement, escharotomy, skin grafting and rehabilitation requires a specialist burns unit.

PAEDIATRIC TRAUMA

The principles of managing the traumatised child are identical to those of adult trauma, but the practicalities of airway management, shock assessment and vascular access may be more difficult. A child's vital signs may remain normal until more than 25% of blood volume is lost; the only sign of severe shock may be poor peripheral perfusion.

The volume of fluid used in adults for the initial bolus resuscitation (2000 mL warm Hartmann's solution) must be adjusted for children according to the following formula: 20 mL per kg body weight.

The Broselow Paediatric Resuscitation Measuring Tape (present in all A&E units) is useful to estimate the child's weight.

For children under 6 years of age, an intraosseous needle in the proximal tibia provides an emergency route for fluid transfusion if venous access is not obtainable.

Young flexible bones are less likely to fracture than adult bones; if fractures are found then the probability of organ damage is higher than for an adult.

TRAUMA IN PREGNANCY

Always involve a senior clinician if there is any suspicion of NAI (non-accidental injury). The well-being of the fetus depends on the mother's state; therefore the mother should be resuscitated first then the baby assessed, before completing the secondary survey of the mother. Surgeon and obstetrician must be involved early.

Blood volume increases in pregnancy and a pregnant patient may lose up to 1500 mL circulating volume before showing signs of hypovolaemia. By this stage the fetus is already severely compromised.

In the supine position the uterus compresses the inferior vena cava (IVC), reducing venous return to the heart and exacerbating the effects of haemorrhage. The pregnant female should therefore be nursed with wedges under the right buttock and shoulder, tilting the mother to the left side without rotating the spine.

Initial X-rays should still be obtained since the benefit to the fetus outweighs the small risk.

Perimortem caesarean section rarely delivers a healthy baby, since by the time the mother suffers cardiac arrest the fetus has already been hypoxic for some time.

CONCLUSION

About 1% of patients who attend A&E have suffered from major trauma. Most major emergency departments have established a 'trauma team' to implement early, targeted treatment to severely injured patients. Application of ATLS and the management of the 'golden hour' in a multidisciplinary team setting will save many lives.

ABDOMINAL PAIN

Abdominal pain is the most frequent presenting complaint on a typical general surgical 'take'. Diagnosis depends more on clinical assessment of symptoms and signs than on special investigations.

History

- Onset (especially exactly where the pain started)
- Site, radiation and progression
- Nature
- Relieving and exacerbating factors
- Past episodes
- Associated symptoms:
  - loss of appetite
  - nausea/vomiting
  - bowel function
  - urinary symptoms
  - gynaecological symptoms.

Past medical history

Special note is taken of past illnesses which may be directly relevant to the presenting problem, for example Crohn's disease in a patient with recurrent right iliac fossa pain, or previous renal stones in a patient with loin pain.

- Medication
- Allergies
- Family history
- Social history (occupation, tobacco and alcohol consumption, home circumstances)
- Systemic enquiry.

Examination

Inspection

- Swellings (bulges at site of hernia orifices)
- Distension
- Scars (beware the scars that are easy to miss, e.g. in the groins, skin creases and loins, laparoscopic scars)
- Discoloration (e.g. bluish colour around umbilicus (Cullen's sign) or flanks (Grey Turner's sign) seen in haemorrhagic pancreatitis)
- Visible peristalsis (obstructed bowel)/pulsation (abdominal aortic aneurysm: AAA).

Palpation

- Tenderness (establish area of tenderness and site of maximum severity)

- Guarding (reflex contraction of the abdominal wall in response to palpation)
- Rebound tenderness (exacerbation of pain on sudden release of the palpating hand; care is needed to avoid excessive discomfort)
- Distension
- Masses (establish site and nature)
- Organs (liver, kidneys and spleen)
- AAA (felt as a pulsatile, expansile swelling in the epigastrium)
- *Check the groins carefully.* Strangulated femoral hernias are quite often missed, especially in elderly women with non-specific symptoms
- Examine the external genitalia

Percussion

A tympanic sound indicates gas, a dull note means solid or fluid beneath. Pain on percussion may also indicate rebound tenderness.

Auscultation

Absent bowel sounds indicate peritonitis or ileus (i.e. inactive bowel following surgery). Tinkling bowel sounds occur in bowel obstruction.

Rectal examination

Look for anal abnormalities (scarring, fissures, skin tags, ulceration, 'Crohn's anus'), whether the rectum is empty or contains gas/faeces, nature of faeces (liquid/constipated/blood/melaena/steatorrhoea), tenderness, rectal mucosal lesions and extra-rectal masses.

Differential diagnosis

At the end of your clinical assessment, write down your differential diagnosis in the patient notes, rather than just the presenting problem. For example, 'epigastric pain' is a problem but not a diagnosis. It is better to write 'epigastric pain, differential diagnosis peptic ulceration, pancreatitis, biliary colic'. Later, when the diagnosis is firmly established, check whether it was included in your differential diagnosis. Your diagnostic skills will become much more accurate if you develop the habit of committing yourself to a differential diagnosis after your clinical assessment.

Investigation

There is no blanket series of investigations which is performed for every painful abdomen. Different tests are required depending on the differential diagnosis.

Urine

- Urinalysis is vital to exclude diabetes, pregnancy and microscopic haematuria
- Any condition causing inflammation in the lower abdomen can cause leucocytes in the urine (e.g. appendicitis and diverticulitis) and this does NOT confirm a urinary tract infection (UTI)
- Bilirubin appears in urine in obstructive jaundice
- Urine microscopy and culture (microscopy may demonstrate numerous organisms in UTI)

Blood tests

Haematology

- FBC is nearly always required
- Clotting studies (selectively)
- Group and save serum (G&S; for patients likely to need operation).

Biochemistry
- U&E
- Glucose
- Amylase.

These are useful in almost all cases. (NB: the amylase is often forgotten: beware since pancreatitis can cause pain all over the abdomen.)

The C-reactive protein (CRP) is a non-specific marker of infection/inflammation. Liver function tests should be performed for jaundiced patients and those with suspected biliary or pancreatic problems. More complex tests such as tumour markers are not usually available in the acute A&E setting and are unnecessary to arrive at most common diagnoses.

Plain X-rays
- Erect CXR – vital to exclude free gas under the diaphragm
- Plain abdominal X-ray (AXR) (Boxes 5.1 and 5.2).

Box 5.1 The plain AXR in the acute abdomen is full of useful information. It is often helpful to re-examine the abdomen after inspecting the AXR

Gas pattern
Gas in small or large bowel
Evidence of small or large bowel obstruction (is there gas in the rectum?)
'Sentinel loop' of distended small bowel in the upper abdomen in acute pancreatitis
Evidence of free gas (intra- or retroperitoneal)
Air in the biliary tree (choledochal fistula, previous biliary surgery)

Abnormal calcification
Renal, ureteric or bladder stones
Calcified gallstones in gallbladder or gallstone ileus
Calcified aorta or AAA
Pancreatic calcification in chronic pancreatitis
Calcified fibroids and phleboliths

Soft tissue shadows
Loss of psoas shadow in ruptured AAA
Masses/fluid displacing normal bowel pattern

Bones
Rib fractures
Spine/pelvic fractures
Bony metastases

Foreign bodies
Clips from previous surgery
Shrapnel
Swallowed
Rectal
Intrauterine contraceptive device

Kumar and Clark's Handbook of Medical Management

Box 5.2 Eponymous signs on plain AXR (both radiologists)

Rigler's sign or 'double-wall' sign – air visible on both sides of
bowel wall

Chilaiditi's sign or pseudopneumoperitoneum – presence of
bowel between liver and diaphragm mimicking intra-abdominal
free air

Table 5.1 Indications for CT scanning in the acute abdomen

Indication	Advantage of CT
Pancreatitis	Demonstrates pancreatic necrosis
Aortic aneurysm	CT scanning is the only reliable way to exclude aortic rupture (ultrasound detects aneurysms but does not exclude rupture)
Severe or non-resolving diverticulitis	Allows differentiation between localised perforation of diverticulum, diverticular abscess, diverticular mass
Large bowel obstruction	Avoids need for water-soluble contrast enema. Usually accurately demonstrates level of obstruction and cause
Small bowel obstruction with no hernia or scars	May detect the cause of the obstruction preoperatively
Suspicion of malignancy	Acute abdominal pain is common in advanced malignancy. CT scanning may confirm extensive metastatic disease, avoiding laparotomy when palliative care is more appropriate
Peritonitis in absence of gas on AXR	CT scanning is very sensitive for small pockets of free gas after perforation of a viscus
Acute abdomen	Standard in many hospitals

CT scanning

When teamed with a good clinical assessment, CT scanning is a tremen-
dously useful examination to diagnose acute abdominal pain. It is sometimes said that a CT scan is unnecessary if there is already an indication
for laparotomy. However, CT may render some operations unnecessary
(e.g. by confirming terminal malignant disease, or demonstrating acute
pancreatitis where perforated duodenal ulceration was expected). Other
operations may be made easier by providing useful information preoperatively (Table 5.1). The risk of ionising radiation and contrast exposure must
always be weighed against these potential benefits.

Ultrasound

Ultrasound reliably detects free fluid, gallstones, intrahepatic duct dilatation and aortic aneurysm. It is less useful for looking at bowel (sound does not penetrate gas-filled structures). It is operator dependent and picture quality is affected by body habitus and presence of bowel gas. Pelvic ultrasound is useful for detecting gynaecological disorders when diagnosing appendicitis in the female.

Contrast studies

Contrast studies including barium meal, follow-through, water-soluble contrast enema and intravenous urography may each be useful in selected settings.

PATTERNS OF ABDOMINAL PAIN

Appendicitis

Pain is initially central, then localises to the right iliac fossa with guarding and rebound tenderness (Fig. 5.1).

Aetiology and pathology

Appendicitis is the commonest cause of the acute abdomen in the United Kingdom. It occurs when there is an obstruction of the lumen either by faecolith or foreign body or enlargement of the lymphoid follicles in its wall. It may affect any age but is rare in the extremes of life.

Rare causes of appendicitis include carcinoma of the caecum, carcinoid tumour or obstructing fibrous bands. A severely inflamed appendix may be walled off by omentum (an appendix mass) which will eventually contain pus (an appendix abscess). Untreated, the condition threatens life in the very young and elderly, mainly because the diagnosis is difficult.

The appendix may be in a number of different positions in relation to the caecum: medial; medial and below; extending over the pelvic brim; retrocaecal; or retroileal.

Clinical features

- Symptoms The pain starts as central abdominal associated with anorexia, nausea and occasional episodes of vomiting. As the organ becomes inflamed, local peritoneal irritation causes more severe right iliac fossa pain. If the appendix ruptures, generalised peritonitis results and the pain becomes spread across the whole abdomen.

    If the appendix is lying close to the ureter/bladder then irritative urinary symptoms may result.
- Signs A coated tongue and *fetor oris* accompanied by mild pyrexia are characteristic. Local tenderness and guarding at McBurney's point (the junction of the middle and outer third of the line which joins the umbilicus to the anterior superior iliac spine) is present. These signs may vary, particularly when the appendix is in the retrocaecal position. Pressure applied to the left iliac fossa causes increased pain in the right lower quadrant (Rovsing's sign) but this is unreliable. Pelvic examination may be helpful in an attempt to localise the site of maximum tenderness.

Investigations

Appendicitis remains mainly a clinical diagnosis but investigations help reduce unnecessary operations to remove normal appendices. This is especially so in females where UTI, salpingitis, ectopic pregnancy and ovarian cysts may mimic appendicitis.

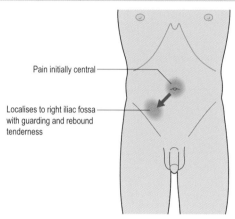

Pain initially central

Localises to right iliac fossa
with guarding and rebound
tenderness

Any age but mainly adults <50 y	
Associated symptoms: Anorexia Vomiting	Associated signs: Pyrexia Fetor oris
Urine: Leucocytes commonly in urine if appendix lying near bladder	PR: High right rectal tenderness Bloods: WBC usually ↑
In males Differential diagnosis: Crohn's disease Gastrointestinal infection NSAP	In females Differential diagnosis wider: Exclude ectopic pregnancy Do pelvic ultrasound to exclude ovarian pathology Consider salpingitis

NB Do not start antibiotics until diagnosis is established

Figure 5.1 Symptoms, signs and differential diagnosis of appendicitis. NSAP, non-specific abdominal pain.

- The WBC is usually raised
- AXR is of no value in appendicitis
- The urine often contains leucocytes, but no organisms
- Pregnancy test in females is mandatory to exclude ectopic pregnancy
- Abdominal/pelvic ultrasound may not diagnose appendicitis but usefully rules out ovarian pathology
- In the older patient, CT detects caecal carcinoma and diverticulitis, and reduces normal appendix removals – becoming standard
- Diagnostic laparoscopy in young females is accurate at identifying gynaecological conditions which mimic appendicitis.

Scoring systems are variably used (e.g. the Alvarado score) but are no substitute for clinical experience and regular re-evaluation of the patient, and may increase the use of cross-sectional imaging.

Treatment (see Box 5.3)

Once the diagnosis has been made, appendicectomy is required. This may be done through a small, transverse incision of the right iliac fossa or laparoscopically. Prophylactic antibiotics reduce the incidence of wound or port site infection.

An appendix mass may be managed non-operatively with parenteral fluids, antibiotics and frequent clinical re-assessment and imaging. The majority of the masses resolve and elective appendicectomy may be undertaken some weeks later. In the elderly, a preliminary barium enema or colonoscopy is advised to exclude carcinoma.

Appendix abscesses may be drained percutaneously by ultrasound with subsequent delayed operation 6 weeks later.

Appendicitis in pregnancy

Pain and tenderness are higher because of the displacement of the appendix by the enlarging uterus. Prompt assessment and intervention are essential. The risk of abortion in the first trimester is considerably higher if treatment is delayed until perforation occurs.

Intestinal obstruction (Fig. 5.2)

Classification and causes

Bowel obstruction may be due to mechanical obstruction or failure of peristalsis. The main clinical issue is to determine whether the obstruction affects the small bowel or the colon, since the causes and treatments are different.

The causes of mechanical obstruction are summarised in Box 5.4. In general, the commonest causes of small bowel obstruction are adhesions

Kumar and Clark's Handbook of Medical Management

> **Box 5.3** History of modern surgery: appendicitis
>
> Described for centuries as 'the iliac passion' the successful removal of an acutely inflamed appendix was first reported in 1887 by the American Surgeon Thomas Morton, who (successfully) resorted to laparotomy only after the failure of poultices, enemas and leeches to produce a cure.

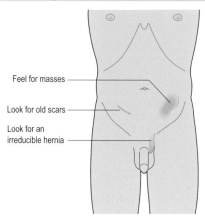

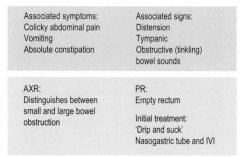

Figure 5.2 Bowel obstruction.

or hernia (Table 5.2), and those of large bowel obstruction are colon cancer or diverticular mass.

Clinical features

The features of bowel obstruction are colicky abdominal pain, vomiting, abdominal distension and constipation.

If the colic is in the lower abdomen it is more likely to be due to colon obstruction. Vomiting follows the pain. For high obstructions, vomiting is more profuse and occurs earlier. In colon obstruction the vomiting occurs much later if at all, especially if the ileocaecal valve remains competent. Initially, food contents are vomited but later the vomit becomes faeculent (brown and foul smelling). Distension is usually evident and more marked the more distal the obstruction. Constipation is absolute (i.e. no faeces or flatus).

The physical findings include dehydration, abdominal distension and sometimes visible peristalsis. The cause of the obstruction may be evident (e.g. scars from previous surgery, a tender irreducible hernia, an

Box 5.4 Causes of mechanical obstruction

Luminal
Gallstone (gallstone ileus)
Food bolus
Meconium ileus

Mural
Stricture   Intussusception
- Congenital
- Inflammatory
- Ischaemic
- Neoplastic

Extramural
Adhesions   Volvulus (twisting)
- Congenital   - Congenital
- Inflammatory   - Acquired
- Malignant
- Ischaemic
Hernia
- External
- Internal

Table 5.2 Causes of small bowel obstruction

Cause	Examination pointers	Requirement for surgery
Adhesions from previous surgery	Look for the abdominal scar (the surgery may have been many years ago)	Likely to resolve with non-operative treatment
Strangulated hernia	Examine hernial orifices carefully: it is easy to miss a small femoral hernia in an obese patient	Unless the hernia can be reduced easily, surgery will be required

abdominal mass). Percussion produces a tympanic note and auscultation high-pitched tinkling bowel sounds.

If the obstruction is advanced there may be signs of bowel strangulation (worsening constant pain, toxic patient, tachycardia and hypotension, pyrexia). Rectal examination must ALWAYS be performed in bowel obstruction. The rectum will be empty unless the cause of the problem is impacted faeces. A pelvic mass may be palpable.

Investigations

Plain abdominal X-rays confirm the diagnosis and distinguish small from large bowel obstruction.

AXR features of small bowel obstruction:
- distended loops of small bowel (over 3 cm)
- no gas is seen in the colon or rectum.

AXR features of large bowel obstruction:
- distended colon (over 5 cm) proximal to the obstructing lesion, collapsed colon distally; this is known as the 'cut-off' sign
- distended small bowel may also be seen if the ileocaecal valve is incompetent.

CT scanning is excellent at confirming diagnosis and identifying the level of the obstruction – use it often.

Small bowel obstruction

Adhesions and hernias are the commonest causes of small bowel obstruction. If there is no abdominal scar or irreducible hernia, consider Crohn's disease, small bowel lymphoma, caecal carcinoma obstructing the ileocaecal valve and internal hernia.

Treatment requires IV fluid replacement and nasogastric decompression ('drip and suck'). Patients with bowel obstruction may be severely dehydrated and may require large volumes of fluid resuscitation (use 0.9% saline, NOT dextrose). Catheterise the bladder, monitor hourly urine output and watch U&E closely. A CVP line may be needed in the elderly.

Most cases of adhesion obstruction resolve with nonoperative management. Surgery is required if there is evidence of bowel strangulation: watch carefully for clinical deterioration, pyrexia, development of localised tenderness or peritonism and rising WBC or acidosis.

Large bowel obstruction

When a diagnosis of large bowel obstruction is suspected on AXR, the next step is to exclude pseudo-obstruction (Box 5.5) and to determine the site of the obstructing lesion. This requires either water-soluble contrast enema or CT scan.

- **Pseudo-obstruction** Pseudo-obstruction has the same clinical features as mechanical colon obstruction but there is no mechanical obstructing lesion. The problem results from failure of peristalsis. The condition is commonly seen in elderly inpatients and is associated with abnormal electrolytes, diuretics, analgesics and antidepressant or antipsychotic therapy. AXR shows dilated colon from caecum to rectum. The rectum is distended with gas or liquid faeces. Colonoscopic decompression may provide relief. Correction of the underlying metabolic abnormality is the priority.

> **Box 5.5** Causes of large bowel obstruction

Pseudo-obstruction
Mechanical obstruction:
    Carcinoma of the colon
    Diverticular stricture
    Diverticular abscess/mass
    Crohn's disease
    Faecal impaction

Neostigmine infusion may be used for refractory cases but ECG monitoring is essential as the drug may induce cardiac arrhythmias.

Pseudo-obstruction may occasionally cause caecal perforation, which requires laparotomy, but most cases resolve with non-operative therapy.

- **Treatment of large bowel obstruction** Treatment of large bowel obstruction depends on the underlying cause. Lesions causing mechanical obstruction require laparotomy and resection of the affected colon. The bowel may be restored in continuity immediately, or a temporary colostomy may be performed.

Acute pancreatitis (see p. 139)

See Figure 5.3.

Diverticulitis (see p. 152)

See Figure 5.4.

Perforated viscus

See Figure 5.5.

Constipated elderly patient (a dangerous diagnosis)

See Figure 5.6.

Ureteric colic (see p. 249)

See Figure 5.7.

Biliary colic (see p. 135)

See Figure 5.8.

Ruptured abdominal aortic aneurysm (see p. 207)

See Figure 5.9.

NON-SURGICAL CAUSES OF ACUTE ABDOMINAL PAIN

A number of medical conditions cause very severe pain, which on occasion may even mimic peritonitis. Some are rare but they should be considered when diagnosis is proving difficult:

- diabetic ketoacidosis
- gastroenteritis (some GI infections cause severe pain, e.g. *Campylobacter*, coxsackie virus (Bornholm disease), typhoid fever, cholera, *Yersinia*, TB)
- irritable bowel syndrome
- acute myocardial infarction
- pneumonia
- sickle cell crisis
- Addisonian crisis
- familial Mediterranean fever (FMF)
- lead poisoning
- acute intermittent porphyria.

Kumar and Clark's Handbook of Medical Management

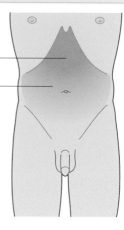

Associated symptoms:
Severe upper abdominal pain
spreading to back and all
over abdomen

Associated signs:
Tenderness and guarding,
worse in epigastrium. May be
jaundiced if gallstones are the
cause. Look for Cullen's +
Grey Turner's signs.

Treatment:
–O₂
–IVI
–catheterise
–analgesia
–antibiotics
–early ERCP
if due to gallstones
–manage on HDU

Imaging:
Erect CXR
AXR
USS abdo (not to diagnose the
pancreatitis but to look for
gallstones and biliary
obstruction)
CT abdo

Blood tests:
Determine the Glasgow
Criteria for EVERY patient
with acute pancreatitis before
they leave A&E

Age >55
WBC >15 x 10^{12}/L
Glucose >7 mmol/L
Urea >7 mmol/L
Albumin < 32 g/L
Calcium <2 mmol/L
PaO_2 <10 kPa

Differential diagnosis:
If amylase is raised but non-diagnostic (i.e. <1000) consider
perforated viscus, ruptured AAA, bowel ischaemia, chronic pancreatitis.
Do early CT abdo.

Serum amylase >1000 is diagnostic
90% of cases are due to either gallstones or alcohol

Figure 5.3 Acute pancreatitis.

PAINFUL TESTICLE

Epididymo-orchitis

In boys, a painful testicle must be assumed to be due to torsion (see below).
After puberty, epididymo-orchitis is more likely. In young men this is

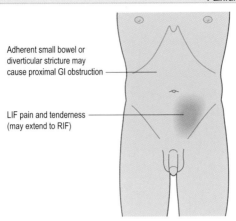

Adherent small bowel or
diverticular stricture may
cause proximal GI obstruction

LIF pain and tenderness
(may extend to RIF)

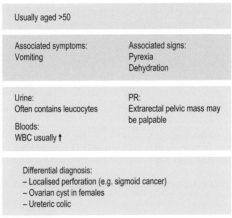

Usually aged >50

Associated symptoms:
Vomiting

Associated signs:
Pyrexia
Dehydration

Urine:
Often contains leucocytes

Bloods:
WBC usually ↑

PR:
Extrarectal pelvic mass may
be palpable

Differential diagnosis:
– Localised perforation (e.g. sigmoid cancer)
– Ovarian cyst in females
– Ureteric colic

Figure 5.4 Diverticulitis.

usually due to sexually transmitted infection, whereas in older men secondary infection due to bladder outflow obstruction is the commonest
cause.

Investigation
- Urine culture
- Scrotal ultrasound (exclude underlying testicular tumour or abscess).

Treatment
Analgesia and antibiotics.

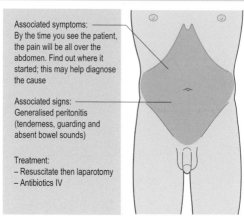

Associated symptoms:
By the time you see the patient, the pain will be all over the abdomen. Find out where it started; this may help diagnose the cause

Associated signs:
Generalised peritonitis (tenderness, guarding and absent bowel sounds)

Treatment:
– Resuscitate then laparotomy
– Antibiotics IV

Generally manifested by peritonitis and free gas under the diaphragm on erect CXR

Imaging:
20% show no free gas on CXR. CT is required if in doubt

Causes:
– Perforated duodenal ulcer (common)
– Perforated gastric ulcer (common)
– Perforated diverticular disease or colon cancer (common)
– Perforated gallbladder (rare)
– Perforated Meckel's/small bowel (rare)

If the perforation has become walled off by omentum, the pain and tenderness may be confined to part of the abdomen

Figure 5.5 Perforated viscus.

Testicular torsion

Torsion of the testicle is a surgical emergency, since the twisting of the spermatic cord cuts off the blood supply to the testes, which will infarct within 6 hours. Torsion occurs in boys at any age and is rare after puberty. There is severe pain in the testicle and iliac fossa. Vomiting is common. The testicle is extremely tender, swollen and drawn up.

The differential diagnosis includes epididymo-orchitis, torted hydatid of Morgagni (appendix testes) and idiopathic scrotal oedema. Immediate exploration of the scrotum is required since no investigation will reliably distinguish torsion from the other causes. Consent must be obtained for

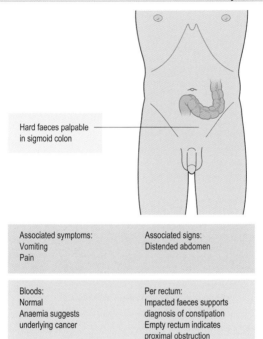

Hard faeces palpable
in sigmoid colon

Associated symptoms:
Vomiting
Pain

Associated signs:
Distended abdomen

Bloods:
Normal
Anaemia suggests
underlying cancer

Per rectum:
Impacted faeces supports
diagnosis of constipation
Empty rectum indicates
proximal obstruction

Differential diagnosis:
High likelihood of underlying colon cancer or diverticular mass
Do not discharge until these are excluded

Figure 5.6 Constipated elderly patient.

orchidectomy in case the testicle is non-viable. The opposite testicle is fixed
at the same operation to prevent torsion on the other side.

URINARY RETENTION

Acute urinary retention

Patients are invariably male, usually over 50. Symptoms are suprapubic
pain of sudden onset, with inability to pass urine. The patient is distressed
and the bladder is tender and palpable.

The commonest causes are benign prostatic hypertrophy, prostate
cancer, bladder cancer, urethral stricture and urinary infection causing
prostatic and urethral inflammation and constipation. About half of
patients have a history of obstructive urinary symptoms due to prostate
hypertrophy. There is often a precipitating event such as cystoscopy,
surgery elsewhere on the body (especially groin hernia) and overdisten-
sion of the bladder (e.g. on a coach journey).

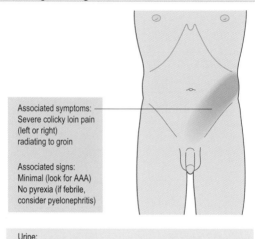

Associated symptoms:
Severe colicky loin pain
(left or right)
radiating to groin

Associated signs:
Minimal (look for AAA)
No pyrexia (if febrile,
consider pyelonephritis)

Urine:
Haematuria (micro or macroscopic)
is usually present (85%)

Differential diagnosis:
– If patient is over age 50, consider ruptured AAA
– Pyelonephritis

Figure 5.7 Ureteric colic.

Treatment requires catheterisation of the bladder, usually per urethra. If urethral catheterisation is unsuccessful (or contraindicated such as in pelvic trauma) then suprapubic catheterisation can be attempted by more specialist practitioners (risk of bowel or vascular injury).

After catheterisation the cause of the retention must be established. Examine the prostate (small/large/hard/irregular). Check FBC, U&E, PSA (though the PSA is always raised just after catheterisation) and send urine for culture and cytology. Renal ultrasound is necessary if there is renal impairment.

A trial without catheter (a 'TWOC') is usually attempted after an interval of up to two weeks (often in the urology outpatient clinic), the patient having been given a course of medication aimed at reducing the degree of prostatic hypertrophy. If this is unsuccessful, prostatectomy is usually offered (see p. 252).

Chronic urinary retention

Chronic retention commonly presents as a non-specific illness and there may be no pain from the bladder at all, which is lax and grossly distended (up to several litres) compared to acute retention. The patient may frequently pass small volumes of urine and is often incontinent (overflow incontinence).

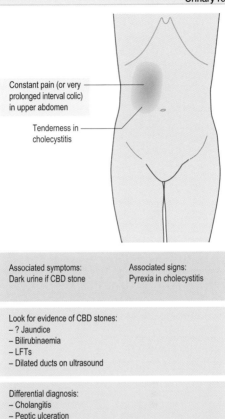

Constant pain (or very prolonged interval colic) in upper abdomen

Tenderness in cholecystitis

Associated symptoms: Dark urine if CBD stone

Associated signs: Pyrexia in cholecystitis

Look for evidence of CBD stones:
– ? Jaundice
– Bilirubinaemia
– LFTs
– Dilated ducts on ultrasound

Differential diagnosis:
– Cholangitis
– Peptic ulceration
– Pancreatitis
(always do amylase)

Figure 5.8 Biliary colic. CBD, common bile duct.

After catheterisation for chronic retention, there may be hypotension (a vagal response) and haematuria due to bleeding from submucosal veins inside the bladder. Decompressing the bladder in stages may help but evidence suggests the severity of damage is correlated to the degree of distension.

Chronic retention is often associated with renal impairment and after bladder decompression severe polyuria may cause hypotension and collapse. Hourly urine measurements must be taken and if polyuria occurs, a safe regimen is to replace urine output with an equal volume of IV 0.9% saline until equilibrium is restored.

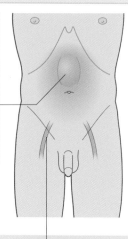

Associated symptoms:
Classically severe epigastric and back pain BUT the pain may be in any part of the abdomen

Associated signs:
Tender, pulsatile expansile mass BUT this can be difficult to feel if patient is large, or the AAA is surrounded by haematoma

Imaging:
USS detects AAAs but does not reliably detect rupture
CT is required

Femoral pulses:
Usually present. 20% of patients also have popliteal aneurysms

Treatment:
Immediate repair by a vascular surgeon
DO NOT over-transfuse the patient or you will convert a contained rupture into a free one

The presentation of ruptured AAA is notoriously variable and many patients die each year due to late diagnosis

BP may be high, normal or low, depending on whether the rupture is contained or free

Epidemiology:
Typically in males >age 60 with a history of smoking

Figure 5.9 Ruptured abdominal aortic aneurysm.

ACUTE LIMB ISCHAEMIA

Lower limb ischaemia

Presentation

Presentation of acute limb ischaemia is characterised by 'the 6 Ps': pain, pallor, paraesthesia, paralysis, pulselessness and perishing cold. The Doppler signal is often undetectable or severely diminished at the ankle (i.e. the ankle-brachial pressure index (ABPI) is at or close to zero).

Untreated, within a few hours such a limb will become mottled with fixed staining of the skin, the paralysis will be complete and the muscles will become tense, tender and swollen. Once these features have developed the limb is non-salvageable and amputation is necessary to save the life of the patient.

Causes

Causes of acute limb ischaemia include:

- thrombosis
  - *in situ* thrombosis of atherosclerotic native vessel
  - *in situ* thrombosis of a normal or minimally diseased artery due to a hyperthrombotic state (often seen in advanced malignancy)
  - thrombosis of popliteal aneurysms
  - occlusion of a bypass graft
- embolism
  - atrial fibrillation
  - cardiac vegetations (in past commonly due to rheumatic mitral valve disease)
  - embolism of mural thrombus of proximal aneurysms
  - embolism from unstable plaque
  - following angiography
- aortic dissection
- trauma
- rarer causes including popliteal entrapment and compartment syndrome.

Management

Time is of the essence. Inform a senior as soon as a patient with acute limb ischaemia is expected. Patients with acutely ischaemic limbs are in great pain and often in poor health, hypoxic, dehydrated with failing heart and kidneys. Treating these conditions appropriately often brings about a marked improvement in the affected limb without any specific vascular intervention, simply by improving circulation of well-oxygenated blood.

Immediate action to be taken is outlined in Box 5.6. The next priority is to obtain imaging to determine the cause of the ischaemia and to plan

---

Box 5.6 Immediate actions to be taken in the event of acute lower limb ischaemia

Oxygen: at least 24–28% via face mask

Take blood for FBC, baseline coagulation studies, G&S, U&E, glucose

Do CXR and ECG

Heparin: give a bolus of 5000 units IV then infuse 1000 units per hour to maintain the APTR at between 2 and 3 (monitor APTR every 6–8 hours and titrate heparin dose)

Rehydration: set up intravenous infusion and catheterise the bladder to monitor fluid balance

Analgesia: morphine 5–10 mg IV with 10 mg metoclopramide

Treat specific co-morbid conditions, e.g. fast atrial fibrillation, cardiac failure or pneumonia

Kumar and Clark's Handbook of Medical Management

treatment. Duplex ultrasound, magnetic resonance angiography, CT angiography and digital subtraction angiography are all useful; the choice of modality depends on the local facilities available.

Many patients present with so-called acute subcritical limb ischaemia. In these patients the pain is of recent onset (less than 2 weeks) but there is no paralysis and the sensory loss is mild. There may even be a weak audible Doppler signal at the ankle.

Treatment options include:

- palliative care
- primary amputation
- urgent surgery (embolectomy or bypass)
- thrombolysis
- endovascular therapy (suction thrombectomy, angioplasty with or without stenting).

Irreversible limb ischaemia requires amputation or palliative care. The acute white bloodless leg needs immediate intervention to save the limb. The distinction between thrombosis and embolism may not be obvious. Pointers towards embolism include no past history of claudication, normal pulses in the opposite leg and a likely embolic source, usually atrial fibrillation. In these patients the best approach is urgent exploration of the groin with balloon embolectomy of the femoral arteries and on-table angiography.

Thrombolysis is achieved by inserting an arterial catheter into the thrombosed artery and infusing the thrombolytic agent (usually tissue plasminogen activator: TPA). This may unblock small and large arteries and reveal the lesion that led to the occlusion (e.g. an arterial stenosis or popliteal aneurysm). The technique is less invasive than surgery but has a high incidence of bleeding complications and stroke, particularly in those over 80 years of age.

Table 5.3 Acutely painful anal conditions

Condition	Treatment	Page reference
Perianal abscess	Examination under anaesthesia including sigmoidoscopy, incision and drainage, culture swab, histology of abscess roof	See p. 165, 360
Anal fissure	Trial of medical treatment (glyceryl trinitrate or diltiazem ointment) and/or examination under anaesthesia, injection of botox to internal anal sphincter or lateral sphincterotomy	See p. 164
Thrombosed haemorrhoid	Usually conservative, analgesics, ice and metronidazole, occasionally emergency haemorrhoidectomy	See p. 162
Perianal haematoma	Evacuation under local anaesthetic provides immediate relief	See p. 164

Upper limb ischaemia

In contrast to the leg, upper limb ischaemia is usually due to embolisation from the heart. Brachial embolectomy may be needed but in many cases heparinisation and hydration are sufficient. The underlying cause must be sought (echocardiography, CXR for cervical rib, upper limb duplex scan).

PERIANAL ABSCESS (SEE P. 165, 360)

Perianal abscess is the commonest of a number of painful anal conditions which present on the general surgical take (Table 5.3). Examination under anaesthetic is usually required so that sigmoidoscopy (exclude Crohn's disease) and adequate drainage of the abscess may be performed.

The surgical specialties

Surgical oncology   6

The management of patients with malignancy involves several specialties. A typical cancer multidisciplinary team (MDT) will include surgeon, radiologist, pathologist, medical oncologist and radiotherapist. Specialist nurses play an increasing important role.

DEFINITIONS

- **Malignancy and cancer** A malignant tumour has the capacity to invade local tissues and produce distant metastases. Cancer used to be a term reserved for a malignant tumour originating from epithelial tissue, but is now used interchangeably to refer to any malignant tumour.
- **Carcinoma** A carcinoma is a malignant tumour arising from epithelial tissue.
- **Sarcoma** Sarcomas are malignant tumours arising from tissues of mesenchymal origin and may thus occur anywhere in the body.
- **Lymphoma** Lymphoma refers to malignancy of the immune system, specifically of lymphocyte cells.

EPIDEMIOLOGY OF MALIGNANCY

Cancer is common and accounts for a quarter of all deaths in Western populations. Carcinomas of the breast, lung and GI tract are the most common causes of death from cancer. Lung cancer causes most deaths in males, and has overtaken breast cancer in females. In both sexes the incidence rises with age, especially over the age of 60.

AETIOLOGY

The causes of malignancy are multifactorial. No single chemical or biological factor has been shown to cause cancer but a combination of factors, for example genetic susceptibility, chemicals, occupation, lifestyle and viruses, may induce malignant change in certain tissues in susceptible individuals (Table 6.1).

PATHOLOGY OF CARCINOGENESIS

Normal processes such as embryogenesis, differentiation, tissue regeneration, wound healing and apoptosis are under tight cellular control. When these control mechanisms go wrong, cellular proliferation goes unchecked and results in tumour formation. Cancers are characterised by abnormal expression of genes which normally regulate cell growth (oncogenes). Three types of gene are important in carcinogenesis. Oncogenes encourage cells to multiply. Tumour suppressor genes stop cell multiplication and when damaged cause loss of control of multiplication (the best known suppressor gene is p53) whilst genes that normally repair damaged DNA may, if defective, promote mutations. Important genes in colorectal cancer

Table 6.1 Examples of causative factors in malignant disease

Causative factor		Tumour
Genetic	Retinoblastoma gene (Rb)	Childhood retinoblastoma
	FAP gene	Familial adenomatous polyposis leading to colorectal cancer
	BRCA1 and BRCA2	Breast/ovarian cancer
	p53 oncogene mutation	Abnormal p53 gene predisposes to several cancers
	Defective DNA mismatch repair genes	Hereditary non-polyposis colon cancer syndrome (HNPCC)
Sunlight	Ultraviolet radiation	Malignant melanoma and basal cell carcinoma
Diet	Alcohol	Oropharyngeal and oesophageal cancer
	Aflatoxins	Oesophageal carcinoma
	Smoked foods	Gastric carcinoma
	High fat intake	Breast and colon cancer
Chemicals	Beta-naphthalene	Bladder carcinoma
	Vinyl chloride	Hepatic angiosarcoma
	Tobacco smoke	Lung cancer; implicated in a third of all other cancer deaths
	Asbestos	Mesothelioma
Ionising radiation		Skin cancers, leukaemia, thyroid malignancies
Infections	Hepatitis B/Hepatitis C	Hepatocellular carcinoma
	Epstein–Barr virus	Burkitt's lymphoma
	Human papilloma virus	Cervical and anal cancer
	HIV	Kaposi's sarcoma and B-cell lymphoma
	Schistosomiasis	Bladder cancer
	Helicobacter pylori	Gastric cancer
Therapeutic immunosuppression	Transplant recipients	Skin cancers, lymphomas

include the APC gene on chromosome 5. In breast cancer the BRCA1 and BRCA2 genes are increasingly recognised as important. Any factor causing abnormal DNA (external radiation, spontaneous or inherited mutations) may result in faulty oncogene expression and subsequent tumour development.

INVASION AND METASTASIS

The difference between a benign and a malignant tumour is the capacity to invade and metastasise. A benign tumour generally grows slowly, is always well encapsulated and may compress, but never invades, local tissues. In contrast, cancers invade surrounding tissues (Fig. 6.1) and spread to form distant tumour deposits (metastases).

Carcinoma *in situ* is a collection of malignant cells confined by their normal basement membrane. These cells are both functionally and structurally altered (dysplasia). The process may be multifocal. Malignant disease advances by local tissue invasion through and beyond the basement membrane and metastasis of cells to form autonomous tumour deposits. Invasion occurs when tumour cells secrete enzymes capable of digesting intercellular stroma, particularly the matrix metalloproteinases. Continued growth encroaches upon and destroys adjacent organs. The resistance to invasion is variable. Arteries and tendons are rarely destroyed but lymphatics and veins are commonly breached.

Metastases occur by three routes (Fig. 6.2):
- lymphatic spread to local and distant nodes
- haematogenous spread (mainly to lung, liver and bone)
- transcoelomic (i.e. across a body cavity, e.g. peritoneum).

Tumour metastases themselves may undergo further malignant progression and bear little resemblance to the primary tumour. The pattern of spread can be predicted for most tumours and may be used to plan surgical removal. Because lymphatics usually accompany the arterial supply to an organ, in many instances the surgical removal of an organ which contains a tumour involves dissection and removal of the arterial supply and the associated lymphatic tissue. Similarly, venous drainage of an organ is an important determinant of spread and many surgical procedures are designed to reduce the chance of spread during surgery by dividing the blood supply before the tumour is palpated.

The distribution of metastases varies with the type of tumour. However, some tumours have a predilection for particular sites, e.g. gastrointestinal malignancy tends to metastasise to the liver whereas kidney and breast carcinomas metastasise to the lung.

Five cancers commonly metastasise to bone; these are thyroid, lung, breast, kidney and prostate.

MICROMETASTASES

Microscopic tumour deposits present at the time of the original diagnosis and treatment are of considerable importance in surgical oncology. They may have escaped detection at the original diagnosis and treatment and may emerge some time later as metastases or recurrent disease. Modern oncological management aims to include adequate treatment to deal with such micrometastases, particularly for example in breast cancer involving the use of systemic therapy in addition to local surgery – adjuvant therapy.

Kumar and Clark's Handbook of Medical Management

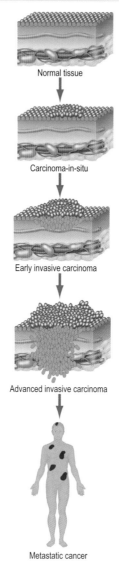

Normal tissue

Carcinoma-in-situ

Early invasive carcinoma

Advanced invasive carcinoma

Metastatic cancer

Figure 6.1 The natural history of the development of malignant disease.

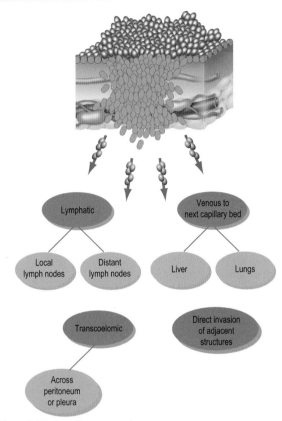

Figure 6.2 Routes of tumour spread.

TUMOUR MARKERS

Some cancers secrete substances into the circulation (Table 6.2).

Unfortunately tumour markers are not often useful in cancer diagnosis because of their low specificity. They may, however, be helpful in monitoring response to treatment and detection of relapse if levels were high to start with. No marker is perfect and they are only used as one of a number of factors guiding management.

MANAGEMENT

Clinical assessment

When taking a history and examining a patient who might have cancer it is useful to remember that the disease may present in several ways (Table 6.3).

Table 6.2 Commonly used tumour markers and their origin

Cancer	Marker
Prostate	PSA (prostate specific antigen)
Colon	CEA (carcinoembryonic antigen)
Hepatocellular carcinoma	AFP (alpha-fetoprotein)
Pancreatic cancer	CA19.9
Choriocarcinoma	Beta-HCG
Ovarian	CA125
Testicular teratoma	AFP, beta-HCG

Table 6.3 Presentations of malignant disease

Presenting	Examples
Problems due to the primary tumour	Haemoptysis from lung cancer
	Tenesmus from rectal cancer
	Visible lump of thyroid cancer
Problems due to a metastasis	Pathological fracture of bone
	Malignant pleural effusion
	Jaundice due to hepatic secondaries
Problems resulting from a substance secreted by the tumour	Syndrome of inappropriate antidiuretic hormone secretion from lung cancer
	Polycythaemia due to erythropoietin from a renal cancer
	Hypertension due to catecholamines from phaeochromocytoma
General features of malignancy	Weight loss
	Cachexia
	Anaemia
	Deep vein thrombosis

Investigation and diagnosis

Investigations should include FBC, U&E, LFTs, urine cytology, plain X-ray, e.g. chest X-ray, serum tumour markers.

Complex investigations, determined by the suspected diagnosis, include ultrasound, CT, MRI, PET, PET-CT and contrast radiology of the GI tract (now superseded by endoscopy, laparoscopy and thoracoscopy).

A pathological diagnosis is essential prior to treatment. This may be achieved by aspiration cytology, done by passing a fine needle into the lesion and applying suction with a syringe. Small fragments are drawn into the barrel and can be extracted and stained for examination under the microscope, giving an assessment of the shape and features of individual cells. Needle biopsy produces a tissue core which is processed and sectioned, providing a histological examination showing the pathological architecture. Open biopsy, either incisional or excisional, confirms the diagnosis. All the above methods may be undertaken under X-ray, ultrasound or CT guidance.

Tumour staging

Staging of a tumour is an attempt to quantify how advanced a cancer has become at the time of diagnosis. Many systems have been devised for different organs and are detailed in the specific chapters. The TNM (tumour, nodes, metastases) system (Box 6.1) is now more widely adopted. This may be divided into a clinical staging or, after pathological assessment, a pathological system (pTNM classification). This system is being constantly updated (the latest revision is TNM7).

Histological grade

Tumour grading is used in conjunction with the TNM to give an assessment of prognosis for the patient (Table 6.4). It also permits evaluation of the efficacy of different treatments on tumours of comparable stage.

Operations for cancer

Definitive elective treatment surgically of a tumour is ideally decided on unequivocal histological confirmation and an accurate pre-operative assessment of stage. However, some patients present as an emergency (e.g. carcinoma of the colon) without this information. The aim of surgical management is either curative or palliative.

Box 6.1 TNM staging system

Tumour
T0: primary unknown (Tis: tumour *in situ*)
T1: tumour <2 cm
T2: tumour >2 cm
T3: tumour >5 cm (or reaching serosa in GI tract)
T4: tumour infiltrating local tissues, e.g. skin, vessels, nerves

Nodes
N0: not involved
N1: local nodes involved
N2: distant nodes involved

Metastases
M0: no metastases
M1: metastases present
Mx: status unknown

Postoperative
R0: no residual tumour
R1: microscopic residual disease
R2: macroscopic residual disease

Table 6.4 Histological classification

Differentiation	Features
Grade 1 – well differentiated	Forms recognisable structures of parent tissue
Grade 2 – moderately differentiated	Some degree of organisation
Grade 3 – poorly differentiated	Architecture totally disorganised; cells not recognisable from parent tissue

Increasingly, patients are having systemic and/or radiotherapeutic treatment (e.g. for advanced carcinoma of the rectum) prior to surgery. This is termed neo-adjuvant therapy; the aim being to downstage the tumour.

A curative procedure involves total excision of all the tumour-bearing tissues with associated lymphatic and venous drainage. Invasion of adjacent vital structures may determine feasibility of removing a tumour (its operability). The determination of how far to place the resection away from the visible growth (the resection margin) is described in appropriate sections of this book.

Reconstruction after surgery is an important aspect of surgical technique which aims to enable most patients to regain as near normal a lifestyle and self-perception as possible. This is particularly important in colorectal disease where a stoma may be required, or breast surgery where reconstructions after mastectomy are important for the restoration of body image and confidence. Fully informed consent is needed after detailed discussion with the patient, and a full understanding of the balance between the need to cure the patient of their cancer and the results of surgery in this context.

Adjuvant therapy

Adjuvant therapy is additional anti-cancer treatment used for some patients thought to have had tumours completely removed by surgery. The aim is to destroy occult micro-metastases by chemotherapy, local radiotherapy or a combination of these. Some patients may not need this treatment and the risks of adjuvant treatment need to be borne in mind in this situation. Adjuvant therapy may be given before (neo-adjuvant therapy) or after surgery (Table 6.5). Useful regression of some tumours (e.g. rectum and breast) can be achieved, converting non-operable into operable disease. Many new trials of different regimes are being performed throughout the world to determine the best treatments.

Radiotherapy

There are three ways of administering radiotherapy to kill cancer cells:
- external beam radiation
- radioactive implants
- systemic administration of radioactive isotopes (e.g. radioactive iodine).

Table 6.5 Adjuvant and neo-adjuvant therapy

Tumour	Adjuvant protocol	Timing
Breast	Cyclophosphamide, methotrexate, 5-fluorouracil	Postoperative
	Methotrexate, mitoxantrone, mitomycin	Postoperative
	Radiotherapy or tamoxifen, or both	Postoperative
Oesophagus	5-Fluorouracil and other agents with or without radiotherapy	Pre- and postoperative
Colorectal	5-Fluorouracil and levamisole	Postoperative
Rectum	Radiotherapy	Pre- and postoperative
Osteosarcoma	Methotrexate, epirubicin with or without radiotherapy	Pre- and postoperative

Radiotherapy acts by inducing chemical changes within the nucleus of the cell that cause damage to DNA. A tumour is therefore depopulated of its malignant cells during mitosis and the number of viable cells present, the intrinsic radiosensitivity of the cells and the mitotic rate determine the efficacy of radiotherapy. Surrounding normal tissues are also damaged by radiation, and those with a high cell turnover are especially susceptible.

The total dose for the tumour is calculated for each individual site and size. Treatment is given in fractions of the total dose, thus minimising unpleasant side effects, for example local soreness, skin changes, lethargy, nausea and vomiting. New super-voltage apparatus is able to deliver increased penetration into deep tissues from various directions, enhancing destruction of tumour cells without damaging surrounding structure.

Side effects of radiotherapy include local soreness, skin changes and burning, lethargy, nausea and vomiting. Pelvic radiotherapy causes cystitis and diarrhoea. Radiation damage to normal tissues may not become apparent for several years (e.g. radiation enteritis, see p. 129).

Cytotoxic chemotherapy

Cytotoxic chemotherapy interferes with cell division in both normal and malignant cells. Success depends on the intrinsic resistance of the tumour cell to the agent and the toxic effects on normal tissues. There are four main types of chemotherapy agents, many of which can be used in combination. Their effects on normal proliferating cells may result in bone marrow and intestinal toxicity.

Alkylating agents

Examples include cyclophosphamide, melphalan and chlorambucil, which combine nucleic acids, enzymes and cell membranes. Damage to the enzymes which link DNA strands disrupts mitosis.

Antimetabolites

Antimetabolites, for example methotrexate, 5-fluorouracil, 6-mercaptopurine, are incorporated into the DNA instead of the normal nucleotide.

Vinca alkaloids

Vinca alkaloids, for example vincristine, bind to intracellular tubulin, inhibiting microtubule formation.

Antimitotic antibiotics

Examples include doxorubicin (adriamycin), epirubicin and dactinomycin (actinomycin D). These compounds intercalate between DNA strands, disturbing DNA function, or inhibit DNA and RNA synthesis, generating oxygen free radicals, which are toxic.

Miscellaneous agents

Miscellaneous agents, for example cisplatin, which reacts with guanine in DNA, forming cross-linkages along the DNA chain or biological agent infliximab.

Endocrine manipulation

Some tumours are dependent on hormones for their normal growth. Endocrine manipulation may effectively inhibit tumour progression. Examples are shown in Table 6.6.

Prognosis

Prognosis is determined by the stage and grade of the cancer at presentation. Survival is usually expressed as percentage of patients alive after 5 or 10 years. Such data is derived from population studies and it is always impossible to predict life expectancy for an individual patient, only the probability of their surviving a specified time.

Palliative care

When cure is impossible, palliative care must be provided. Full and frank discussion about the prognosis with the patient when treatment for cure fails is essential. Early referral to a team which can provide palliative care

Table 6.6 Examples of endocrine manipulation which may inhibit tumour progression

Cancer type	Drug	Mechanism of action
Breast	Tamoxifen	Blocks oestrogen receptor binding
	Anastrazole	Aromatase inhibition (peripheral conversion of oestrogen)
	Herceptin	Monoclonal antibody inhibiting cell-membrane receptor protein HER2
Breast/Prostate	Gonadotropin releasing hormone analogues	Suppression of LH and FSH

helps address the fear of death. Terminal care alleviates the psychological disturbance associated with impending death whilst counselling of the patient and family can help greatly. The aim of terminal care is to try to keep the patient in familiar surroundings, preferably home, whilst providing adequate facilities for analgesia and nursing care.

SCREENING FOR MALIGNANT DISEASE

For a screening programme to be effective, the following points are essential.

- The disease should be common or have defined high-risk groups
- The natural history should be known
- The screening method must be sensitive and specific and able to detect disease early
- Detection methods should be cheap, easy to use and have a high patient compliance
- Effective treatment for early disease should be available
- The screening procedure must not involve hazard to the population tested.

Examples include mammography for breast cancer, faecal occult blood testing for colorectal cancer, and cervical smear testing for cervical cancer.

Upper gastrointestinal disease and disorders of the small bowel

OESOPHAGUS – DYSPHAGIA

Many conditions of the oesophagus present with dysphagia. If chronic there is nearly always associated weight loss. Dysphagia may be progressive, suggesting a malignant growth or stricture, or non-progressive, suggesting a disorder of function. Conditions of the oesophagus may be divided into causes in the lumen, in the wall or outside the lumen. In addition, some neurological conditions may also cause dysphagia (Box 7.1).

Foreign body

This condition usually presents in young children accidentally (e.g. coins, buttons) or occasionally deliberately in the mentally disturbed (e.g. razor blades, spoons). Impaction usually occurs at the narrowest point (the commencement or the crossing of the left main bronchus or at the diaphragm). In general, once a foreign body has passed below the diaphragm, it will pass through the rest of the GI tract without causing problems.

Small smooth objects often pass into the stomach and may safely be left to pass through the GI tract. Serial radiography is not indicated for young children. Irregular and sharp objects may impact or perforate and need to be retrieved.

Clinical features

There is usually a short history of painful dysphagia. Psychiatric patients may give a history of previous episodes.

Investigations

- CXR is a useful investigation to determine whether the object is stuck in the mediastinum, and whether perforation has occurred
- Barium swallow is rarely needed, and may result in aspiration
- Oesophago-gastro-duodenoscopy (OGD).

Treatment

Most foreign bodies can be retrieved endoscopically with grasping forceps. Laparoscopic thoracotomy or open thoracotomy is indicated for perforation.

OESOPHAGEAL PERFORATION

Causes include:
- iatrogenic following therapeutic dilatation
- foreign body
- corrosive liquids
- penetrating injury
- Boerhaave's syndrome (perforation due to violent vomiting).

> **Box 7.1** Causes of dysphagia
>
> In the lumen
>   Foreign body
> In the wall
>   Carcinoma
>   Stricture (inflammatory)
>   Achalasia
>   Scleroderma
>   Plummer–Vinson
>   Atresia (congenital)
>   Post radiotherapy
> Outside the wall
>   Bronchial carcinoma
>   Mediastinal
>   lymphadenopathy
>
> Rolling hiatus hernia
> Retrosternal goitre
> Thoracic aortic aneurysm
> Pharyngeal pouch
> Vascular ring (dysphagia
>   lusoria)
> Neurological
>   Myasthenia gravis
>   Bulbar palsy
> Polio
> Psychological

Clinical features

These include sudden/gradual onset of chest, neck and upper abdominal pain, pyrexia, shock, surgical emphysema (in neck or suprasternal notch). Mediastinitis has a high mortality in the elderly.

Investigations

Urgent chest X-ray (CXR) is required looking for air in the mediastinum or neck, and pleural effusion. Confirm with water-soluble contrast swallow to delineate site of perforation.

Treatment

- Resuscitate if shocked
- Broad-spectrum antibiotics
- Nothing by mouth
- Small leaks may be conservatively treated
- Do not pass a nasogastric tube
- Large leaks can be repaired by thoracotomy or laparoscopic thoracotomy with drainage
- Stents occasionally used.

CORROSIVE OESOPHAGITIS

Common substances ingested either accidentally or intentionally include caustic soda, sulphuric acid and household bleach. Severe damage (bleeding/perforation) is caused not only to the oesophagus, but to the mouth, pharynx, larynx and stomach. Aspiration of corrosive liquid can also occur, giving rise to severe respiratory problems. In the longer term, stricture may occur.

Clinical features

- History of ingestion
- Severe pain from mouth to stomach

- Signs of shock, pyrexia, respiratory distress
- Oedema of lips, mouth, pharynx, lung.

Treatment

Immediate

- If the ingestant is known, immediately give a buffering solution, e.g. milk
- Do not induce emesis; this may rupture the oesophagus.

Urgent

- Endoscopy to assess extent of damage (may need general anaesthetic)
- Broad-spectrum antibiotics/steroids/total parenteral nutrition.

Long-term

- Dilatation of early strictures
- Surgery required for severe strictures
- ENT/respiratory support may also be needed.

Long-term results depend on the degree of stricture formation. Prompt early treatment gives better outcome.

GASTRO-OESOPHAGEAL REFLUX (GORD)

Gastric acid may reflux through an incompetent gastro-oesophageal sphincter. The most common cause is a sliding hiatus hernia. Rarer causes include previous surgery (e.g. for achalasia, Ivor Lewis oesophago-gastrectomy, prolonged nasogastric intubation).

Not all patients with sliding hiatus hernia have reflux and vice versa. Oesophageal pH monitoring and manometry is vital to confirm significant reflux if surgery is being considered after medical treatment has failed. Significant reflux is confirmed when the pH is <4 for >4% of the 24-hour period.

Long-standing reflux may lead to Barrett's oesophagus – a precursor of malignancy or stricture. Barrett's oesophagus is inflamed 'salmon pink' epithelium in the distal oesophagus which has undergone gastric metaplasia in response to chronic reflux. Complications include bleeding, stricture, ulceration and malignancy. Once Barrett's oesophagus has been identified, regular endoscopic surveillance, and biopsy is required if dysplasia. Development of severe dysplasia indicates a high risk of malignancy and oesophagectomy may be required.

HIATUS HERNIA

Two types of hiatus hernia are described: sliding (90%) and rolling (para-oesophageal). In the latter, the gastrooesophageal sphincter remains intact and reflux does not occur (Fig. 7.1). The common sliding hiatus hernia disrupts and changes the oesophago-gastric junction, giving rise to reflux.

Long-term complications include ulceration, Barrett's oesophagus, bleeding and stricture.

Clinical features

Retrosternal burning pain, worse on lying, bending or stooping ('heartburn'), relieved by antacids. Waterbrash (reflux of fluid up into the mouth). Many cases present to ENT departments with a hoarse voice.

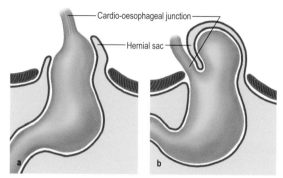

Figure 7.1 (a) The oesophago-gastric anatomy in a sliding hiatus hernia. (b) The anatomy in a para-oesophageal hernia.

Investigations

- OGD to assess degrees of inflammation and exclude malignancy by biopsy
- Barium swallow
- pH monitoring.

Treatment

- Weight loss in the obese
- Elevate head of the bed to avoid nocturnal reflux
- Alginate antacids
- Reduce gastric acidity with either H_2 receptor antagonists or proton pump inhibitors (PPIs).

Surgery is indicated if conservative measures fail and reflux is considerable. Nissan's fundoplication is now performed laparoscopically. Rolling hiatus hernias should be repaired due to risk of incarceration, strangulation (high mortality) and gastric volvulus.

ACHALASIA

The cause is unknown but the result is a failure of the lower sphincter to relax in response to oesophageal contraction. This leads to retention of the bolus and ultimate dilatation and elongation of the whole oesophagus. Aspiration pneumonia may result. There is an increased risk of malignancy due to chronic inflammation of the mucosa. Pathologically there is loss of ganglion cells in Auerbach's plexus.

Clinical features

There is intermittent dysphagia in the 30–40-year age group. This gets progressively worse (for liquids rather than solids) and there is a slowing down of ingestion of food – the patient gets left behind at meals.

Investigation

Barium swallow shows 'rat's tail' stricture in chronic cases. OGD is essential in the elderly to exclude malignancy and other causes of stricture.

Treatment

Medical treatment with anti-spasmodics is unrewarding. Balloon dilatation is successful in 80%. Heller's operation (longitudinal myotomy) via laparoscope in the abdomen or chest is very effective. Injection with botulinum toxin is increasingly being used.

CARCINOMA OF THE OESOPHAGUS

The incidence in Europe is 2–8 cases/100 000. It is much higher in the Far East (100–150/100 000). Males are more commonly affected. The aetiology of oesophageal cancer is summarised in Figure 7.2.

Pathology

Cancers of the upper two-thirds of the oesophagus are usually squamous, the lower third adenocarcinoma. Both spread by local invasion, lymphatic and blood-borne metastases.

Clinical features

The main symptom is progressive dysphagia to solids then liquids. Other features are regurgitation, weight loss, anorexia, anaemia, painful cough, hoarse voice (recurrent laryngeal nerve palsy), supraclavicular lymph nodes and palpable liver metastases.

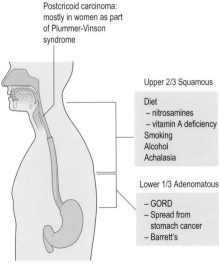

Postcricoid carcinoma: mostly in women as part of Plummer-Vinson syndrome

Upper 2/3 Squamous

Diet
– nitrosamines
– vitamin A deficiency
Smoking
Alcohol
Achalasia

Lower 1/3 Adenomatous

– GORD
– Spread from stomach cancer
– Barrett's

Figure 7.2 The aetiology of oesophageal cancer. GORD, gastro-oesophageal reflux disease.

Kumar and Clark's Handbook of Medical Management

Investigation

- Barium swallow – demonstrates stricture and provides a road map for surgery
- CXR
- OGD and biopsy
- FBC, U&E, LFT, clotting studies
- CT scan of chest and abdomen (the main staging investigation)
- Endoluminal ultrasound – to assess depth of invasion and nodal spread (increasingly important to determine operability)
- Occasionally thoracoscopy and PET scan.

Treatment

The only prospect for cure is surgery. Most tumours are advanced and palliation of dysphagia remains a common goal (palliative resection may still be an option even in the advanced case). The stomach is mobilised, brought into the thorax and anastomosed to the remaining oesophagus in the neck or chest (Ivor Lewis oesophagectomy). This high morbidity/mortality operation is reserved for patients who are in good condition. Patients often receive two cycles of chemotherapy (cisplatin and 5-FU) prior to surgery.

If surgery is not possible then radiotherapy for squamous carcinoma with or without chemotherapy can be used, with variable results. Oesophageal stenting with expanding metal stents is often performed endoscopically in addition to laser ablation techniques for palliation.

Prognosis

Prognosis is poor, although early tumours can result in 60% 5-year survival. Overall 5-year survival is <10%.

PLUMMER–VINSON SYNDROME (PATERSON–BROWN–KELLY SYNDROME)

An iron-deficiency anaemia with formation of a postcricoid web, this is a premalignant condition. Treatment is by dilatation of oesophagus and screening for development of malignancy. It occurs, rarely, in middle-aged women.

PEPTIC ULCERATION

Peptic ulceration includes ulceration of the stomach, duodenum, lower oesophagus and Meckel's diverticulum related to excess acid production and *Helicobacter pylori*. Predisposing factors include smoking, NSAIDs, poor socioeconomic conditions and *H. pylori* infection. The causes of peptic ulceration are summarised in Table 7.1.

Clinical features of duodenal (DU) and gastric (GU) ulcers

- Epigastric pain (eating sometimes exacerbates GU pain and relieves DU pain)
- Radiates to back
- Heartburn
- Gastric outflow obstruction due to chronic ulceration may cause vomiting.

Table 7.1 Contributing factors in peptic ulceration

Factor		Site of ulcer	Presumed mechanism
H. pylori infection 1	>90%	Duodenum, stomach	Hypergastrinaemia, mucosal injury
Non-steroidal anti-inflammatory drugs (NSAIDs)		Stomach, duodenum (usually acute)	Imbalance between mucosal regeneration and acid-pepsin digestion (speculative)
Genetic susceptibility		Duodenum	Non-secretors of blood group 0 into gastric secretions
Hyperchlorhydria		Duodenum	Increased number of acid-secreting cells in stomach (increased parietal cell mass – ? also genetic)
Hyperparathyroidism		Duodenum	Hypercalcaemic stimulation of acid secretion
Benign or malignant gastrinoma (Zollinger–Ellison syndrome)		Stomach, duodenum	Unchecked gastrin hypersecretion

Signs may be minimal though the epigastrium may be tender. Outflow obstruction causes gastric dilatation, which may result in succussion splash (splashing sound heard on rocking the patient).

Investigation

OGD is the principal investigation for peptic ulcer disease. Duodenal ulcers are invariably benign but gastric ulcers must be biopsied to exclude cancer. Barium meal examination is sometimes used.

Treatment

Uncomplicated peptic ulcers require H. pylori eradication (e.g. amoxicillin and clarithromycin) and reduction of acid secretion with H_2 blockers or proton pump inhibitors.

GUs require repeat endoscopy after 6 weeks to check healing and exclude malignancy.

Surgery is only required for complications, e.g. bleeding, perforation and obstruction. Failure of medical treatment for symptoms is rare.

The principal aims of duodenal ulcer surgery are to reduce acid production by reducing parietal cell mass or abolition of cephalic phase of acid secretion (vagotomy) (Table 7.2). Indications for gastric surgery are shown in Box 7.2.

Kumar and Clark's Handbook of Medical Management

Table 7.2 Operative procedures to reduce acid-pepsin secretion, all rarely used

Operation	Mechanism	Severity	After effects
Partial gastrectomy	Reduces parietal cell mass and antral gastrin secreting cells	Major procedure, for malignancy only	Destroys pylorus and may result in dumping syndrome with weight loss and diarrhoea Gastric atrophy may predispose to late gastric cancer
Total vagal pyloric section (vagotomy)	Removes cephalic phase of acid secretion	Less severe procedure than gastrectomy	Requires destruction (pyloroplasty) or bypass (gastroenterostomy): dumping may result
Highly selective vagotomy	As total vagotomy	Benign procedure. Possible by laparoscope	Minimal side effects; procedure of choice

(from Henry & Thompson 2001 *Clinical Surgery*, Elsevier, Edinburgh, with permission)

Box 7.2 Indications for surgical intervention in peptic ulcer

Urgent complications
   Bleeding
   Perforation
Obstruction – usually by inflammation and fibrosis at the outflow of the stomach
Malignancy – gastric ulcers may be malignant and require biopsy if they fail to heal

GASTRIC CARCINOMA

Epidemiology and aetiology

Stomach cancer is the fourth most common cause of death from cancer in women and third in men (10 000 deaths in UK per year). The overall incidence is decreasing but there is a significant increase in incidence in carcinoma of the oesophago-gastric junction. Gastric cancer is more common in China and Japan. The peak age distribution is 50–70 years and men are more commonly affected.

Predisposing factors include *H. pylori* infection, blood group A, atrophic gastritis, pernicious anaemia, smoking and previous gastric surgery. Screening occurs in Japan, but not in the West.

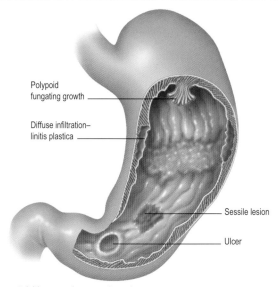

Polypoid
fungating growth

Diffuse infiltration–
linitis plastica

Sessile lesion

Ulcer

Figure 7.3 Macroscopic types of gastric cancer.

Pathology

The four main types of gastric cancer are shown in Figure 7.3.

Gastric cancer spreads by direct local invasion, transcoelomic spread throughout the peritoneal cavity (e.g. Krukenberg tumours: ovarian metastases from a gastric primary), lymphatic and blood-borne metastases.

Clinical features

Early diagnosis is the key to cure. Any patient >40 years old with persistent dyspepsia should have an OGD. Onset of symptoms is insidious and quiet. Weight loss, pain, nausea/vomiting, abdominal discomfort, dysphagia, and upper GI bleeding are the most common presenting features. Signs include:

● weight loss (26%)
● epigastric mass (17%)
● hepatomegaly (13%)
● ascites (3%)
● supraclavicular node involvement (Virchow's node – Troisier's sign (4%))
● possible succussion splash.

The best sign is no sign, since more advanced tumours are usually incurable.

Investigation

● OGD and biopsy is the most sensitive investigation
● CT scan for staging

Kumar and Clark's Handbook of Medical Management

- Ultrasound is more sensitive for liver metastases
- Laparoscopy for detection of peritoneal seedlings not seen on CT and to determine operability.

Treatment

The only curative treatment is surgery, aided by neo-adjuvant chemotherapy. Seventy per cent of growths may be 'resectable', but in the UK only 30–40% are suitable for an attempt at cure. Principles of surgery are wide excision and regional lymph nodes (N2). Palliation may be achieved by resection or bypass, laser ablation or chemotherapy (cisplatin based). Radiotherapy is of no benefit.

Prognosis

The relationship between stage and prognosis is shown in Table 7.3.

ACUTE UPPER GI BLEEDING

This is a common life-threatening emergency. The most frequent causes are peptic ulceration, oesophageal varices and gastroduodenal erosions. GUs are more dangerous than DUs and mortality can be as high as 30%.

Clinical features

Haematemesis and melaena are the commonest presentations of upper GI bleeding. The blood may be altered and result in so-called 'coffee ground' vomitus. Some blood travels through the gut and becomes partially digested, resulting in black tarry stool (melaena).

Significant bleeding (>500 mL) causes fainting, pallor, sweating, tachycardia, hypotension and tachypnoea. A brisk upper GI haemorrhage (UGIH) can result in bright red rectal bleeding.

Management

In a hypovolaemic patient, treatment and investigation occur simultaneously. A multidisciplinary team approach reduces mortality. Urgently:
1. establish bleeding has occurred
2. assess how much and rate of bleeding
3. determine cause of bleeding.

Prompt resuscitation requires intravenous access, urinary catheterisation and early administration of blood to maintain a haemoglobin (Hb) >10 g/dL. CVP monitoring may be necessary for the resuscitation of elderly

Table 7.3 Staging treatment and survival in carcinoma of the stomach

UICC stage	TNM stage	Method of treatment	5-year survival (%)
I	T1 N0 M0	Radical resection	70
II	T2 N0 M0	Radical resection	30
III	T0–4 N1–3 M0	Radical resection	10
IV	T4 N3 M0–1	Palliation	1–2

patients. The plasma/serum urea (but not creatinine) is invariably raised in UGIH because of digestion of blood; this is a useful test if unsure of the diagnosis. The urea is not raised in a colonic bleed.

Requirements for blood are shown in Table 7.4. When the patient is stable a detailed history and examination may be obtained to establish the cause (Table 7.5). OGD is essential to achieve a diagnosis within 24 hours.

Treatment depends on cause and may be conservative or operative. Patients with Hb >12 g/dL are unlikely to re-bleed. Increasingly endoscopic interventions are used (e.g. injection of adrenaline (epinephrine) into ulcer base, clipping of the artery, thermocoagulation and banding of varices).

Peptic ulcer

Many bleeds are self-limiting. Withdrawal of NSAIDs and treatment with PPIs or H_2 receptor antagonists is effective. Patients more likely to re-bleed are elderly, with a large ulcer with endoscopic stigmata of visible vessel, adherent clot, black spot in the ulcer crater or actively bleeding vessel (Table 7.6). The decision to operate should be made in a multidisciplinary setting (Table 7.7). Absence of *H. pylori* is confirmed by ^{13}C urea breath test or by stool sample.

Operatively, for DU the bleeding vessel is under-run with a suture. Definitive operations for peptic ulceration (vagotomy and pyloroplasty) are rarely required, since medical therapy is so effective. Gastric ulcers may be excised locally and sent for pathology to exclude malignancy. If malignancy is confirmed, elective radical surgery may be contemplated.

Oesophageal varices

Oesophageal varices are increasingly common, especially in alcoholic liver disease. Fifty per cent of patients with varices have a bleed and 70% will have another within 1 year. Mortality is higher according to the amount of blood lost, inability to control the bleeding and the severity of the liver damage. Treatment aims to reduce portal pressure (intravenous infusion of vasopressin and betablockade) and to tamponade the oesophageal varices with a Sengstaken-Blakemore tube. Further treatment may include sclerosant injection or rubber band ligation via the endoscope.

Table 7.4 Guidelines for cross-matching and transfusion of blood in upper GI bleeds

Clinical state	Action
Without haemodynamic problems	None
With haemodynamic problem	4 units
Anaemic (Hb <10 g/dL)	1 unit of blood for every 1 g deficit below 10 g/dL
Continued bleeding	Guided by clinical features but at least 4 units
Re-bleed if under 60 years	No action unless there is haemodynamic instability
Re-bleed if over 60 years	4 units

Table 7.5 Salient historical features in common causes of haematemesis

Cause	Mechanism	Historical features
Mucosal tear at cardia (Mallory–Weiss syndrome)	Forceful attempted vomiting	Acute inebriation Initial clear vomit Bright red haematemesis
Oesophageal varices	Rupture or erosion of mucosa over varix	Past liver disease Absence of peptic ulcer history Dark red haematemesis
NSAID-induced erosions	Breakdown of mucosal barrier to acid	Pain-producing associated disorder (e.g. rheumatoid arthritis) Intake of NSAID, including low-dose aspirin
Peptic ulcer	Peptic digestion of vessel in base of ulcer Fibrinoid necrosis of vessel holding lumen open Exacerbation of ulceration by NSAIDs	Previous episodes of dyspepsia Diagnosed ulcer Recent worsening of symptoms Blood of variable colour with or without clots
Angiodysplaslas	Rupture or mucosal digestion of a surface lesion	No history on initial occurrence
Other causes to consider	Varies with cause	Examples: History of anticoagulant intake Haematological disorders

Transjugular intrahepatic portosystemic shunting (TIPSS) is replacing gastric transection and surgical portosystemic shunts as a means of reducing variceal pressure. Variceal bleeding has a high mortality and is best treated in a specialist unit.

Gastric erosions

Gastric erosions associated with liver or multi-organ failure as a cause of upper GI bleeding are managed conservatively with proton pump inhibitors and occasionally sucralfate. Operation (gastrectomy) is rarely contemplated.

Table 7.6 Re-bleeding in peptic ulcer

Class of evidence	Features
Haemodynamic evidence of continued blood loss after resuscitation	Persistent – low or falling CVP; tachycardia; hypotension
Clinical evidence of continued or repeated bleeding	Further fresh haematemesis (not old blood) Melaena
Re-endoscopy	Visible fresh bleeding
Haematological	Progressive haemodilution beyond 24 hours

Table 7.7 Indications for surgery for a bleeding duodenal ulcer

Timing	Age (years)	Basis of decision
Immediate	Any	Uncontrollable spurting vessel at endoscopy Clinical exsanguination
Delayed	Over 60	More than 4 units of blood required for haemodynamic stabilisation or more than 8 units over 48 hours
	Under 60	More than 8 units necessary for stabilisation or more than 12 units needed over 48 hours
On rebleeding	Over 60	One re-bleed after initial successful control but while still in hospital
	Under 60	Two re-bleeds after initial successful control but while still in hospital

Mallory–Weiss tear

The Mallory–Weiss syndrome is bleeding from an incomplete lower oesophageal tear due to severe vomiting. The blood loss is usually self-limiting.

Aortoenteric fistula

This is a rare cause of UGIH unless the patient has had previous aortic surgery (e.g. AAA repair), in which case it must be the presumed diagnosis until proved otherwise. A major bleed may be preceded by a number of minor ones (the 'herald bleed') which may lull doctors into a false sense of security. CT scanning should be performed before OGD (look for inflammation between the duodenum and the aortic graft). OGD usually shows bleeding but not the source. Treatment usually requires removal of the

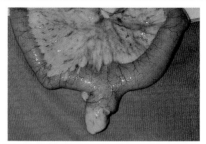

Figure 7.4 Meckel's diverticulum.

aortic graft which is infected and extra-anatomic reconstruction (axillo-bifemoral bypass). This carries a high mortality (over 40%).

DISORDERS OF THE SMALL BOWEL

Meckel's diverticulum

This is a remnant of the vitello-intestinal duct of the embryo which classi-cally occurs in 2% of patients, is 5 cm long and 60 cm from the ileocaecal junction. It occurs on the antimesenteric border of the terminal ileum (Figure 7.4).

Clinical features

Most Meckel's diverticula are an incidental finding at laparotomy although, because of the presence of ectopic gastric mucosa, symptoms typical of appendicitis may occur if the mucosa is inflamed. Alternatively, chronic lower GI bleeding from ulceration ulceration can lead to anaemia. Intesti-nal obstruction due to a volvulus of small bowel around the band from the apex of the diverticulum to the back of the umbilicus may occur. Investigations include a technetium scan for GI bleeding or a red cell scan if bleeding is severe. Excision of the diverticulum is curative.

Tuberculosis

Aetiology

The organism enters the gut via the lymphoid follicles of the ileum. Both human and bovine strains of *Mycobacterium tuberculosis* may be the cause but the latter is uncommon. In patients with immunodeficiency, unusual strains (e.g. *M. avium-intracellulare*) may be found. TB infection of the small bowel is uncommon but remains a feature of communities with poor nutrition.

Pathology

Typically, tuberculosis causes ulceration, lymph node enlargement and subsequent caseation and healing with the formation of strictures. Tuber-culous peritonitis involving the peritoneum produces characteristic miliary nodules and the development of ascites.

Clinical features

Weight loss, low grade pyrexia, anaemia, diarrhoea, vague abdominal pain and rectal bleeding may all be present. Inflammatory masses and strictures can cause obstructive symptoms. Abdominal TB and Crohn's disease may be difficult to distinguish one from another.

Investigations

MRI enteroclysis can provide functional pictures. Barium follow-through may show distortion of the caecum and is difficult to distinguish from Crohn's disease. Laparoscopy may be helpful in this situation. Half of patients with abdominal TB also have an abnormal chest X-ray.

Treatment

The primary treatment of abdominal TB is the same as TB of other organs, i.e. with antibiotics (usually a combination of rifampicin and isoniazid) for up to six months.

Radiation enteritis

Radiotherapy, increasingly used for the treatment of malignancy, can damage small and large bowel. Radiation enteritis may not develop until many years after the treatment. The end effect is an endarteritis in the small blood vessels of the wall of the gut, leading to mucosal atrophy and fibrosis, strictures, ulceration and obstruction. Surgical excision of the damaged loops may be required. Care must be exercised in using healthy un-irradiated bowel for one side of the anastomosis. Poor healing and anastomotic breakdown are common.

Small bowel neoplasms

Primary tumours in the small bowel are uncommon. Small bowel tumours are associated with polyposis coli, Peutz–Jeghers syndrome and Gardner's syndrome. Immunocompromised patients are prone to small bowel malignancy including Kaposi's sarcoma and lymphomas. Lymphomas are more common in the Middle East than in Western society. Secondary metastases to the small bowel can occur, especially in malignant melanoma and small-cell carcinoma of the lung.

Carcinoid tumours

See Chapter 11, p. 192.

Typhoid

This is caused by *Salmonella typhi*. Two hundred cases occur in the UK per year. It may occur in the immigrant population or those who have travelled to endemic countries. The organism enters Peyer's patch and may result in perforation or bleeding during the third week of the disease. Patients present urgently with signs of peritonitis and perforation. Surgical closure of the perforation is required. Chloramphenicol is given intravenously for 2 weeks postoperatively.

CROHN'S DISEASE

Aetiology

This chronic inflammatory condition may affect any part of the GI tract from the mouth to the anus, though the most commonly affected area is the terminal ileum. The cause of this condition is not known, although tuberculosis-type organisms (mycobacteria) have been implicated.

Pathology

There is transmural inflammation with oedema, fissures and non-caseating foci of epithelioid and giant cells leading to fibrosis. Skip lesions can occur

Kumar and Clark's Handbook of Medical Management

throughout the bowel (i.e. there may be normal segments of bowel between affected areas). Oedema and fibrosis lead to intestinal obstruction and internal fistulae may form between loops of bowel, retroperitoneum or the skin.

Clinical features

Acute

There are three main acute presentations of Crohn's disease: right iliac fossa (RIF) pain mimicking appendicitis, small bowel obstruction and perianal suppuration in the form of abscess and fistula. All these are common on general surgical takes and Crohn's disease is always in the differential diagnosis of these problems.

Chronic

Crohn's colitis resembles ulcerative colitis (p. 149, p. 152); the clinical features are similar. There may be symptoms of ill health, weight loss, abdominal pain and diarrhoea. A mass may be present in the RIF. There may be signs of the 'Crohn's anus': skin tags, fissuring and scarring from previous perianal abscess. Other clinical signs that may suggest the diagnosis include clubbing, erythema nodosum, pyoderma gangrenosum and uveitis.

Investigations

Imaging

Barium meal and follow-through demonstrates mucosal irregularities and ulceration, strictures (the string sign of Kantor), skip lesions and internal fistulae.

Radiolabelled white blood cell imaging identifies active foci of disease in patients suspected of having recurrent disease.

Increasingly MRI enteroclysis and capsule endoscopy are increasingly useful for diagnosis.

Biopsy

Biopsies obtained endoscopically from the rectum and terminal ileum may be diagnostic even if the macroscopic appearance is normal. If Crohn's disease is diagnosed at laparotomy, a biopsy of the lymph node is helpful in distinguishing the condition from tuberculosis but open biopsy of bowel should be avoided because of the risk of fistula formation.

Management

There is no specific treatment for Crohn's disease and patients are managed symptomatically, usually with steroids, sulfasalazine or mesalazine to maintain remission. Immunosuppression (azathioprine) may reduce steroid requirement. Metronidazole is useful for perianal sepsis and antidiarrhoeal agents may reduce bowel frequency. Newer agents are increasingly used in the management of Crohn's disease. Antibodies to TNF-alpha (infliximab and adalimumab) exert complex immunosuppressive effects.

Surgery is required for obstruction, abscess or fistula and involves resection of the diseased segment. Patients with multiple small bowel patches of disease may require stricturoplasty to enlarge narrow lumens, rather than resection. Conservative resection is the rule. Fifty per cent of patients who have surgical treatment will require further procedures within 10 years. There is a small risk of carcinoma of the colon in a patient with chronic Crohn's disease.

Hepatobiliary disease 8

JAUNDICE

Classification

Jaundice is due to elevated bilirubin in blood (upper limit of normal is 17 µmol/L). Jaundice may be pre-hepatic, hepatic or post-hepatic (Table 8.1).

Investigations

Blood tests

See Table 8.2. Liver function tests (LFTs) comprise:

- bilirubin
- alkaline phosphatase
- alanine transferase and aspartate transferase
- albumin
- PT clotting
- alpha-fetoprotein
- gamma-glutamyl transferase (indicative of cell damage caused by alcohol).

Serum albumin is a good indicator of hepatic function along with vitamin K dependent clotting factors (prothrombin time). Alpha-fetoprotein is a tumour marker of hepatocellular carcinoma.

Imaging

Ultrasound is most useful and is non-invasive, inexpensive and repeatable. It reliably detects biliary dilatation, gallstones and pancreatic lesions. CT scan provides more precise anatomy. MRI scan (magnetic resonance cholangiopancreatography MRCP) is being increasingly used instead of endoscopic retrograde cholangiopancreatography (ERCP) to delineate common bile duct anatomy/abnormality.

Percutaneous transhepatic cholangiography (PTC) is used when other methods of imaging fail. PTC and ERCP can obtain cytological material for analysis and may proceed to interventions such as biliary stenting. Endoscopic ultrasound (EUS) is increasingly used for diagnosis and obtaining cytology.

Arteriography demonstrates pathological circulation of tumours and helps to determine operability of malignant lesions.

Surgery in jaundice

Jaundiced patients are prone to significant postoperative morbidity. Preoperative correction of as many factors as possible is mandatory prior to surgery. Infective complications are common so antibiotic prophylaxis is essential (also used prior to invasive radiology). Jaundice is also associated with poor wound healing with delayed angiogenesis and reduced collagen synthesis. Clotting is corrected by vitamin K. This takes time and levels

Table 8.1 Classification and causes of jaundice

Type	Causes	Examples	Comments
Pre-hepatic	Haemolysis	Malaria Septicaemia Any haemolytic anaemia	Red cell breakdown produces bilirubin faster than liver can take up Circulating bilirubin unconjugated and not excreted by kidney, so urine of normal colour
Hepatic	Congenital defect of hepatocyte function Infections Toxins	Gilbert's syndrome (harmless unconjugated bilirubin) Crigler–Najjar syndrome Dubin–Johnson–Rotor syndrome Viral hepatitis Paracetamol poisoning	Uptake, conjugation or secretion of conjugated bilirubin is impaired Causes dark-coloured urine
Post-hepatic (also called obstructive/cholestatic jaundice)	Bile duct obstruction	Gallstones Cholangiocarcinoma Carcinoma of the head of pancreas Liver metastases Biliary atresia (in the neonate)	Causes dark-coloured urine/pale stool

Table 8.2 Liver enzymes in jaundice

	Alkaline phosphatase	Aspartate and alanine transferases
Hepatocellular damage	↑	↑↑↑
Extrahepatic biliary obstruction	↑↑↑	↑

Box 8.1 Causes of liver abscess

Cholangitis
Portal pyaemia secondary to
    abdominal infection, e.g.
    appendicitis, diverticulitis,
    peritonitis
Biliary disease
Trauma

Empyema of gallbladder
Septicaemia
Infected liver cyst
Cryptogenic

---

should be checked just prior to surgery. Preoperative biliary decompression by stenting the common bile duct endoscopically can be helpful. Hepatorenal syndrome is prevented by adequate preoperative hydration, to avoid hypotension (set up an intravenous infusion (IVI) and urinary catheter 24 hours preoperatively to ensure good hydration and urine output).

Biliary atresia

Mild jaundice is not uncommon in the neonatal period but persistent or worsening jaundice after 2 weeks is abnormal and suggests biliary atresia. The cause is unknown. Without surgery, death from liver failure results within 6 months. Treatment requires hepatic portoenterostomy or liver transplantation.

LIVER INFECTIONS

Pyogenic liver abscess

Liver abscess is rare. Common organisms include *Streptococcus milleri*, *E. coli, Enterococcus faecalis, Staphylococcus aureus* and *Bacteroides* (see Box 8.1 for causes).

Symptoms and signs are variable and may reflect underlying disease – fever, rigors, jaundice and upper abdominal pain.

Investigations include WBC, LFTs, blood cultures, ultrasound, CT scan and white cell scan. Differential diagnosis includes tumour and amoebic abscess.

Management requires IV antibiotics. Percutaneous drainage may be used and the collection followed ultrasonically. Sometimes open surgical drainage is required. Morbidity and mortality are high if abscesses are multiple or inadequately drained.

Amoebic liver abscess

Due to infection with *Entamoeba histolytica* as a complication of parasitic colitis, the amoeba enters the portal circulation through an ulcer in the colonic mucosa. Abscesses due to the parasite may be single (common) or multiple. They may be extensive and are more common in the right lobe of the liver. The pus formed is thick and contains small quantities of blood – the description often used is that it resembles anchovy sauce. Extension of the abscess may lead to pleural effusion, bronchopleural fistula and lung abscess.

Clinical features

There may be a history of colitis. More usually there is progressive, painful right upper quadrant pain with sweating, rigors and pyrexia. Respiratory symptoms may occur. Physical findings include right upper quadrant tenderness, hepatomegaly and jaundice.

Investigation and management

Investigations include ultrasound or CT scan with aspiration and culture of pus, stool examination, serology testing (negative almost excludes abscess).

Metronidazole is specific with or without percutaneous drainage. Open surgery is unusual.

Hydatid disease

This is a common condition in the Mediterranean and Middle East, due to the parasite *Echinococcus granulosus* (tapeworm). The tapeworm develops in the dog intestine after the dog eats contaminated sheep or cattle offal. The ova are shed in the faeces which contaminate grass or vegetables and are then eaten by sheep, cattle or humans. The ova pass to the liver and develop into hydatid cysts. The cysts usually occupy the upper pole of the right lobe and are slow growing. Many become inactive and calcify.

Clinical features are a symptomless mass, abdominal pain and jaundice.

Investigations include plain X-ray, which may show calcification, ultrasound and CT.

Calcified cysts require no treatment. Drug therapy includes albendazole. Obstructive jaundice due to daughter cysts or cholangitis is managed by endoscopic sphincterotomy. Open surgery is rarely needed.

LIVER TUMOURS

Benign tumours

Benign tumours are common and are usually haemangiomas, focal nodular hyperplasia or hepatic adenomas (occasionally associated with oral contraceptives). CT or MRI scan facilitates diagnosis. Biopsy is contraindicated for haemangioma and no treatment is needed. Distinguishing between a benign adenoma and a well-differentiated hepatocellular carcinoma may be difficult.

Malignant tumours

Hepatocellular carcinoma

Hepatocellular carcinoma is common in Africa but rare in the UK. Widespread Hep-B vaccination is reducing incidence in the Far East. Predisposing factors include alcoholic cirrhosis and chronic liver disease caused by hepatitis B or C, or haemochromatosis. The disease is frequently multifocal with metastatic spread to the lungs.

Presenting features are vague or superimposed on a background history of previous liver disease. Malaise, weight loss and abdominal discomfort are common. Hepatomegaly and signs of metastatic disease may be obvious.

Investigation includes liver function tests and alpha-fetoprotein. CT scan and angiography confirm the presence of tumour and vascular anatomy.

Surgical resection offers the only hope of cure, with a 45% 5-year survival rate. Palliative treatment includes embolisation of tumour blood supply, chemotherapy, alcohol injection and CT-guided cryotherapy.

Cholangiocarcinoma

Cholangiocarcinoma may be intra- or extrahepatic (Klatskin tumours). There is an association with primary sclerosing cholangitis, liver flukes and anabolic steroids.

Clinical features may include progressive jaundice, weight loss, cholangitis and palpable mass in the right upper quadrant.

A combination of ultrasound, CT or MRI combined with ERCP/PTC demonstrates the site of the lesion. Fine-needle aspiration cytology may confirm the diagnosis.

The prognosis is poor; surgical reconstruction may be possible with up to 40% 5-year survival, dependent upon appropriate selection of patients. Biliary enteric bypass and endoscopic biliary stenting provide other palliative options.

Liver metastases from distant primary cancer

Almost any cancer may metastasise to the liver but the commonest are colon, breast, lung, pancreas and stomach. Most metastases are asymptomatic. Large lesions may cause pain, jaundice and anorexia. CT scan and MRI are used to assess resectability, particularly for colorectal primary lesions with increasing prospects of cure combined with chemotherapy. Most other metastatic lesions are treated with palliative chemotherapy.

GALLSTONES (CHOLELITHIASIS)

Epidemiology and aetiology

Gallstones occur in 10% of the population over 50. They are more common in females but can affect anyone. Cholesterol is the principal constituent of the majority of stones, usually combined with bile pigment, especially bilirubin. Stones composed of pigment alone account for 5% of the total. Eighty per cent of stones are asymptomatic. Gallstones are caused by a combination of excess cholesterol concentration in bile, stasis or increased bilirubin secretion in bile. Bacterial infection may also play a role. Symptoms of gallstones are related to the complications they cause (Box 8.2).

Stones in the gallbladder

Biliary colic (see p. 95)

When a gallstone becomes impacted in Hartmann's pouch or the cystic duct it causes biliary colic. The cycle of the colic is long and the pain may be felt as a constant pain in the epigastrium and right upper quadrant, radiating through to the back. Attacks may be precipitated and exacerbated by eating fatty food. Vomiting is common. The pain spontaneously

> **Box 8.2** Complications of gallstones
>
> **Gallbladder**
> Biliary colic (p. 95)
> Acute cholecystitis
> Empyema
> Mucocele
>
> **Common bile duct**
> Obstructive jaundice
> Cholangitis
> Pancreatitis
>
> **Small intestine**
> Gallstone ileus

settles when the stone disimpacts, or passes into the common bile duct. Physical findings may be minimal.

LFTs and WBC are normal. Plain X-ray reveals only 10% of gallstones and is not a useful test. Ultrasound detects 98% of gallbladder stones but is less reliable for bile duct stones.

Management requires analgesics and bed rest (antibiotics are not required for biliary colic), then elective cholecystectomy.

Acute cholecystitis

If a stone impacts in the cystic duct preventing gallbladder drainage, a chemical cholecystitis ensues often with secondary bacterial infection. The pain is more severe and persistent than in biliary colic. Fever is usually present. There is tenderness and guarding in the right upper quadrant (positive Murphy's sign). Hyperaesthesia of the skin over the ninth to eleventh right ribs posteriorly (Boas' sign) may be present. Omentum and small bowel adhere to the inflamed gallbladder and may be palpated as a mass in the right upper quadrant.

The WBC is raised and LFTs often mildly deranged due to partial obstruction of the hepatic duct. Ultrasound confirms stones in the gallbladder with a thickened wall, often surrounded by fluid. Initial treatment is nonoperative with analgesics, antibiotics and intravenous fluids. Failure to settle may result in empyema formation or perforation of the gall bladder. Cholecystectomy prevents further attacks, and should either be performed early (within 2–3 days) or after 6 weeks when inflammation has subsided.

Chronic cholecystitis

This is due to recurrent attacks of obstruction and inflammation; a history of intolerance of fatty foods is common. Diagnosis is confirmed on ultrasound, which reveals a shrunken gallbladder with a thick, fibrotic wall. Cholecystectomy results in cure.

Stones in the bile duct (choledocholithiasis)

Common bile duct stones may cause obstructive jaundice, acute cholangitis and acute pancreatitis. The majority of stones originate from the gallbladder but some may form within the duct system de novo. Common bile duct stones are usually removed prior to cholecystectomy at ERCP and sphincterotomy. This is performed using baskets or sweeping the duct with a balloon.

Obstructive (cholestatic) jaundice

A history of preceding biliary colic is common. The main complaints are jaundice, pruritus, dark urine and pale stools. Abdominal signs are minimal (Courvoisier's law: a palpable gallbladder in the presence of jaundice is NOT due to stones).

Ultrasound confirms dilatation of the bile and intrahepatic ducts and may show ductal stones. MRCP is the best non-invasive test to visualise stones in the bile duct. ERCP confirms the diagnosis, and extraction of stones and sphincterotomy are carried out at the same procedure. Cholecystectomy is required to prevent recurrence.

Acute cholangitis

Ductal stones are the commonest cause for organisms entering the biliary tree from the GI tract. The causative organism is usually *E. coli*. Cholangitis is potentially fatal, due to septicaemia and hepatorenal failure. Liver abscess, secondary biliary cirrhosis, liver failure and portal hypertension are long-term complications.

Clinical features include abdominal pain, fever, rigors and jaundice (Charcot's triad) with a tender, enlarged liver. Investigations may reveal leucocytosis, deranged LFTs and positive blood culture. Gas may be seen in the biliary tree on abdominal X-ray. Ultrasound shows stones and a dilated bile duct.

Treatment requires intravenous fluids, broad-spectrum antibiotics, urgent ERCP and/or stenting. Elective cholecystectomy is required once the acute episode has resolved.

Gallstone ileus

Occasionally in elderly patients a gallbladder containing stones erodes into the duodenum and stones migrate into the GI tract. A stone that has a greater diameter than the narrowest part of the small bowel (terminal ileum) may impact to cause small bowel obstruction (see p. 88). Biliary symptoms may be minimal.

Abdominal X-ray shows air in the biliary tree, small bowel obstruction and possibly a gallstone in the right iliac fossa. Laparotomy confirms the diagnosis and the stone is extracted via an enterotomy. The gallbladder should be left alone (it is usually buried in adhesions by this stage anyway).

Cholecystectomy (see Fig. 25.8)

Cholecystectomy remains the treatment of choice for patients with proven symptomatic gallstones and is described on page 368-9.

Before operation, consideration should always be given to the possibility of gallstones in the common bile duct, which are only reliably detected by MRCP, preoperative ERCP or perioperative cholangiography. Factors which indicate the possibility of gallstones in the bile duct include a history of jaundice or pancreatitis, abnormal liver function tests or a dilated bile duct greater than 10 mm on ultrasound.

ACALCULOUS CHOLECYSTITIS

Acute cholecystitis may develop in the absence of gallstones. It usually occurs in the very ill, often diabetic patient, on the intensive care unit.

Aetiological factors include gallbladder stasis secondary to analgesia or parenteral nutrition. The condition is severe and may progress to gangrene and perforation, with a mortality approaching 15%.

Clinical features

The diagnosis may be difficult in an unconscious patient but should be remembered in a critically ill patient with developed signs of an acute abdomen. Ultrasound may demonstrate oedema in the gallbladder wall which may be dilated. Drainage may be considered percutaneously with ultrasound unless perforation has occurred, in which case laparotomy is required.

GALLBLADDER TUMOURS

Benign

Gallbladder adenoma is uncommon but can predispose to gallbladder cancer. Adenomas less than 1 cm found on ultrasound can be left but larger adenomas should be removed by cholecystectomy.

Carcinoma of the gallbladder

The incidence of carcinoma of the gallbladder is less than 1% in all gall-bladders removed in the UK. Peak incidence occurs in the 60–80-year age range and most are associated with gallstones (male to female ratio 1:4); 90% are adenocarcinomas, 10% are squamous carcinomas. The disease infiltrates locally into the adjacent liver and has a poor prognosis due to inoperability, with a 5-year survival rate of between 2% and 5%. In early T1-stage disease surgery is potentially curative.

PANCREATIC DISEASE

Developmental anomalies

- Pancreas divisum – most of the pancreas drains into the duodenum through the accessory duct of Santorini
- Annular pancreas – a rare cause of extrinsic compression of the second part of the duodenum, from failure of the two developing pancreatic ducts to fuse
- Heterotopic pancreas – accessory budding of the primitive duodenum results in nodules of pancreatic tissue in abnormal positions, for example stomach, duodenal wall or jejunum.

Physiology

The pancreas is an endocrine and exocrine organ. Acinar cells, which synthesise exocrine pancreatic enzymes, drain via intra-glandular ductules into the main pancreatic duct. Secretin and cholecystokinin (produced from the APUD group of cells in the duodenum and upper jejunum) control pancreatic secretion.

Secretin is released into the bloodstream when acid gastric contents enter the first part of the duodenum. This produces a secretion of watery, alkaline pancreatic juice rich in electrolytes. Cholecystokinin (CCK) is released when fatty acids and amino acids enter the duodenum, stimulating contraction of the gallbladder and bile ducts and secretion of pancreatic juice rich in enzymes. These products break down carbohydrates, fats and proteins.

The endocrine portion of the pancreas is arranged as islands (the islets of Langerhans) of endocrine tissue. These have a rich blood supply. The endocrine cells secrete hormones directly into the portal blood.

Investigation of pancreatic function is shown in Box 8.3. The imaging methods for the pancreas are shown in Table 8.3.

Pancreatitis

Pancreatitis may be classified as either acute or chronic, based on presentation, aetiology (e.g. gallstones or alcohol) or pathology (e.g. necrotising or oedematous).

- *Acute pancreatitis* Both endocrine and exocrine function, as well as structure of the gland, return to normal after resolution of the attack unless complications occur. The aetiology of pancreatitis is shown in Table 8.4.
- *Chronic pancreatitis* Permanent structural changes occur, leading to a small, fibrotic gland with either exocrine or endocrine dysfunction. Patients with chronic pancreatitis (i.e. with structural changes including calcification, strictures, stones or cysts) may have episodes that are pain-free but also acute exacerbations of the chronic condition.

Acute pancreatitis

- Pathology Mild pancreatitis is characterised by oedema and exudates which, in the more severe forms, can lead to necrosis which may involve surrounding pancreatic tissues. Infection is a common complication. Acute pancreatitis may range from mild and self-limiting to a rapidly fatal disorder with multi-organ failure.
- Clinical features Abdominal pain (mild or severe) localised to the epigastrium, radiating to the back between the scapulae. Nausea and vomiting are common. The patient may be acutely ill and in shock. Variable

---

Box 8.3 Investigation of pancreatic function

Exocrine
Serum amylase concentration
Duodenal enzyme concentrations after:
    stimulation with CCK and/or secretin
    food stimulation (Lundh meal)
PABA test
Faecal fat estimation
$^{14}CO_2$ breath test

Endocrine
Glucose tolerance test
Plasma levels of:
    insulin
    glucagon
    pancreatic polypeptide

CCK, cholecystokinin; PABA, p-aminobenzoic acid.
Better pancreatic imaging is replacing these conventional tests.

Table 8.3 Methods of visualisation of the pancreas

Technique	Purpose
Abdominal X-ray	Calcification
	Sentinel loop in acute pancreatitis
Ultrasound	Gland size
	Presence of gallstones
	Cysts
	Calcification
	Tumour
	Duct dilatation
	Venous encasement/obstruction
CT	As for ultrasound and is better to define vascular involvement in malignant disease
MR	MRI similar to CT but MRCP gives good images of the bile and pancreatic ducts
Angiography	Tumour detection
	Anatomical definition and vascular involvement
Endoscopic ultrasound	Becoming gold standard to give additional information and permit guided biopsy
Laparoscopy with or without ultrasound	Valuable for detection of small liver and peritoneal metastases

Note: percutaneous biopsy under image control can be done to determine the nature of pancreatic swellings.

MRCP, magnetic resonance cholangiopancreatography.

degrees of tenderness, guarding and rigidity may be present. Body wall ecchymoses around the umbilicus (Cullen's sign) or in the flanks (Grey Turner's sign) are due to haemorrhagic fluid tracking from the retroperitoneum. A serum amylase concentration in excess of 1000 IU per litre is highly suggestive of acute pancreatitis (although a number of other acute abdominal emergencies, particularly bowel ischaemia and perforated ulcer, can elevate the levels).

- **Assessment of severity** Clinical assessment at presentation is unreliable at predicting the course of the illness. Remarkably well-looking patients with serum amylase >1000 can deteriorate suddenly, and desperately sick-looking individuals can recover quickly. For this reason scoring systems have been developed which allow low- and high-risk patients to be identified. The most commonly used scoring system is the Glasgow method, summarised in Table 8.5. All patients with a serum amylase over 1000 should have their Glasgow criteria established and repeated daily to monitor recovery.
- **Imaging** Plain abdominal X-ray and chest X-ray may exclude perforated viscus and demonstrate a sentinel loop of small bowel in the pancreatic region. Ultrasound and CT scan more particularly are used to identify underlying causes, for example gallstones, and to monitor the progress of the disease.

Table 8.4 Known and suspected causes of pancreatitis

Cause	Possible mechanism
Gallstones	Duodenopancreatic reflux Ampullary obstruction with infected bile reflux into pancreatic duct
Alcohol	Unknown
Iatrogenic: – ERCP – Operation at or around the major papilla	? Hypertonic contrast injury ? High-pressure injury ? Obstruction to duct
Neoplasm	Obstruction
Pancreas divisum	
Choledochocele	
Duodenal cysts	
Viral infection: – Coxsackie B – Mumps – ECHO – Epstein–Barr – Cytomegalovirus	Pancreatic cell infection
Bacterial infection: – *Mycoplasma pneumoniae*	Pancreatic infection
Trauma – usually ruptured	Direct trauma ± ductal obstruction in body of gland (over vertebral column)
Hyperparathyroidism	Hypercalcaemia
Sarcoidosis	
Malignancy	
Hyperlipidaemia	Unknown but occurs in Fredrickson's types I, III, IV, V
Drugs: – Corticosteroids – Azathioprine – Thiazides – Tetracycline – Antiretroviral agents – Valproate – Furosemide – Sulphonamides	Unknown
Cushing's syndrome	Unknown
Hypothermia	Unknown
Hereditary – trypsinogen gene mutations	Presumed enzyme activation within pancreas
Pregnancy	Unknown

Table 8.5 The Glasgow criteria to gauge severity of pancreatitis

Factor	Level
Age	>55 years
Leucocytosis	>15 × 10^9/L
Blood urea concentration	>16 mmol/L (no response to fluid administration)
Blood glucose concentration	>10 mmol/L in the non-diabetic
Serum albumin concentration	<32 g/L
Serum calcium concentration	<2.0 mmol/L
Lactate dehydrogenase	>600 IU/L
Aspartate aminotransferase	>100 IU/L
Arterial PO$_2$	<60 mmHg (8.0 kPa)

If more than three of the above are positive, the attack is severe.

Acute pancreatitis due to gallstones requires early ERCP (within 72 hours) and removal of gallstones from the bile duct. Cholecystectomy is required once the attack has settled to prevent recurrence.

- **Prognosis** The overall mortality lies between 8 and 10%. Specific treatment for pancreatitis is supportive, with management of complications if and when they occur. Parenteral fluid replacement, nil by mouth and analgesia are the mainstays of treatment, often with antibiotics to prevent super-infection. Large amounts of fluids may be lost into the retroperitoneum and intensive support may be necessary. This may include ventilation and treatment of renal failure. Long-term intravenous nutrition may not be necessary as some studies suggest early enteral nutrition with a nasojejunal tube is more beneficial.

Complications include hypovolaemia, hypoxia, hypocalcaemia, hyperglycaemia and disseminated intravascular coagulation (Table 8.6). Very occasionally, dead infected areas within the pancreas may be treated by surgery (necrosectomy), which can carry a high mortality rate. Pancreatic lavage is sometimes used.

- **Pseudocysts** These arise as a result of fluid collections which mature after 4 weeks as a wall of granulation and fibrosis is formed. They usually occur in the lesser sac and often resolve spontaneously. Large pseudocysts (greater than 6 cm in diameter) more often communicate with the ductal system and require internal drainage either percutaneously, laparoscopically or open (cyst gastrostomy or cyst jejunostomy).

Chronic pancreatitis

Alcohol consumption is a common association with this disease, leading to blockage of the small pancreatic ducts with plugs of protein which then become obstructed and dilated. Atrophy of acini then occurs with or without inflammatory infiltrate. Fibrosis as a result leads to paucity of acinar and islet cells with widely dilated pancreatic ducts with or without stones.

- **History** There is chronic abdominal pain in the epigastrium often punctuated by acute exacerbations of pancreatitis. Some attacks may be precipitated by a bout of heavy drinking.

Table 8.6 Complications of acute pancreatitis

System or site	Nature and cause
Cardiovascular	Circulatory failure: hypovolaemia
Respiratory	Hypoxia and respiratory failure (ARDS): abdominal distension cytokine release bacterial translocation
Renal	Acute renal failure – hypovolaemia
Haematological	Disseminated intravascular coagulation
Metabolic	Hypocalcaemia – calcium deposition in areas of fat necrosis Hyperglycaemia – islet cell dysfunction Acid-base disturbance from tissue necrosis
Nutritional	Muscle wasting/catabolism
Sepsis in damaged tissue	Infected retroperitoneal slough – bacterial translocation
	Pancreatic abscess – infected fluid collection
Retroperitoneum	Fat necrosis – enzyme release
Pseudocyst	Effusion with or without duct damage
Gastrointestinal	Prolonged paralytic ileus – retroperitoneal inflammation Gastrointestinal bleeding – necrosis of gut wall Colonic necrosis Duodenal obstruction
Hepatobiliary	Jaundice/obstruction of common bile duct
Vascular	Portal/splenic vein thrombosis
	Haemorrhage from arterial rupture
SIRS multiorgan dysfunction	Severe pancreatitis causes multiple system failure

ARDS, acute respiratory distress syndrome; SIRS, systemic inflammatory response syndrome.

There may be weight loss and anorexia. Regular analgesic consumption may lead to opiate addiction. When pancreatic lipase secretion is reduced by 90%, steatorrhoea occurs along with the development of diabetes. There is an increased risk for the development of pancreatic cancer. Less commonly, obstructive jaundice and cholangitis may occur as complications. Obstruction of the splenic vein may lead to portal hypertension.

- **Examination** There may be malnourishment, depression and signs of alcoholic liver disease.
- **Investigation** The amylase may be normal or only slightly raised. Plain X-ray, ultrasound and CT scan may show atrophy of the gland and duct

dilatation with or without calcification. Anatomical abnormalities may be confirmed by ERCP, MRCP or endoscopic ultrasound.

- **Treatment** Cessation of alcohol and control of pain are mainstays of treatment. Pancreatic supplements may help steatorrhoea with acid suppression. Control of diabetes is important. Indications for surgery include correction of obstructed pancreatic duct, relief of obstructive jaundice or relief of intractable pain. Duodenal-preserving pancreatectomy is occasionally performed. Results are variable. Complications include pancreatic cysts and ascites.

Pancreatic carcinoma

Epidemiology

Pancreatic carcinoma is the fifth most common cause of cancer death in the Western world. Men are more commonly affected than women. The incidence increases with age (peak in the seventh decade). Putative aetiological factors include Western lifestyle, cigarette smoking, high-fat diet and working in chemical industries. Coffee and caffeine have been linked to pancreatic cancer but the connection is uncertain, as is the role of alcohol consumption.

Pathological features

In the pancreas, 95% of cancers are adenocarcinomas arising from the pancreatic ducts; 70% of tumours occur in the pancreatic head. Their appearance may mimic chronic pancreatitis, making histological diagnosis essential. Spread occurs by direct invasion of neighbouring tissues, lymphatic involvement, blood-borne metastases to the liver and beyond or by transcoelomic spread in the peritoneal cavity. Carcinomas in the head often obstruct the lower end of the common bile duct to cause obstructive jaundice (see below). In addition, direct invasion may obstruct the duodenum, resulting in gastric outflow obstruction and vomiting. Local infiltration (particularly portal venous encroachment) determines resectability.

Clinical features

Patients may present with obstructive jaundice and pruritus. There may be weight loss and epigastric pain radiating through to the back. A diagnosis of diabetes may have been made recently. Gastric outlet obstruction presents with vomiting. Carcinoma of the body or tail presents later and may be associated with non-specific symptoms of malaise, weight loss and epigastric pain. The prognosis is extremely poor. The differential diagnosis includes peptic ulcer, oesophagitis, angina and biliary colic.

Physical findings include jaundice and scratch marks secondary to pruritus. Weight loss is common. Other findings include Virchow's gland in the left supraclavicular fossa, ascites, a palpably enlarged gallbladder (Courvoisier's law). Differential diagnoses include drug-induced cholestasis, carcinoma of the duodenum, carcinoma of the bile duct, Mirizzi's syndrome (cholecystitis and gallstone in Hartmann's pouch causing compression of the common bile or hepatic duct or a stone in the lower end of the common bile duct).

Investigations

LFTs, full blood count, coagulation studies, ultrasound (excluding gallstones, confirming dilated intra- and extrahepatic biliary tree, a mass in the head of the pancreas). ERCP ± EUS may be used in addition to confirm the diagnosis with cytological brushings or biopsy, and therapeutic stenting may be done at the same time. Percutaneous transhepatic cholangiography is performed when ERCP has failed. MRC cholangiography is increasingly being used. CT scan is valuable for determining operability, demonstrating the relationship of the tumour to the superior mesenteric vessels and portal vein. Visceral angiography may show encasement of the portal vein by tumour, suggesting irresectability. Laparoscopy is used to exclude peritoneal spread before an attempt at resection. Serum tumour markers (CEA and CA19–9) are both elevated in pancreatic cancer and may support a clinical diagnosis.

Treatment

Resection of the primary lesion for cure is possible in less than 20% of patients and therefore management is most often palliative to alleviate the jaundice, control pain and treat exocrine and endocrine failure, often combined with radiation and chemotherapeutic palliation. Whipple's operation (pancreatico-duodenectomy) should only be carried out in specialist centres. Tumours irresectable at operation are treated by palliative biliary bypass. Alleviation of obstructive jaundice is achieved by stenting at ERCP or, if unsuccessful, a percutaneous cholangiogram (PTC) can be performed. Surgical decompression may be undertaken using cholecysto-jejunostomy or hepatico-jejunostomy, often combined with a gastro-enterostomy to manage duodenal obstruction. Intractable pain from invasion of the coeliac plexus is managed by plexus nerve block and opiate analgesics. Chemotherapy, including doxorubicin (adriamycin), epirubicin and mitomycin, has demonstrated some palliative response (10–30%). Less toxic derivatives of platinum-based compounds and metalloproteinase inhibitors are being evaluated. External beam radiotherapy has been shown to prolong survival but is not curative.

Prognosis

Overall prognosis is dismal, with a median survival after diagnosis of 6 months.

THE SPLEEN

The spleen is situated in the left hypochondrium and is the largest lymphoid organ in the body. Its main functions include phagocytosis of all red blood cells, immunological defence and acting as a 'pool' of blood from which cells may be rapidly mobilised. In fetal life, the spleen makes red cells but in adults this function is reactivated only in myeloproliferative disorders that impair the ability of the bone marrow to produce sufficient red blood cells. An increased susceptibility to severe infection after splenectomy (overwhelming post-splenectomy infection – OPSI) has highlighted the major role the spleen plays in both humoral and cell-mediated immunity.

Splenomegaly

The spleen must be enlarged to three times its normal size before it becomes clinically palpable. The lower margin may feel notched to palpation. Massive splenomegaly in the United Kingdom is likely to be due to chronic myeloid leukaemia, myelofibrosis or lymphoma. Splenomegaly may lead to hypersplenism (pancytopenia) due to cells being trapped and destroyed in an over-active spleen; anaemia, infection and haemorrhage result.

Causes of hypersplenism and possible indications for splenectomy are shown in Table 8.7. Other indications for splenectomy include trauma or

Table 8.7 Causes of hypersplenism; possible indications for splenectomy

Condition	Mechanism	Blood disorder	Splenomegaly
Inherited haemolytic anaemias: Spherocytosis Elliptocytosis	Increased red cell fragility	Anaemia	Variable but rarely large
Autoimmune haemolytic anaemias	Antibodies to red cells	Anaemia	Usual
Thalassaemia Sickle cell disease	Abnormal haemoglobins	Anaemia	Variable
Immune thrombocytopenic purpura (primary or secondary)	Antibodies to platelets	Thrombocytopenia	Rare
Portal hypertension	Raised splenic venous pressure with delayed transit of blood	Pancytopenia	Always
Rheumatoid arthritis (Felty's syndrome)	Uncertain	Leucopenia or pancytopenia	Always

as part of other operative procedures, for example gastrectomy, tumours, cysts or more rarely diagnostic procedures such as colonoscopy.

Clinical features

These are often non-specific and generally painless. Features include anaemia, purpura or respiratory infections. Physical findings vary with the underlying cause. A mass in the left upper quadrant, characteristic of splenic origin, has the following characteristics: it is dull on percussion; it moves downwards with respiration; it may have a notch; the upper margin cannot be palpated. The differential diagnoses include gastric or colonic tumours, or masses arising from the pancreatic tail, for example pseudo-cyst or tumour or renal masses.

Management

Infections are treated with appropriate antimicrobial agents. Occasional massive tropical enlargements may require splenectomy because of pain and/or secondary hypersplenism. Hereditary spherocytosis, thalassaemia major, sickle cell disease and elliptocytosis, if there is a high rate of haemo-lysis, may respond to splenectomy. Splenectomy is indicated for patients with idiopathic thrombocytopenic purpura who fail to respond to steroid treatment.

Ruptured spleen

The immediate management of traumatic ruptured spleen (resuscitation) is covered in Chapter 4, p. 66-68. The majority of ruptures are associated with blunt trauma, although splenic hypertrophy may make injury more likely. In the haemodynamically unstable patient laparotomy and splenec-tomy are indicated, but there is a trend towards conservative management in the stable patient. A CT grading system has developed (see American Association for the Surgery of Trauma guidelines) with Grade 1 = <10% area, subcapsular haematoma to Grade V = 'Shattered spleen'. Stable patients >55y with isolated Grade 1 or 2 injury can often be managed with close observation.

Overwhelming post-splenectomy infection (OPSI)

OPSI is a serious late complication of splenectomy. Patients are prone to severe infection from encapsulated organisms such as pneumococci and meningococci and *Haemophilus influenzae*. Post-splenectomy sepsis may start insidiously but can rapidly develop into a fulminant infection with fever, vomiting, dehydration and collapse. Early treatment with antibiotics is essential. Prophylactic immunisation should take place before an elective splenectomy and within two weeks after an emergency splenectomy. Pro-phylactic antibiotics should be taken after an emergency operation, and usually are continued for life (a typical regimen would be penicillin V 250 mg b.d.). All UK hospitals have guidance available for patients who have undergone splenectomy. Any patient who develops a viral or bacte-rial illness should have antibiotic treatment without delay.

Colorectal disorders 9

ULCERATIVE COLITIS

This is a chronic, inflammatory disease which involves the whole or part of the colon. Colitis may be caused by a number of different conditions, including infection (Boxes 9.1 and 9.2). Ulcerative colitis is common in the UK, North America and Scandinavia, with a slightly increased incidence of familial occurrence. The inflammation is confined to the mucosa and nearly always involves the rectum (Fig. 9.1).

Aetiology is unknown but immunological, dietary and genetic factors and transmissible agents may be involved. The inflammatory changes are most marked in the rectum and spread to a varying degree proximally into the colon. The disease does not extend proximal to the ileocaecal valve. The histological features are shown in Box 9.3.

Clinical features

- Diarrhoea
- Rectal bleeding
- Abdominal pain
- Fever
- Weight loss.

Advanced cases may demonstrate malnutrition and abdominal distension. Extra-abdominal manifestations include erythema nodosum, pyoderma gangrenosum, arthritis, uveitis and sclerosing cholangitis.

Physical findings in mild cases are few or absent. Severe cases demonstrate weight loss, anaemia, dehydration, abdominal distension and tenderness.

Complications of ulcerative colitis

Toxic megacolon

Severe inflammation may cause the transverse colon, in particular, to dilate. There is severe systemic disturbance including toxaemia, anaemia, water and electrolyte depletion and progressive distension. Perforation of the colon, which has a high mortality, may ensue.

Colorectal cancer (p. 157)

The risk increases in patients who have had total colitis, approaching 20% risk at 20 years of the disease. Dysplastic change in the glands is thought to be a marker for the risk of malignant change. Regular colonoscopy is required yearly in longstanding colitis to exclude development of carcinoma.

Investigations

- Rigid sigmoidoscopy
- Biopsy
- Colonoscopy

Box 9.1 Non-infective causes of colitis/proctitis

Ulcerative colitis   Ischaemic colitis
Crohn's disease   Irradiation colitis

Box 9.2 Infective causes of colitis/proctitis

Bacterial
Salmonella
Shigella
Mycobacterium tuberculosis
Staphylococcus
Gonococcus
Campylobacter
Clostridium difficile

Viral
Enteroviruses
Cytomegaloviruses
Herpes

Spirochaetal
Treponema pallidum

Chlamydial
Lymphogranuloma venereum

Protozoal
Entamoeba histolytica

Metazoal
Schistosoma mansoni

Mycotic
Histoplasma capsulatum

- Stool cultures to exclude infective causes of colitis
- Barium enema, rare now in UK
- FBC, U&E, LFTs
- AXR in the acute situation to watch for development of toxic megacolon.

Treatment

Medical

The majority of patients have limited disease and are managed by a combination of prednisolone suppositories and a 5-ASA preparation, e.g. mesalazine. Chronic severe cases may respond to immunosuppressive therapy. Acute severe disease causes severe systemic illness and requires admission to hospital. Treatment of acute colitis requires:

- parenteral steroids
- blood transfusion

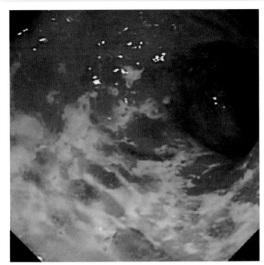

Figure 9.1 A patient with ulcerative colitis.

Box 9.3 Histological features of ulcerative colitis

Lymphocyte and neutrophil infiltration of lamina propria
Crypt abscess formation
Goblet cell depletion
Destruction of surface epithelium (ulceration)
Mucosal oedema
Dysplasia (serious sign – precedes malignancy)

- intravenous fluid replacement
- daily AXR (risk of colon perforation high as caecal diameter approaches 10 cm)
- close collaboration between gastroenterologist and surgeon.

Surgical

Indications for surgery are listed in Box 9.4.

In acutely ill patients who have not responded to maximal medical therapy, the best operation is subtotal colectomy with end-ileostomy, leaving the rectum in situ. In elective cases, the conventional treatment is proctocolectomy (i.e. removal of colon and rectum) with permanent ileostomy. In younger patients, restorative proctocolectomy with ileal pouch to prevent lifelong ileostomy is often performed. In elderly patients, ileorectal anastomosis or continent ileostomy are alternatives. Ileostomy complications include hernia, prolapse, renal calculi, electrolytic imbalance, psychological/sexual problems and parastomal dermatitis.

Kumar and Clark's Handbook of Medical Management

> **Box 9.4** Indications for surgery in ulcerative colitis
>
> Severe exacerbations of colitis
> Toxic colon/acute dilatation
> Chronic colitis refractory to medical treatment
> Development of premalignant changes (dysplasia) in colon/rectum
> Development of carcinoma of colon/rectum

CROHN'S DISEASE OF THE COLON (SEE P. 129)

Crohn's disease may involve the large bowel, either in isolation or in combination with small bowel disease. Symptoms include diarrhoea, indistinguishable from ulcerative colitis. In addition, perianal problems (perianal abscess, fissure and fistula) may occur (see later).

Clinical findings

A high incidence of anal lesions is seen. Sigmoidoscopy and biopsy or colonoscopy confirm the histological diagnosis. Colonoscopy will demonstrate segmental disease and the presence of fissures and fistulas in the bowel. Medical treatment is similar to ulcerative colitis but colectomy may be required, particularly for bowel obstruction; pouch or continent ileostomy is not performed due to risk of anastomotic breakdown and fistulas.

Surgical procedures for colitis

See Figure 9.2a, b and c.

ISCHAEMIC COLITIS

This is uncommon under the age of 50 years. It usually occurs at the splenic flexure at the junction of the mid- and hind-gut arterial supply. Patients often present with acute left-sided abdominal pain and dark red rectal bleeding. Clinical features include fever, hypotension and abdominal distension. Diagnosis is confirmed by colonoscopy and biopsy. Spontaneous resolution is the rule. Anticoagulation may be beneficial (therapeutic-dose LMWH). Occasionally, surgery is required for progressive ischaemia and gangrene. Late complications include stricture.

DIVERTICULAR DISEASE

The main manifestations of diverticular disease are listed in Box 9.5.

Epidemiology and pathology

Diverticular disease comprises outpouching of the mucosa through the bowel wall associated with an increased intraluminal pressure. The most common site is the sigmoid colon. Diverticular disease is rare under the age of 35 years, but reaches a prevalence of 50% among those in their eighth or ninth decade. It is common in Western countries and rare in China, India and Africa. Lack of roughage in the diet appears to be the most common risk factor.

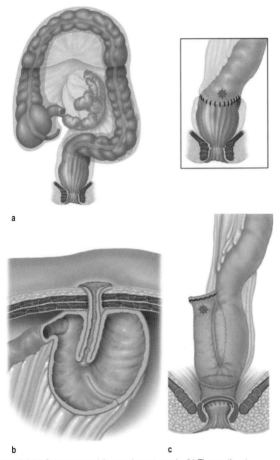

a

b   c

Figure 9.2 (a) Colectomy and ileorectal anastomosis. (b) The continent ileostomy. (c) Ileal pouch with ileo-anal anastomosis.

Inspissated faeces may accumulate within the narrow neck of a diverticulum and inflammation of the sac may lead to perforation, leading to a diverticular abscess or peritonitis. Fistula formation may occur to adjacent organs, for example the bladder. Diverticular disease may be asymptomatic. Acute diverticulitis presents as lower abdominal pain localising to the left iliac fossa. Changes in bowel habit and abdominal distension may occur.

Chronic diverticular disease may cause lower abdominal pain, alternating constipation and diarrhoea with excessive flatus. Findings in the

> **Box 9.5** Manifestations of diverticular disease
>
> Chronic LIF pain, altered bowel habit
> Acute diverticulitis (p. 91)
> Diverticular abscess or mass
> Rectal bleeding
> Perforation causing acute peritonitis
> Fistula formation (into bladder or vagina)

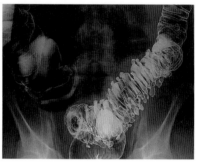

Figure 9.3 Barium enema in a patient with diverticular disease.

chronic case may be minimal. Acute diverticulitis (p. 91) has been called left-sided appendicitis in terms of physical findings. A perforated diverticulum may cause generalised peritonitis, or become walled by omentum and small bowel to form an abscess surrounded by inflamed tissues: this is termed a diverticular mass.

Investigations

Full blood count, colonoscopy (electively) and CT scanning are the usual methods of confirming the diagnosis. Coexistent carcinoma of the colon is not uncommon, and it may be difficult to distinguish a diverticular mass from a cancer.

Treatment

- Uncomplicated diverticular disease may respond to bulking agents (e.g. ispaghula). If pain or complications occur, resection of the affected segment may be considered. Barium enema assists assessment of the extent of bowel to be resected (Fig. 9.3)
- Acute diverticulitis requires bed rest, fluids only, and antibiotics (e.g. cefuroxime, metronidazole). Perforated diverticulum requires laparotomy and resection of the perforated bowel. Rejoining the bowel is risky in the presence of peritonitis and the proximal bowel is usually brought out as an end colostomy (Hartmann's procedure: resection of the sigmoid colon, oversewing of the rectal stump and LIF end colostomy). This may be performed laparoscopically

- Haemorrhage – rectal bleeding due to diverticular haemorrhage can be profuse and require significant transfusion. The distinction between upper and lower GI bleeding can be difficult (Table 9.1) and OGD is usually required to exclude UGIH. Most diverticular bleeds stop spontaneously. Urgent colonoscopy and angiography ± embolisation may be required. If haemorrhage is life-threatening, a colectomy with ileostomy may be considered.

Diverticular mass/abscess/fistula (Table 9.2)

The surgery required for such problems can be complex and difficult. Antibiotics may help reduce some of the inflammation preoperatively. Simple defunctioning ileostomy may be very helpful. Exclusion of cancer is mandatory.

VOLVULUS

This is a loop of bowel twisted around its mesenteric axis, resulting in partial or complete obstruction. Gangrene may occur due to occlusion of the arteries at the base of the mesentery. The sigmoid and caecum may be involved, the former being more common.

Volvulus occurs more commonly in the elderly patient. Features are of large bowel obstruction, often with previous episodes. If infarction occurs, the presentation is acute with signs of shock. A grossly distended abdomen is characteristic and a plain abdominal film is diagnostic (omega sign). Further confirmation may be obtained with a water-soluble enema and/or CT. Caecal volvulus results in a closed loop obstruction and operation is immediately undertaken with right hemicolectomy. Sigmoid volvulus may be managed non-operatively by sigmoidoscopy and a widebore flatus

Table 9.1 Upper versus lower gastrointestinal bleeds

	Upper gastrointestinal	**Colonic**
Haematemesis	Common	Never
Stool	Melaena, or dark blood with clots, fresh blood for a brisk major bleed	Bright red bleeding or dark red with clots
Plasma urea	Elevated (due to partial digestion of blood)	Normal
Pain	No	No

Table 9.2 Hinchey grading system: classification of perforations of colon due to diverticular disease (and current management strategy)

Grade	Definition	Treatment
I	Localised abscess	Medical ± radiological
II	Pelvic abscess	Medical + radiological
III	Purulent peritonitis	Surgical (laparoscopic or open)
IV	Faeculent peritonitis	Surgical (open)

Box 9.6 Classification of colorectal polyps

Neoplastic
Adenoma
   Tubular
   Tubulovillous
   Villous

Non-neoplastic
Hamartoma
   Juvenile
   Peutz–Jeghers
Inflammatory
   Lymphoid
   Inflammatory
Miscellaneous
   Metaplastic
   Connective tissue polyps

---

tube passed into the sigmoid loop for decompression. Once decompression has been achieved, a decision for surgical excision may be made because recurrence is common.

COLONIC POLYPS

Classification of the different types of polyps is shown in Box 9.6. Many benign large bowel polyps are associated with a number of different conditions, many of which have a genetic component. The most common and important neoplasm is an adenoma arising from the glandular or epithelial cells. Polyps most often have a stalk but flat lesions can occur.

The histology of the polyp is important because adenomas are a premalignant condition and may lead to the development of carcinoma. The polyp-cancer sequence is most likely in lesions over 1 cm diameter. Most polyps are asymptomatic but may present with rectal bleeding or the diagnosis may be made as a coincidental finding at a screening programme or investigations for other symptoms. If a polyp is found, the bowel should be completely examined by colonoscopy and all lesions removed endoscopically. Those that cannot be removed at colonoscopy require surgical resection. Techniques such as EMR have reduced this number.

Familial adenomatous polyposis

This is an important autosomal dominant condition. Multiple polyps develop in the colon and small bowel between the ages of 13 and 30 years. Progression through the cancer sequence is inevitable. A family history is often present. Rectal bleeding is the most common finding. Total colectomy is essential because of the universal progression to cancer. Ileo-anal pouch reconstruction is the treatment of choice for younger patients.

Hereditary non-polyposis colorectal cancer (HNPCC)

HNPCC is a hereditary syndrome, caused when a person inherits a mutation in one of five genes. People with HNPCC have a high risk of developing colorectal cancer (up to 80%); 2–5% of all colorectal cancers are attributed to HNPCC, or 'Lynch Syndrome'. HNPCC also puts patients at risk of other forms of cancer (e.g. endometrium, ureter or renal pelvis).

It is an autosomal dominant condition, so family history is crucial in detecting potential cases, guided by the Amsterdam II criteria: at least three members of the family has a diagnosed HNPCC-associated cancer, one of the three must be a first-degree relative, at least two successive generations should be affected and at least one must have been diagnosed before age 50. Screening for colorectal cancer in this group is essential and should start at an early age (after 20 years).

COLORECTAL CANCER

Colorectal cancer is the second most common type of carcinoma in the UK. The disease is uncommon in Asia, Africa and South America. The disease develops from any age from the second decade but the peak incidence occurs in the sixth and subsequent decades.

Aetiology and pathology

A diet rich in animal fat is a major risk factor. This may predispose gut bacteria to convert bile salts to carcinogens. Adenomatous polyps, genetic factors and inflammatory bowel disease are other well-known risk factors. The distribution of colorectal cancer is most common in the rectum and sigmoid. Up to 5% of patients have synchronous cancers and 75% of patients have coexistent benign adenomas. Tumours are classified as polypoid, ulcerative, annular or a combination.

Spread may occur by direct local invasion, by lymphatic, haematogenous or transcoelomic routes, and by direct implantation of exfoliated cells.

Staging

A conventional method of staging is the Dukes classification (Fig. 9.4):
- A: cells are confined to the mucosa (5-year survival: 95%)
- B: the tumour has extended through all muscle layers (5-year survival: 65%)
- C: lymph node metastases (5-year survival: 30%)
- D (added to Dukes later on): disseminated metastatic disease (5-year survival is now approaching 20% after surgery).

Many centres now use the TNM staging system as a basis for further decisions about adjuvant radio- or chemotherapy (Box 9.7).

Screening

Increased numbers of Dukes stage A cancers can be detected by screening patients with either a known increased risk of cancer or first-degree relatives who have had polyps or cancers (Amsterdam criteria). Faecal occult blood estimations have also been shown to detect earlier cases of stage A disease. In the UK a national screening programme for colorectal cancer was started in 2007. Thus far the number of Duke's A tumours has increased from 10% in the symptomatic group to 50% in the screened group.

Clinical features

The most important of these are shown in Box 9.8.

Right-sided tumours have non-specific complaints (e.g. malaise, weight loss, vague abdominal pain and occasionally a mass in the abdomen).

Kumar and Clark's Handbook of Medical Management

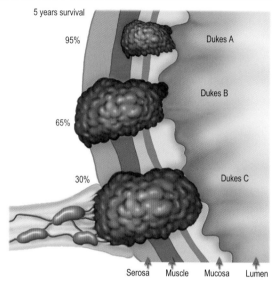

Figure 9.4 The Dukes staging of colonic carcinoma.

Box 9.7 TNM staging system for colorectal cancer

Tumour

T1: Tumour invades submucosa

T2: Tumour invades muscularis propria

T3: Tumour invades through the muscularis propria into the subserosa, or into the pericolic or perirectal tissues

T4: Tumour directly invades other organs or structures, and/or perforates

Node

N0: No regional lymph node metastasis

N1: Metastasis in 1–3 regional lymph nodes

N2: Metastasis in 4 or more regional lymph nodes

Metastasis

M0: No distant metastasis

M1: Distant metastasis present

Iron-deficiency anaemia is a common presentation. Intestinal obstruction is unusual for carcinomas of the right side, due to the liquid nature of the faeces.

Left-sided tumours are more likely to present with obstructive symptoms due to the solid stool and decreased calibre of bowel. Colicky

Alteration in bowel habit
Rectal bleeding and/or
  mucus
Abdominal pain

Malaise
Weight loss
Tenesmus

abdominal pain and a change in bowel habit, which is usually loose or more frequent stool or alternating constipation and diarrhoea, occur. Mucus is another common symptom.

Rectal tumours present with rectal bleeding, mucus discharge and tenesmus. Advanced tumours may spread locally, causing faecal incontinence, back pain and urinary infections due to fistulas. Physical findings are often absent but a mass may be palpable per abdomen or rectally. Associated signs of disseminated disease include weight loss, ascites and hepatomegaly.

Investigations

All patients should have a rectal examination and a sigmoidoscopy and biopsy. Full visualisation of the bowel requires colonoscopy or CT colonography if colonoscopy cannot be completed. Once diagnosed, patients with colonic tumours are additionally imaged with CT of the chest, abdomen and pelvis for staging purposes. Patients with rectal cancer will have an additional MRI of the pelvis to better delineate whether the mesorectal envelope is threatened. If it is then preoperative adjuvant radiotherapy/ neo-adjuvant chemoradiotherapy will be considered.

Treatment

Colonic carcinoma is treated by surgery (Fig. 9.5) following preoperative staging with CT scans, colonoscopy to exclude metachronous lesions and general fitness for a general anaesthetic. Bowel preparation is usually mechanical with Picolax or Klean-Prep. Colostomy is avoided.

Rectal carcinomas present different preoperative problems and many patients are entered into trials of adjuvant radio/chemoradiotherapy (e.g. the CRO7 trial comparing preoperative radiotherapy and selective postoperative chemoradiotherapy for rectal cancer). Radiotherapy may be either a short course (5 days) or a long course, depending on stage of tumour, usually assessed by MRI of the rectum. Rectal cancers are surgically treated by anterior resection or abdominoperineal excision (Fig. 9.6). Complications of colorectal surgery are listed in Box 9.9.

Advanced disease

Local recurrence remains a serious problem for the patient and is most unlikely to be resectable. Palliation is the rule of treatment. Hepatic metastases, if they are solitary or less than four in number, can be resected, which has resulted in some improvement in survival. Multiple hepatic secondaries are treated palliatively by chemotherapy or radiofrequency ablation.

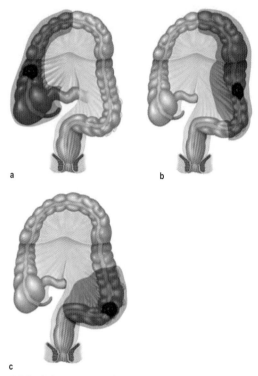

a   b

c

Figure 9.5 Surgical management of colectomy. Shaded areas are resected: (a) right hemi-colectomy, (b) left hemi-colectomy, (c) sigmoid colectomy.

ANAL AND PERIANAL DISORDERS

Anal disorders usually present with bleeding at the time of defecation, pruritus (itching), pain on defecation, perianal swelling or discharge. Discharge may be subdivided into faecal, mucus or pus.

Clinical examination is an essential feature of assessment of any patient with symptoms attributable to the anal canal and the rectum must always be examined to make certain that the underlying cause is not proximal. The causes of rectal bleeding as a symptom are shown in Box 9.10. The patient is placed in the left lateral position. The examination comprises three components: inspection, palpation and endoscopy (sigmoidoscopy and proctoscopy). If investigation is impossible in the outpatients department, it can be done under anaesthetic (EUA), particularly when pain and discomfort prevent digital palpation.

Further investigations include flexible sigmoidoscopy or colonoscopy and intraluminal ultrasound (which provides accurate information about

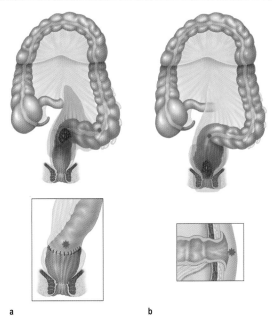

Figure 9.6 Surgical management of rectal carcinoma. (a) Anterior resection of the rectum. (b) Abdominoperineal excision of the rectum and anus. Shaded areas are resected.

Box 9.9 Complications of colectomy and rectal excision

Haemorrhage
Ureteric damage (left-sided
  resections)
  Urinary leakage
  Ureteric stricture
Damage to bladder function
  Acute retention
  Urinary incontinence
Damage to sexual function
Damage to duodenum (right
  hemicolectomy)
Damage to spleen (left
  hemicolectomy/anterior
  resection)

Anastomotic complications
  Stenosis
  Leakage
Complications of stoma
  Parastomal hernia
  Prolapse
  Electrolyte imbalance
  Ischaemia
  Stenosis
Diarrhoea/constipation

Box 9.10 Causes of rectal bleeding

Haemorrhoids	Solitary rectal ulcer
Diverticular disease	Anal conditions
Colorectal cancer	Fissure
Colorectal polyps	Fistula
Arteriovenous malformations	Thrombosis
Ischaemia	Squamous carcinoma
Trauma	Warts
Colitis	

Table 9.3 Bacteriological examination of anorectal material

Condition	Examination	Finding
Acute abscess	Standard cultures	Intestinal organisms – ? fistula
Gonorrhoea	Fresh swab and culture	*Neisseria gonorrhoeae*
Syphilis	Dark ground examination	Spirochaetes
Fungal infection	Direct microscopy of scrapings of perianal skin Culture	Pathogenic organism
Tuberculosis	Histopathological examination Culture for *Mycobacterium tuberculosis*	Caseating granulomas Organisms on Ziehl–Neelsen stain Organism and sensitivity

the anal canal and sphincters and localising perianal sepsis/fistulas). MRI scanning can accurately identify primary and secondary fistulous tracks and abscess and may provide additional data about the extraluminal spread of rectal cancer (particularly useful in patients with early rectal cancer, who are being considered for TEMS.) Fistulography and evacuation proctography are rarely used in general practice. Examination of pus may be helpful in determining whether or not anal fistula is present (Table 9.3). Anorectal physiology studies are widely used to evaluate patients with faecal incontinence. These tests measure the anal canal pressure, the anorectal reflex, the ability to expel a faecal bolus and electromyographical assessment of the external sphincter and its response to pudendal nerve stimulation.

Haemorrhoids

These are engorgements of the haemorrhoidal venous plexuses with redundancy of their coverings. The anal cushions may remain in their usual position in the anal canal (first degree), descend to involve the skin

Table 9.4 Conditions related to (and which may be confused with) haemorrhoids

Condition	Position
Anal skin tags	Anal margin
Fibrous anal polyps	Line of the anal valves
Prolapse of rectum	Similar to haemorrhoids but circumferential
Thrombosis in perianal skin (perianal haematoma)	Distal to mucocutaneous junction
Fissure	Primarily at the mucocutaneous junction but may have a distal skin tag
Benign tumours of the rectum	Within the rectum at sigmoidoscopy
Varices	Rare but almost impossible to distinguish
Haemangioma	Rare congenital abnormality

of the distal anal canal so that they prolapse on defecation but reduce spontaneously (second degree), or become of such a size that they are always partly outside the anal canal (third degree). Classical positions are the left lateral, right posterior and right anterior positions, although secondary haemorrhoids can occur in between these anatomical sites. The diagnosis of haemorrhoids is shown in Table 9.4. Constipation and straining at the time of defecation may be a factor in the development of haemorrhoids. In women, pregnancy is a common risk factor.

Clinical features

Bleeding – usually at defecation – bright red in nature, dripping or spurting into the toilet pan or onto toilet paper may occur afterwards. This is painless. Minor faecal soiling or mucus leak is common along with pruritus, occasional discomfort and palpable swelling. Pain only occurs upon thrombosis or the development of coexistent anal fissure. On examination, haemorrhoids vary from a slight increase in the normal anal cushion size, visible only at proctoscopy, to large third degree internal/external haemorrhoids apparent on inspection of the anal verge.

Treatment

Reassurance that this is a benign condition is very helpful to alleviate the fear of more sinister pathology. Regulation of the bowels, particularly relief of constipation by an increased intake of fluids, fruit, vegetables and bulking agents, and the avoidance of prolonged straining at stool are often recommended. Proprietary medications and suppositories may also be helpful for the relief of pruritus.

Several treatments are available. Injection sclerotherapy and Barron banding (with or without the use of suction) are treatments used in the outpatient department. Cases requiring general anaesthesia include standard haemorrhoidectomy, THD and, more recently, stapled

Kumar and Clark's Handbook of Medical Management

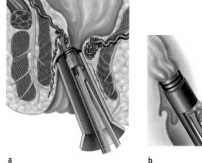
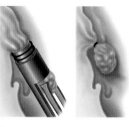

a   b   c

Figure 9.7 Band ligation for haemorrhoids. (a) The haemorrhoid is grasped (or held by suction). (b) The haemorrhoid is drawn further within the instrument (and thus within the elastic band held outside). (c) The strangulated haemorrhoid with the elastic band at its base (which necroses and is later shed, sometimes accompanied by bleeding).

haemorrhoidopexy. The latter are generally reserved for resistant cases or third-degree haemorrhoids. Manual dilatation of the anus is rarely used for fear of irreversible damage to the anal sphincter. Injection sclerotherapy may need to be repeated. Barron-band ligation (Fig. 9.7) has a serious complication of pain and haemorrhage after the application of the bands. Cryotherapy and lateral anal sphincterotomy are rarely used for the treatment of haemorrhoids today. Haemorrhoidectomy aims to excise as much redundant epithelium and vasculature as possible and may be carried out by a variety of methods.

Thrombosed haemorrhoid

Thrombosis may develop within haemorrhoidal veins and commonly presents as a surgical emergency. The episode is best managed conservatively with the application of ice, non-constipating analgesics and lubricant laxatives. Resolution takes place over the following 7–10 days. Urgent haemorrhoidectomy is occasionally used but runs the risk of postoperative anal stenosis.

Perianal haematoma

This condition, also known as thrombosed external pile, is a discrete, painful swelling in the perianal margin that looks like a small blackcurrant. There is often a history of straining 2 or 3 days prior to the episode of acute rectal pain. If severe, the haematoma may be deroofed under local anaesthetic with immediate relief.

Fissure in ano

Aetiology

Often idiopathic, other risk factors include constipation (adults and children), traumatic childbirth and anal intercourse leading to pain, sphincter spasm and constipation and occasional anal bleeding. The pain characteristically occurs during defecation and continues for some time after the passage of stool. Constipation may be a consequence of the patient's unwillingness to defecate because of pain. Pruritus ani and a discharge of small quantities of pus occur.

Clinical findings

Separation of the buttocks and palpation of the anal verge reveals the site of tenderness and fissure, which is usually in the midline (the majority posteriorly). Digital examination may not be possible. In chronic lesions, a sentinel tag is visible. The fibres of the internal sphincter may be visible. Other causes, apart from idiopathic fissure, include Crohn's disease, primary syphilitic chancre, herpes simplex, lymphoma and leukaemia. Basal and squamous cell carcinomas and excoriation of the perianal skin may simulate the condition.

Management

For acute fissure, local anaesthetic gel and bulk laxatives may help. More recently, topical glyceryl trinitrate 0.2% and diltiazem 2% ointment have been tried for the acute fissure with some success but are more often used for chronic anal fissure. More recently botulinum toxin injection to the internal anal sphincter has been tried. If this fails, a lateral internal sphincterotomy carries a 95% chance of cure but the patient must be counselled about the risk of passive flatus incontinence. Most clinicians use a trial of GTN or diltiazem for a variable period, then botulinum toxin injections. If this fails, surgery is the next step but entails the risk of permanent damage to the internal sphincter.

Perianal sepsis

A variety of anal conditions present with suppuration, as shown in Table 9.5. The spread of sepsis begins in the intersphincteric space and may

Table 9.5 Conditions associated with perianal sepsis	
Condition	**Usual finding**
Non-specific infection	Acute abscess Fistula in ano
Tuberculosis	Chronic infection Occasionally fistula
Crohn's disease	Chronic intractable infection Complex fistula
Hidradenitis suppurativa	Skin abscesses Anal canal rarely if ever involved
Skin sepsis	Usually *Staphylococcus aureus* Abscesses are often multiple
Trauma	External: sexual intercourse; accidental injury Internal: foreign body (ingested bone)
Intrapelvic sepsis	Diverticular disease Crohn's disease
Sepsis in developmental cysts	Usually dermoid cysts
Malignant disease	Sepsis is an uncommon complication

Kumar and Clark's Handbook of Medical Management

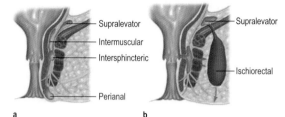

Figure 9.8 Spread of infection. (a) Vertical spread. (b) Horizontal spread.

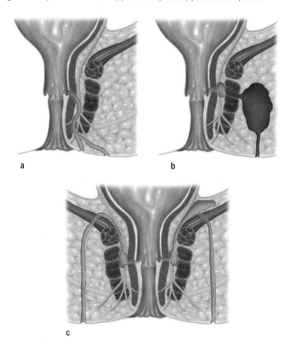

Figure 9.9 Types of fistula. (a) Trans-sphincteric. (b) Suprasphincteric. (c) Extrasphincteric.

spread vertically, horizontally or circumferentially (Fig. 9.8). Five anatomical sites of abscess are classified into intersphincteric, perianal, intermuscular, supralevator and ischiorectal. The formation of a fistula occurs as a result of pus spreading along a track to emerge distal to the mucocutaneous junction, and an internal and external track is formed. Fistulas are classified according to their intersphincteric/trans-sphincteric nature. Other types of fistula include superficial, suprasphincteric and extrasphincteric (Fig. 9.9).

Clinical features

Clinical features are abscess and fistula. There may be a history of similar episodes of intermittent discharge, starting as an abscess prior to discharge. Signs of an abscess include acute pain, inflammation of the perianal area or an obvious fistula. The management of perianal abscess is surgical incision and drainage and the pus is sent for microbiology. If gut organisms are cultured, a fistula may be suspected. Superficial fistulas are laid open without damage to the external sphincter. The majority heal without difficulty. Trans-sphincteric and suprasphincteric fistulas require specialist care and may be carried out in stages (the insertion of a seton suture is placed through the primary tract to act as a drain or tightened to bring the fistula to the surface). Expert nursing care is required for wound dressings to ensure that the wounds heal from their depth to the surface. Crohn's disease may be considered as a cause of fistulas if there are oedematous skin tags, a bluish hue to the perianal margin, sepsis and ulceration. Tuberculosis is the differential diagnosis.

Pilonidal disease

This is common, and usually occurs in the natal cleft but can occur in the umbilicus and in the webs of the fingers. Aetiology is unclear. It presents as a sepsis resulting in pain, tenderness and discharge, often with a history of previous recurrent episodes. There are one or more openings in the midline or to either side with protruding tufts of hair. The management is usually surgical. Orthodox treatment is excision of the pits and the wound is left to heal by secondary intention. Post-treatment shaving of the skin is necessary for 6 months – failure to do so is the commonest cause of recurrence.

Hidradenitis suppurativa

The apocrine sweat glands, usually in the perineum, inguinal regions and axilla, become the site of a mixed bacterial infection. Obesity, poor hygiene and hormonal imbalance are contributory factors. Various degrees of sepsis occur, with tracks running widely in the subcutaneous tissue. In the perianal region, these may be confused with anal fistula. The treatment is to control the contributory factors and to lay open the septic areas. Long-term prophylactic antibiotics and occasionally plastic surgery procedures are necessary.

Pruritus ani

Pruritus ani is a common symptom which may be caused by inadequate hygiene, anal disorders, as part of a skin infection, local infection, infestation by parasites or an allergic reaction to pharmaceuticals or as part of a generalised pruritus in obstructive jaundice or in faecal incontinence due to a sphincter defect. Itching in the perianal skin is the initial symptom. If the causative factor persists, soreness and pain even on walking occur. The perianal skin commonly shows evidence of abrasion or the presence of one of the specific factors described.

The key to successful management is the accurate determination and treatment of the cause. Ointments for symptomatic management should only be used when a precise diagnosis has been made. Short courses of topical steroids may be given. Threadworms should be treated. Strict instruction in anal hygiene should be given to avoid faecal soiling.

Kumar and Clark's Handbook of Medical Management

Faecal incontinence

This may occur either as the inability to defer defecation for more than a few minutes or as passive incontinence defined as the loss of stool without the patient being immediately aware. Aetiology may include sphincter inadequacy due to large third-degree haemorrhoids, rectal prolapse or a large faecal mass in the rectum, or anal canal tumour. Damage to the sphincter from previous surgery or overstretching (previous surgery or unusual sexual practices) or obstetric injury (third-degree perineal tear) or loss of the motor innovation to the internal sphincter, e.g. diabetes, spina bifida or prolonged, complicated obstetric delivery, may all contribute. Loss of cerebrospinal regulation and fistula between rectum and vagina may also be factors.

Clinical features

An accurate past history is essential to determine the cause of the incontinence. Clinical findings will depend on the cause, ranging from obvious scarring of the perineum from previous surgery or obstetric trauma, to evidence of anal disease.

Investigation and management

Digital rectal examination and proctosigmoidoscopy are essential. Anorectal physiology studies will measure the pressure in the anal canal at rest (internal sphincter) and on maximum voluntary contraction (external sphincter) to establish which muscle group is at fault.

Management depends on the cause. Faecal impaction is dealt with by manual evacuation. Minor incontinence may respond to an anti-motility drug (e.g. loperamide). Biofeedback uses the recording of the patient's pressure trace to encourage increased tone. Surgery is only indicated where there is a known cause which can be corrected by anatomical and physiological reconstruction. Central nervous conditions may require a stoma to divert the faecal stream but this may not be the only alternative to incontinence. Anterior anal sphincter repair is successful for the trauma from obstetric injuries. Posterior anal repair is occasionally used for neuropathic problems to restore the anorectal angle and the length of the anal canal. Gracilis muscle neosphincters have been used in specialist centres. Increasingly, SNS is achieving good results for idiopathic faecal incontinence. The mechanism of action is not clear. Similar outcomes are being recorded for patients with chronic constipation.

Tumours of the anal canal

Perianal warts caused by the human papilloma virus are common, most often sexually transmitted by both sexes. They are common in HIV infection. Bowen's disease, basal cell and squamous cell carcinomas of the anus have all been described. Their presentation is similar to all other anal diagnoses and a careful examination must be undertaken to establish the diagnosis. Perianal warts are treated by excision under a general anaesthetic, as are keratoacanthoma and Bowen's disease. Basal cell carcinomas and squamous cell carcinomas may respond to either local excision or radiotherapy with or without chemotherapy.

Breast disease 10

Breast symptoms are common but only one in ten patients referred to surgical clinics has a carcinoma. The remainder have a variety of conditions labelled benign breast disease. Many conditions are not truly pathological but aberrations of normal development that occur between puberty and old age.

Patients with breast symptoms are best assessed in a one-stop breast clinic where so-called triple assessment, i.e. clinical examination, fine-needle aspiration cytology and imaging (ultrasound or mammography), allows rapid diagnosis of most breast conditions.

BENIGN BREAST DISEASE

Mastalgia (breast pain)

This is usually cyclical. Pain occurs early in the menstrual cycle and worsens to reach a peak just before menstruation, easing with the start of the period. Mild pain may affect the upper outer quadrants of the breast, causing minor symptoms. In severe cases, the breast may be engorged, tender and heavy.

Pain occasionally occurs in postmenopausal women, often related to hormone replacement therapy (HRT). Pain may be in one or both breasts. Clinical findings, apart from tenderness and occasionally nodularity, may be normal.

Management

Breast cancer is hardly ever painful and this reassurance may help. In women under 35 years, mammograms are of no diagnostic help since the breast tissue is too dense. Ultrasound may exclude a discrete lump.

A diary chart may determine if the problem is cyclical or non-cyclical. The most important aspect of management is reassurance. Patients with severe disease may be treated with gamma-linoleic acid (evening primrose oil), danazol or bromocriptine. Evening primrose oil is an essential fatty acid which may work by making the breast cells less sensitive to sex hormones. Sixty per cent of patients respond to the treatment if taken in a full dose (320 mg per day for 3–4 months). Danazol affects the action of oestrogen on the breast tissue. Side effects which are similar to those experienced in the menopause may make compliance low. Bromocriptine blocks the pituitary production of follicle-stimulating hormone (FSH) and luteinising hormone (LH).

Breast lumpiness and lumps

It is vital, but sometimes difficult, to distinguish whether a breast lump is part of a diffuse lumpiness or a discrete, isolated lump. The diagnosis may be influenced by whether the lump is painful and/or the age of the patient (Table 10.1).

Table 10.1 Likely diagnosis of discrete breast lumps at different ages

Young adult	Fibroadenoma
Middle-aged	Cyst
Elderly	Carcinoma

The triple approach (physical examination, mammography/ultrasound and fine-needle aspiration cytology) enables a diagnosis to be made in most patients. Mammography is unhelpful in women under 35 years of age because the breasts are frequently too dense for small lesions to be seen.

Lumpiness

Lumpiness is frequently associated with cyclical breast pain and is also known as fibroadenosis, cystic mastopathy, fibrocystic disease and cystic mastitis. These terms are now discouraged since their use suggests the breast condition is pathological, but in fact these changes are part of normal breast development throughout life which is more pronounced in some individuals. Lumpiness may be very localised and lead to difficulty in deciding whether a discrete lump is present.

Discrete single lump

The common benign causes are localised fibroadenosis, cyst, fibroadenoma and trauma.

● **Localised fibroadenosis** Usually the upper outer quadrants are affected or it may be unilateral. Patients are often young and the findings may be single or multiple lumps in either breast which may be tender premenstrually.

Investigation requires mammography in the over-40s combined with ultrasound and fine-needle aspiration cytology (FNAC). Treatment is by reassurance.

● **Fibroadenoma** This affects younger women. Fibroadenoma may remain of a small size but some regress or increase in size. Pain is not a usual feature. The lump is well-defined, rubbery or firm to hard, and may be mobile and difficult to find, hence the nickname 'breast mouse'.

If triple assessment supports the diagnosis of fibroadenoma, small lesions may be left alone, but removal by excision should be advised for larger lesions in older women.

● **Breast cysts** Breast cysts occur at a later stage of life (35 through to the menopause). They may represent an involution of other cyclical breast changes. Multiple recurrent cysts may be associated with an increased risk of breast cancer.

The findings are of a tense, discrete, mobile lump which then may be aspirated, yielding a straw-coloured fluid and causing collapse and disappearance of the lump. If the cyst does not completely disappear, repeat examination is advised and the lump evaluated by triple assessment. The aspirate is usually straw-coloured but a bloodstained aspirate (which may be traumatic) should be sent for cytological examination and possible excision biopsy. Multiple cysts may be treated with danazol, which helps reduce the incidence of clinical recurrence. Follow-up mammography is advised.

● **Trauma (fat necrosis)** Trauma to the breast is uncommon but may damage local blood supply and cause fat necrosis. This results in a hard, painful lump with irregularity over the overlying skin, mimicking a carcinoma. Triple assessment is required for diagnosis but no specific treatment is recommended.

Nipple discharge

Green or milky discharge is usually harmless. Clear or bloodstained discharge may indicate a duct papilloma and occasionally an underlying malignancy.

Mammary duct ectasia and periductal mastitis

The ducts adjacent to the nipple become dilated and engorged with breast secretion. Secondary infection and abscess may form. Subsequent fibrosis may cause nipple retraction. The condition mostly affects women in their 30s who smoke.

The discharge may be milky or dirty green and may be bilateral. Acute infection causes pain and swelling. The breasts may be lumpy. There may be a characteristic retraction of the nipple mimicking carcinoma. Untreated abscess formation may result in a mammary fistula.

Patients over 40 should have a mammogram and the discharge sent for cytology. If the discharge is very troublesome, excision of the duct system (Hadfield's operation) may provide relief.

Duct papilloma

A serous or bloodstained discharge from a single aspect of the nipple is common. The breast may be clinically normal although pressure on a specific segment may reproduce the discharge.

A triple assessment and, in a bloodstained discharge, excision of the involved system and histological examination establish that a papilloma is present.

Galactorrhoea

This is a rare cause of milky discharge following lactation, caused by a persistent elevation of prolactin. It is treated by bromocriptine until the discharge subsides. Persistent discharge, despite treatment, may suggest a prolactinoma, but this is rare.

Breast abscess

This condition is a complication of breastfeeding caused by *Staphylococcus aureus*. The bacteria may get into the breast through cracks in the nipple during feeding. Initially a segment of the breast becomes inflamed with cellulitis. There is then a rapid build-up of pus with necrosis of local breast tissue, producing an abscess in a short space of time. A tender segment is found in the lactating breast, often with surrounding cellulitis. If detected early, antistaphylococcal antibiotics (e.g. flucloxacillin) may prevent abscess formation.

Once an abscess has formed, the pus must be released. It is usually possible to treat lactational breast abscesses by aspiration (repeated if necessary), though incision and drainage is sometimes required.

BREAST CANCER

Epidemiology and aetiology

Breast cancer was, until recently, the commonest cancer to affect women in the Western world. In the UK, there were 47 695 new cases in 2008.

Table 10.2 Risk factors for breast cancer

Factor	High risk	Low risk
Age (years)	Greater than 50	Less than 35
Country of birth	Northern Europe, North America	Asia or Africa
First-degree relative affected	Yes	
Age at first pregnancy	>30 years	<20 years
Nulliparity	Yes	
Previous breast cancer	Yes	
History of atypical hyperplasia	Yes	

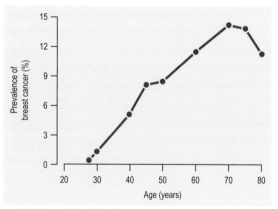

Figure 10.1 Age and risk of breast cancer.

There is variation within various ethnic cultural groups with American Jews and nuns having a higher incidence than, for example, Mormons and American Indians. Breast cancer incidence is increasing, with approximately one woman in eight in 2008 developing the disease in the UK.

The risk factors for breast cancer are listed in Table 10.2.

Age
Breast cancer is rare under the age of 35 (Fig. 10.1).

Country of birth
Breast cancer is less common in the Far East compared to the West. Immigrants assume the same risk as the host community within two generations, suggesting there is a large environmental influence on cancer risk.

Genetic factors
Hereditary and familial breast cancer appears to be increasing (up to one-third of patients will have a family history of the disease).

Early identification of patients at risk may be improved with the discovery of definitive markers of the disease. Two breast cancer genes have been identified: BRCA1 on chromosome 17Q and BRCA2 on chromosome 13Q. BRCA1 is associated with breast and ovarian cancer. BRCA2 is associated with breast and other malignancies. These genes account for a high proportion of hereditary breast cancers but only a small proportion of all breast malignancies.

Hormonal and other factors

Women who have an early menarche and a late menopause are at increased risk of developing the disease. A woman who has a child before the age of 18 has a decreased risk compared to a woman who has a first child after the age of 35. Infertility and nulliparity increase risk. Breastfeeding seems to protect against breast cancer. The role of dietary fat remains controversial. Obesity is a definite risk factor and there may be a slight risk of developing the disease with high-dose oestrogen oral contraceptives and possibly hormone-related therapy.

If a woman has had a previous breast cancer, there is an increased risk of developing a second primary breast carcinoma. Previous ovarian or endometrial cancers also elevate risk.

Natural history

It takes several years for most breast cancers to become palpable, and blood-borne dissemination occurs at an early stage. Nearly one-quarter of patients who have no tumour in regional lymph nodes at the time of removal still relapse later due to distant metastatic disease. This figure rises to half to three-quarters if regional nodes are involved. This provides the rationale for detecting early cancers by screening.

Staging and prognosis

The TNM classification of breast cancer is shown in Table 10.3, and the prognosis in Table 10.4.

The nodal status in the axilla may be established at operation, either by complete clearance or by lymph node sampling. The use of sentinel node biopsy is becoming increasingly common to define whether complete clearance of the axilla is required, thereby preventing long-term complications. Apart from stage and nodal status, the following factors favourably affect prognosis:

- low tumour grade
- high degree of elastosis
- reactive changes in the regional lymph nodes
- positive oestrogen receptor status.

Adverse factors include:

- vascular and lymphatic invasion by tumour
- extensive angiogenesis
- expression of the proto-oncogene C-erb B2 and loss of expression of the suppressor P53 gene.

Screening

It has been shown by studies in New York and Scandinavia that screening for breast cancer can improve long-term survival. In the UK, women between the ages of 50 and 70 are called every three years for a screening

Table 10.3 TNM classification of breast cancer

TNM stage	Pathological description
Tis	Carcinoma in situ (pre-invasive)
	Paget's disease (no palpable tumour)
T0	No clinical evidence of primary tumour
T1	Tumour less than 2 cm
T2	Tumour 2–5 cm
T3	Tumour greater than 5 cm
T4	Tumour of any size but with direct extension to chest wall or skin: (a) Fixation to chest wall (b) Oedema, lymphocytic infiltration, ulceration of skin or satellite nodes (c) Both (a) and (b)
N0	No palpable ipsilateral axillary lymph nodes
N1	Palpable nodes not fixed: (a) Inflammatory only (b) Containing tumour
N2	Fixed ipsilateral axillary nodes
N3	Ipsilateral supraclavicular or infraclavicular nodes or oedema of arm
M0	No evidence of distant metastasis
M1	Evidence of distant metastasis

Table 10.4 Stage and prognosis according to TNM classification

UICC stage	TNM	Category	5-year survival
I	T1, N0, M0	Early cancer	84%
II	T1, N1, M0 T2, N0–1, M0	Early cancer	71%
III	Any T, N2–3, M0 T3, any N, M0	LABC	48%
IV	Any T, any N, M1	Metastatic	18%

LABC, locally advanced breast cancer; UICC, International Union against Cancer.

mammogram. The frequency of screening may increase and extend to other age groups but at present this is under evaluation, particularly for woman under the age of 50. Screen-detected cancers are usually smaller and axillary lymph node involvement is less common, with an approximate 30% reduction in long-term mortality.

Table 10.5 Relative frequency of histological types of breast cancer

Type	Frequency (%)
Ductal	80 (non-specific 50%)
Lobular/ductal combined	5
Medullary	6
Colloid	2
Other less common specific types (tubular, papillary)	2
Sarcoma and lymphoma	0.5

Breast cancer pathology

Invasive breast cancer

The histological types of invasive breast cancer are summarised in Table 10.5.

Most breast cancers are associated with fibrous tissue proliferation (scirrhous). Consequently, the tissues surrounding the growth contract clinically. Dimpling of the skin and indrawing of the nipple may be seen. The majority of breast cancers are adenocarcinomas arising from the epithelium of the ducts and lobules (ductal and lobular types). The degree of differentiation of the tumour determines the grade:

- grade I – well differentiated
- grade II – moderately differentiated
- grade III – poorly differentiated.

Most breast cancers tend to express oestrogen receptors, which can be measured by immunohistochemistry, and cancers are labelled either oestrogen receptor positive or negative. Receptor positive cancers tend to respond to hormonal therapy and have a better prognosis. Some cases have receptors for HER2. Treatments with biological therapies may be used in this case.

Carcinoma in situ

There are two forms:

- lobular – LCIS
- ductal – DCIS.

DCIS is subdivided into commode, solid, cribriform and micropapillary patterns.

Commode DCIS is associated with micro-invasive foci and lymph node metastases. Because necrosis and microcalcification are common and seen on mammography, DCIS is detected increasingly commonly. LCIS has no microcalcification and therefore may not be detected early. 10–30% of patients with LCIS and 30–50% of those with DCIS go on to develop invasive cancer. LCIS may occur in either breast and is a marker of increased risk of diffuse bilateral disease, compared with DCIS, which remains in the ipsilateral breast and is confined to the same quadrant from which the biopsy that yielded the diagnosis was taken.

Table 10.5 shows the relative frequency of the histological types of breast cancer. Ductal with productive fibrosis is the commonest form. Lobular carcinomas have a high propensity for bilaterality, multicentricity

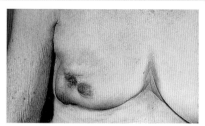

Figure 10.2 Ulceration overlying cancer of the breast.

and multifocality and have a particular propensity for metastasising to membrane structures, for example the peritoneum, pleura and meninges.

Clinical features

Most breast cancers present as a solitary, painless lump. Other symptoms may include pain, nipple or skin retraction, nipple discharge and axillary lump. Metastases may be symptomatic at presentation (breathlessness from malignant effusions, bone pain from bony secondary).

The lump is solitary, firm, non-tender and may be tethered to the skin or pectoral fascia. In advanced cases, the lymphatic channels are blocked and the skin becomes oedematous with thickening (peau d'orange). Very advanced tumours may ulcerate (Fig. 10.2). Axillary lymph nodes may be palpable.

Diagnosis

Triple assessment comprising clinical evaluation, imaging and cytological examination is required to diagnose breast cancer.

History

A detailed history should be taken which should include known risk factors, namely family/menstrual and reproductive history, hormonal use and previous breast cancer or breast disease.

Examination

Inspection and palpation of the entire breast and lymph node areas is mandatory. The breast is examined with the patient sitting facing the examiner with the arms first at the side then raised above the head and then placed on the hips to both relax and contract the pectoral muscles. The doctor assesses asymmetry, visible lumps, erythema, peau d'orange, contour flattening, skin tethering (puckering), abnormal fixation, retraction and altered axis of the nipples or obvious gross ulceration. Skin retraction may also be determined by asking the patient to lean forward (Fig. 10.3). The supraclavicular, infraclavicular and axillary lymph nodes should be examined with the examiner taking the weight of the patient's arm, either on the shoulder or opposite arm (Fig. 10.4). Palpation of the breast is performed in the supine position with the patient's hand behind the head initially and then at the side. Examine the whole breast, from sternum to clavicle, latissimus dorsi to rectus sheath. Examination occurs one quadrant at a time with the flat of the hand followed by the nipple/areola area. The breast lump should be categorised by its position, size, consistency and any fixation to deep or superficial structures. Mobility should be

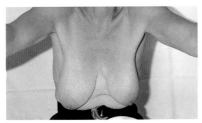

Figure 10.3 Leaning forward to demonstrate any skin retraction.

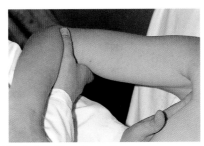

Figure 10.4 Examination of the axillary nodes.

Table 10.6 Models of presentation of breast cancer	
Symptom/sign	**Frequency (%)**
Lump	76
Pain	5
Nipple retraction	4
Nipple discharge	2
Skin retraction	1
Axillary mass	1

assessed. If the patient complains of discharge, an attempt to reproduce this should be made (Table 10.6).

Imaging

- **Mammography** Two views are usually taken (mediolateral oblique and craniocaudal). Abnormalities include microcalcification, stellate densities, architectural distortion and change from previous mammogram. These require further investigation. False negative rate is between 10% and 15%.

- **Ultrasound** This is useful in discriminating solid from cystic masses. Biopsies or needle localisation may be used with this technique and it is particularly useful in younger women where breast density reduces the usefulness of mammography. Blood flow assessment by Doppler ultrasound may provide additional information.

Kumar and Clark's Handbook of Medical Management

- **MRI** MRI may be useful in evaluating indeterminate breast masses or post-treatment. Breast cancers may enhance rapidly in contrast to benign tumours.

Tissue diagnosis

- **Fine-needle aspiration cytology** This is performed with a large needle. The aspirate is expressed onto a slide, fixed and smeared for cytological examination.
- **Wide-bore core biopsy** Wide-bore core needle biopsy under local anaesthetic provides a sample of tissue for histological analysis.
- **Surgical biopsy** Open biopsies may be either excisional or incisional for diagnosis or treatment. Mammographic-guided wire-localisation biopsy enables excision of impalpable lesions, with further imaging done after surgery to confirm that the lesion has been removed.

Treatment of breast cancer

Surgery, radiotherapy and chemotherapy (multidisciplinary approach) all have important roles. Treatment depends on the stage of the cancer.

Carcinoma in situ

Treatment varies from segmental excision with or without radiotherapy to simple mastectomy for multifocal disease and patients who are at risk of local recurrence. Patients are followed up regularly by mammography and clinical examination. If, after local treatment, recurrent disease occurs, mastectomy is advised. LCIS is often multicentric and bilateral. Patients can either be observed closely as the risk of invasive ductal cancer is low, or undergo a curative bilateral mastectomy.

Stages I–II invasive cancer

Radical surgical resection does not enhance long-term survival because of micrometastases. The aims of surgery are therefore local control and, where possible, breast conservation. Local control is achieved by complete removal of the tumour and adjuvant local radiotherapy with or without systemic therapy. Breast-conserving surgery involves removal of the tumour but leaving a better cosmetic result (wide local excision or quadrantectomy). For centrally placed lesions greater than 4 cm in diameter, mastectomy is recommended.

Assessment of the axillary lymph nodes is essential for management and is a marker of prognosis. The presence of nodal metastases implies systemic dissemination of the cancer and adjuvant chemotherapy or hormonal therapy should be considered. The axilla can be cleared surgically (therapeutic) or nodes simply sampled. Axillary sampling has the advantage of being a lesser operation than clearance. However, if the nodes are positive, a cleared axilla needs no further treatment but a sampled axilla will require radiotherapy. See also sentinel node biopsy.

Stage III disease

Preoperative neo-adjuvant chemotherapy may reduce tumour size before mastectomy for stage III disease and for inflammatory carcinoma. Further treatment depends on the menopausal state of the patient.

Adjuvant therapy

- **Cytotoxic therapy** Methotrexate and adriamycin are given intravenously, often combined with cyclophosphamide and 5-fluorouracil. Therapy is considered for all women at high risk of relapse. Maximal benefit is obtained for premenopausal women with node positive and oestrogen receptor negative disease.

- **Hormonal manipulation** Oestrogen receptor positive tumours exhibit a 50–60% response rate compared with 10% of oestrogen receptor negative tumours. Tamoxifen is an anti-oestrogen that binds to the oestrogen receptor, thus blocking the effect of endogenous oestrogen. Thirty per cent of all breast cancers respond to tamoxifen, rising to 60% if they are receptor positive. Maximal benefit is obtained by taking 20 mg of tamoxifen for 5 years. Long-term complications include a 2–6 times increase in endometrial carcinoma, but this is rare. Tamoxifen may have a role in prevention of breast cancer and is now recommended for high-risk groups in the United States. Alternative anti-oestrogens have been developed, including Faslodex and aromatase inhibitors. The inhibition of the aromatisation of androgen to oestrogen has resulted in two major types of inhibitors being developed: type I (formestane and exemestane) and type II (anastrozole and letrozole).

- **Trastuzumab (Herceptin)** Trastuzumab (Herceptin) is one of a new group of cancer drugs called monoclonal antibodies. Herceptin works by attaching itself to the HER2 protein (human epidermal growth factor) found on the cell surface of some breast cancer cells, stopping them from dividing and growing. It only works in patients with high levels of HER2 protein (1 in 5 women with breast cancer will have tumours sensitive to its action). If given with some chemotherapy drugs, notably paclitaxel (Taxol) and docetaxel (Taxotere), it increases the effectiveness of the chemotherapy and may improve survival.

Herceptin was also licensed in the UK in 2006 as a treatment for patients with early breast cancer. NICE produced guidance for its use in this situation stating that its use should be considered for women with HER2-positive tumours following surgery and adjuvant chemotherapy (and radiotherapy if appropriate). Herceptin should be given every 3 weeks for 1 year.

- **Hormonal castration** Castration can be achieved by surgical or pharmacological means. Oophorectomy can be achieved surgically or with radiotherapy or by utilising gonadotrophin-releasing hormone (GnRH) agonists. Adrenalectomy and hypophysectomy have now largely been abandoned.

Metastatic disease

Surgery and radiotherapy are used for local control. Combination chemotherapy, principally the CMF (cyclophosphamide, methotrexate and fluorouracil) regime, may produce remission in up to 70% of patients. Seventy-three per cent of patients with metastatic disease have skeletal metastases, which may present as bone pain or pathological fractures, particularly the femur. These should be orthopaedically treated and followed by radiotherapy. Pain from metastases can be controlled by radiotherapy. Treatment with bisphosphonates may reduce the progression and morbidity associated with bony metastases, even if not associated with hypercalcaemia. Pleural and lung metastases may cause symptomatic pleural effusions managed by aspiration and occasional pleurodesis for reaccumulations. Pleural irritant, for example tetracycline or bleomycin, may be instilled into the pleural cavity to produce pleurodesis. Prognosis is poor, with a median survival between 6 and 15 months. Cerebral metastases, causing symptoms of raised intracranial pressure or focal

Kumar and Clark's Handbook of Medical Management

neurological problems, may be treated with combined therapy which may include surgery, radiotherapy or chemotherapy, with some success. Spinal cord compression resulting in hemiparalysis requires early diagnosis and urgent treatment. Surgical decompression may be appropriate for patients with posteriorly placed lesions or continued progression of disease in spite of radiotherapy.

Breast reconstruction

Reconstruction is considered as a functional restoration of appearance and self-image. Potential patients are usually younger and reconstruction may be carried out at the same time as mastectomy. Techniques include latissimus dorsi flaps, which may allow radiotherapy and chemotherapy to begin shortly after surgery. Reconstruction can also be achieved using implanted expanders and prostheses. The aims of reconstructive surgery are to reproduce symmetry of breast form, including consistency and size, with a lasting result with no detrimental effects on treatment and outcome of the primary disease. See also Chapter 18.

OTHER MALIGNANT DISORDERS OF THE BREAST

Male breast cancer

This occurs in less than 1% of all cases and is associated with high endogenous levels of oestrogen, preceded by gynaecomastia in 20% of patients. Risk factors include testicular feminisation, Klinefelter's syndrome (XXY), oestrogen therapy, irradiation and trauma. The prognosis is the same as for female breast cancer although it tends to present late. Treatment options are similar.

Paget's disease

Paget's disease presents as a chronic, eczematous eruption of the nipple confused with eczema and is almost always associated with underlying carcinoma.

Inflammatory breast carcinoma

This is a rare variant. It is rapidly progressive and characterised by erythema, peau d'orange and skin ridging with or without any mass. Unlike other cancers, it presents with pain. Dissemination of cancer cells through the lymphatics results in a diffusely enlarged breast. If these cells remain within the superficial lymphatics and blood cells, telangiectatic carcinoma may arise with numerous purple papules and haemorrhagic, vesicle-like lesions covering the breast. If associated with fibrosis, a diffuse, thickened lesion occurs (carcinoma en cuirasse).

Malignant phylloides tumour

The name is derived from its fleshy, leaf-like appearance. Histologically, malignant phylloides tumours provide a spectrum of disease from sarcomatous malignancy to fibroadenoma. Despite histological confirmation, the behaviour is difficult to predict but prognosis is generally good. Clinically, they are often large, painless and mobile within the breast, which develops, with enlargement, a characteristic teardrop appearance. Treatment is wide excision but local recurrence can occur.

Endocrine surgery

Most surgical endocrine disorders are neoplastic, autoimmune or genetic. These conditions may or may not result in endocrine dysfunction depending on whether there is abnormal hormone secretion. The principles of endocrine surgery have been crystallised by John Lynn and are summarised in Table 11.1.

THE THYROID

Embryology
The thyroid is derived from the foramen caecum at the junction of the anterior two-thirds and posterior third of the tongue. The gland migrates downwards in front of the foregut to lie anterior to the trachea but occasionally may descend lower to the superior mediastinum. It leaves behind the thyroglossal duct which may persist and form a thyroglossal cyst.

Surgical anatomy
The thyroid is fixed to the trachea by the pretracheal fascia so it moves up on swallowing. Aberrant thyroid tissues may be found anywhere along the embryological descent of the gland. Blood supply is from the superior and inferior thyroid arteries. Thyroid operations may damage important structures, highlighted in Table 11.2.

Thyroid function
The thyroid produces two types of hormones:
- T_3 and T_4, which regulate metabolic rate
- calcitonin, a calcium-regulating hormone which acts to decrease serum calcium by increasing bone uptake and renal excretion of calcium.

Thyroid pathology
The commonest thyroid disorders are:
- goitre (enlarged thyroid)
- hyperthyroidism (overproduction of T_3 and T_4 causing thyrotoxicosis)
- hypothyroidism (underproduction of T_3 and T_4 causing myxoedema)
- thyroid nodules
- thyroid cancers
- thyroiditis.

Goitre

A goitre is a diffuse enlargement of the whole thyroid gland. The patient may be hypothyroid, euthyroid or hyperthyroid, depending on the cause of the goitre. Causes include iodine deficiency, pregnancy, goitrogens, genetic abnormalities, Graves' disease and Plummer's syndrome.

Clinical features
Most goitres simply present as neck swelling. Larger goitres cause dysphagia, discomfort and stridor. The goitre may be smooth or nodular.

Table 11.1 Principles of endocrine surgery

Principle	Example
Be convinced of the biochemical diagnosis	In Cushing's syndrome, is the primary problem of pituitary or adrenal origin?
Make the patient safe	Control thyrotoxicosis in Graves' disease, or hypertension in phaeochromocytoma
Localise the tumour(s)	In Conn's syndrome, which side is the adenoma? CT and renal vein sampling may be necessary
Is an operation necessary?	Sometimes medical therapy is more effective, e.g. radioiodine for hyperthyroidism
Decide best technique	Open versus laparoscopic adrenalectomy

Table 11.2 Structures easily damaged during thyroidectomy

Structure	Result of injury
Recurrent laryngeal nerve	Paresis or paralysis of vocal cord: unilateral – hoarseness bilateral – stridor; change in voice; risk of aspiration
Parathyroid glands	Hypocalcaemia – severity depends on amount of tissue that remains
External laryngeal nerve	Paresis or paralysis of cricothyroid muscle – inability to achieve high-pitched notes

Extrathyroid signs of thyroid disease (i.e. thyrotoxicosis/myxoedema) should be sought.

Investigation

The aims of investigation are twofold:

- determine thyroid function (serum thyroid-stimulating hormone (TSH) and T_3/T_4)
- exclude malignancy (by thyroid ultrasound and fine-needle aspiration cytology (FNAC)).

CXR ± CT may be useful to determine extent of larger goitres extending into the chest (Fig. 11.1).

Treatment

The indications for thyroidectomy for goitre are:

- pressure symptoms (discomfort, dysphagia, stridor)
- cosmetic appearance
- suspicion of malignancy
- rarely, control of hyperthyroidism (as alternative for medical treatment or after relapse).

Other goitres can be left alone once the underlying cause has been addressed.

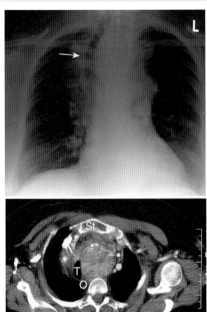

a

b

Figure 11.1 (a) Chest X-ray showing mediastinal mass with displacement of the trachea to the right arrow. (b) CT scan of same patient, demonstrating calcified goitre behind the sternum (St) displacing trachea (T) and oesophagus (O) to the right.

Thyrotoxicosis

This is a common problem affecting 2% of females and 0.15% of males. The three main causes are:
- diffuse toxic goitre – Graves' disease
- multinodular toxic goitre – Plummer's syndrome
- toxic solitary nodule or adenoma.

Graves' disease

This is the commonest cause of thyrotoxicosis, usually occurring between the ages of 20 and 40 years. Women are affected five times more often than males. Graves' disease is due to an autoimmune process characterised by abnormal autoantibodies directed against thyroid TSH receptors. The natural history of Graves' disease is one of intermittent remission and relapse. The thyroid is uniformly enlarged, firm and smooth, not nodular. Eye problems are common (Table 11.3). Thyroid function tests confirm an elevated T_3 and T_4 and reduced TSH. Anti-thyroglobulin and anti-microsomal antibodies are present when the cause is autoimmune.

Table 11.3 Eye abnormalities in Graves' disease

Symptoms	Signs
Poor sight for both near and distant objects	Ophthalmoplegia
Double vision	
Grittiness in the eye	Conjunctival oedema (chemosis)
Exophthalmos – protrusion of the globes	Exophthalmos Lid retraction Lid lag

Multinodular toxic goitre (Plummer's syndrome)

A goitre that has been present for several years may subsequently become overactive. This is known as secondary toxic goitre (Plummer's syndrome). Eye disease is unusual but cardiac arrhythmias and heart failure are common presenting features. The goitre is nodular and may displace the trachea, distinguishing it from Graves' disease where the goitre is smooth and symmetrical. Thyroid autoantibody levels are normal.

Toxic solitary adenoma/nodule

This is a solitary autonomous adenoma occurring in 5% of cases of hyperthyroidism. A single nodule in the gland becomes overactive, causing suppression of all surrounding tissue, and may be diagnosed on an isotope scan because the nodule takes up the isotope but the surrounding gland does not. Eye disease is unusual.

Management of thyrotoxicosis

The underlying cause must be established since the definitive treatments depend on the underlying diagnosis. However, initial treatment is the same.

First, control the thyrotoxicosis with drugs. A combination of antithyroid drugs and beta-blockade is effective. Carbimazole is the initial antithyroid agent of choice. Agranulocytosis is a complication and the drug must not be used in pregnancy. Beta-blockade with propranolol reduces the effects of T_4 on the sympathetic nervous system and controls tachycardia and agitation.

Treat eye complications (seek ophthalmology opinion); see Table 11.4.

Once the acute thyrotoxic state is controlled, definitive treatment is with radioactive iodine or surgery.

Radioactive iodine (^{131}I) achieves definitive control in most cases and is used for older and younger patients or where surgery is contraindicated. Hypothyroidism may result and replacement therapy must be given if necessary. ^{131}I is effective for toxic nodules since the isotope is concentrated in the diseased hyperactive nodule but not in the suppressed normal gland.

Surgery is preferred for younger patients or when medical therapy has failed. For a solitary toxic nodule, only the affected lobe need be removed. For Graves' disease and toxic goitre, the options are total thyroidectomy followed by thyroxine replacement therapy, or subtotal thyroidectomy and monitoring for hypothyroidism or recurrent hyperthyroidism. In all

Table 11.4 Management of eye complications in Graves' disease

Problem	Treatment
Exposed cornea with drying	Methylcellulose eye drops for lubrication
Failure of lid closure in marked exophthalmos	Tarsorrhaphy
Inflammation	Systemic steroids
Deterioration in sight from compressive optic atrophy	Surgical decompression of both orbits
Severe diplopia	Corrective surgery to eye muscles

Box 11.1 Causes of a clinical solitary nodule

Dominant nodule of multinodular goitre
Cyst
Localised Hashimoto's disease
Non-functioning adenoma
Functioning adenoma
Primary malignant tumour
Metastatic deposit

cases the patient must be rendered euthyroid by medical means before surgery to avoid a thyrotoxic crisis. Preoperative iodine therapy reduces the vascularity of the gland and makes excision easier.

Clinical solitary thyroid nodule

The causes of a clinical solitary nodule are shown in Box 11.1.

Approximately 10% of solitary thyroid nodules are malignant.

Risk factors include previous exposure to irradiation, iodine deficiency and a family history of thyroid carcinoma. The clinical features are of a lump in an otherwise normal gland.

Investigation

● *Thyroid function* tests exclude toxicity
● *Ultrasound* determines if the nodule is solitary or multiple (a dominant nodule in a multinodular goitre is the commonest cause of clinical solitary nodule). A cystic lump can be distinguished from a solid one
● *Isotope scanning* determines if the nodule is 'hot' or 'cold'. Hot nodules are almost always benign; 15% of cold nodules are malignant
● *Fine-needle aspiration cytology* confirms the diagnosis in most cases.

Treatment

Benign nodules may be left alone. If the diagnosis is in doubt, the affected lobe is removed and examined by frozen section. If the result is benign, the operation is terminated. If malignant, completion thyroidectomy is performed.

Kumar and Clark's Handbook of Medical Management

Thyroid cancer

Carcinoma of the thyroid causes less than 0.5% of all deaths from malignant disease. The aetiology is unknown. Predisposing factors include genetic (medullary carcinoma of the thyroid is familial and associated with neoplasms in other endocrine organs), radiation from external beam radiotherapy, high natural levels or from nuclear explosions (Hiroshima and Nagasaki) or accidents (Chernobyl). Carcinoma is more common in regions where endemic goitre exists. Pathological classification includes:

- papillary
- follicular
- medullary
- anaplastic
- lymphoma.

Presentation

The patient notices a painless lump in the neck and examination reveals a solitary thyroid nodule. Signs of local invasion may be hoarseness (recurrent laryngeal nerve invasion), stridor or clinical fixity of the lump. Enlarged cervical lymph nodes may be the first sign of the disease, as may distant spread to lung, bone or brain.

Papillary carcinoma

This accounts for two-thirds of all thyroid malignancies and is slow growing. Histologically, finger-like tumour papillae are present. The growth is multifocal. Psammoma bodies are typical. Spread is via lymphatics and 50% of patients have cervical node involvement at the time of presentation. Patients are euthyroid. FNAC is the investigation of choice, with ultrasound demonstrating a solid lesion.

Follicular carcinoma

These are well-encapsulated solid tumours, comprising 20% of all thyroid malignancies. The diagnosis of cancer as distinct from follicular adenoma is dependent on the presence or absence of extracapsular or venous invasion. FNAC is unreliable in distinguishing between follicular adenoma and carcinoma. The tumour spreads by the bloodstream and cervical involvement is found in 5%. Removal of the involved lobe for histological examination establishes the diagnosis.

- **Treatment of papillary and follicular carcinomas** The minimal procedure for differentiated carcinomas (papillary and follicular) is total thyroid lobectomy. Total thyroid excision or ablation by surgical removal or therapeutic doses of ^{131}I or thyroid suppression by T_4 is the subject of debate. Cervical lymph node metastases may be resected. Distant metastases, which tend to be functional, may be treated with radioactive iodine. Follow-up includes clinical examination and measurement of thyroglobulin on an annual basis.

Medullary carcinoma

These account for 5–10% of thyroid malignancies and are derived from the C cells, which produce calcitonin that can be detected in the bloodstream. Some cases are inherited in an autosomal dominant manner. Medullary carcinoma is often multifocal and can be associated with other endocrine disorders, e.g. phaeochromocytoma and parathyroid hyperplasia. Relatives of patients with medullary carcinoma must be screened at the time of diagnosis, usually by measurement of plasma calcium concentrations and 24-hour urinary excretion of vanillylmandelic acid (VMA). Genetic tests are available. Total thyroidectomy and thyroid replacement therapy comprise the initial treatment. The prognosis is favourable if diagnosed early.

Anaplastic carcinoma
These are believed to arise from previously unrecognised differentiated tumours, more common in areas of endemic goitre. Clinical features include a goitre which may have been present for some time but has recently increased in size. Physical findings include hard, woody mass with fixation and can be confused with Reidel's thyroiditis or lymphoma. FNAC or, if equivocal, open biopsy confirms the diagnosis. Lung metastases are frequently found on chest X-ray. Surgical excision, if possible, with adjuvant external beam radiotherapy is the treatment of choice but these carcinomas have a poor prognosis, with few patients surviving more than one year.

Lymphoma
This is a rare growth, affecting elderly females. Longstanding Hashimoto's thyroiditis is the only known risk factor. The diagnosis is made on histology. Treatment is specialised, using a combination of debulking of the tumour with radiotherapy. Advanced disease is managed by chemotherapy.

Thyroiditis

Hashimoto's thyroiditis
This is an autoimmune disease of unknown cause. The thyroid is diffusely infiltrated by lymphoid and plasma cells with the formation of germinal centres and destruction of follicles. Clinical features include early thyrotoxicosis but with progression there is hypothyroidism. A goitre may be present, causing pressure symptoms. A diffuse goitre is characteristic on examination, with a firm and irregular surface.
- **Investigation and management** Autoantibodies directed against thyroglobulin and thyroid microsomes are elevated. The biochemical pattern of hypothyroidism (raised TSH and low T_4) is present. Management is by lifelong thyroid suppression. Most goitres shrink to a minimal size. Occasionally, thyroidectomy is required.

De Quervain's thyroiditis
This is uncommon and is caused by viral infection with an acute inflammatory reaction in the gland with histiocytes, multinuclear giant cells and granuloma formation. Clinically, acute pain in the neck is observed accompanied by malaise and pyrexia with a tender goitre.
- **Investigation and management** The ESR is raised and there may be hyperthyroid elevation of T_4 with a low TSH. The condition is self-limiting and aspirin analgesics suffice. Steroids for severe.

Riedel's thyroiditis
This is a rare condition of unknown cause with dense fibrosis extending into the surrounding soft tissues of the neck. It may occur in association with other disorders, for example retroperitoneal fibrosis, sclerosing cholangitis and mediastinal fibrosis.
- **Clinical features** A rapidly increasing goitre is noticed with features of tracheal and oesophageal compression. A hard, woody goitre is palpable. Decompression of the neck structures may be required with occasional tracheostomy.

Table 11.5 Specific complications of thyroidectomy

Complication	Clinical features	Treatment
Bleeding into the neck	Acute airway obstruction with neck swelling, bruising and haematoma. The venous return from the head is also compressed, causing facial congestion and oedema	Give oxygen, sit upright, call surgeon and anaesthetist and immediately remove skin and strap muscle sutures to release the haematoma
Hypocalcaemia due to parathyroid gland injury	Typically 24–48 hours postoperatively. Paraesthesia round mouth and digits, then muscle spasm and tetany. Tapping the facial nerve below the ear causes facial spasm	Oral calcium usually adequate, IV calcium gluconate if necessary
Recurrent laryngeal nerve (RLN) injury	Unilateral palsy causes hoarseness of the voice. Bilateral partial RLN palsy causes severe airway obstruction	Usually conservative as most will recover Speech therapy may help
External laryngeal nerve injury	Inability to sing, or project voice	Conservative
Thyroid crisis (thyrotoxic storm) caused by massive release of thyroxine into circulation during manipulation, e.g. gland in surgery	Severe thyrotoxicosis, restlessness, confusion, tachycardia, atrial fibrillation, hypotension, hyperpyrexia, cardiac arrest	Control of thyrotoxicosis preoperative is the best way of avoiding the problem. Treatment is urgent using propylthiouracil and beta-blockade, and potassium iodide

Thyroidectomy

Thyroidectomy is described on page 382. Complications of thyroidectomy are potentially life-threatening and are summarised in Table 11.5.

HYPERPARATHYROIDISM

Hyperparathyroidism is the commonest cause of hypercalcaemia in the community (Box 11.2). Three subtypes are recognised.

1. Primary hyperparathyroidism whereby the parathyroid glands secrete inappropriately raised amounts of parathyroid hormone (PTH). Serum calcium is raised, negative feedback abolished and the level of PTH is inappropriately high for the level of calcium. The most common cause is adenomatous change in one parathyroid but there may be hyperplasia of all four or a carcinoma of one.

> **Box 11.2** Causes of hypercalcaemia
>
> Hyperparathyroidism
> Multiple myeloma
> Bony metastases
> Sarcoidosis

2. Secondary hyperparathyroidism occurs in chronic renal failure, which causes a reduction in plasma concentration of calcium, thereby leading to hyperplasia of all four glands. If the cause of hypocalcaemia can be corrected, the parathyroids return to normal.
3. Tertiary hyperparathyroidism occurs if the stimulus in secondary hyperparathyroidism continues unchecked and parathyroid over-activity may become autonomous. It may occur following renal transplantation.

Primary hyperparathyroidism

This is the commonest subtype to present to the surgeon. Hypercalcaemia is often discovered by chance on blood samples sent for other reasons. It occurs at any age with peak incidences between 20 and 50 years. Women are more commonly affected. Eighty per cent of patients have a solitary adenoma. Patients with multiple gland hyperplasia may suffer from multiple endocrine adenoma syndrome (MEN).

Clinical features of hyperparathyroidism

The adage 'moans, bones, stones and abdominal groans' summarises the main symptoms, though most have none. Depression is common. Bone decalcification causes pain and pathological fractures. Ureteric colic and other abdominal pains are often seen. Severe cases may present with vomiting, dehydration and coma.

The diagnosis is established by detecting PTH in the presence of hypercalcaemia. X-rays of the hands may show subperiosteal bone erosion.

Treatment

Parathyroid exploration reveals the enlarged gland in 95% of cases but, if the parathyroid adenoma is not discovered, accurate localisation must be achieved before repeat operation (CT and isotope scanning). Surgical removal offers the only cure.

ADRENAL DISORDERS

The adrenal glands, situated above the kidneys, are derived from two components, the cortex and medulla. The cortex has three zones, each secreting a different hormone (Table 11.6).

Primary hyperaldosteronism

This is a rare condition occurring in less than 2% of patients with hypertension. There are two types:
- idiopathic hyperaldosteronism
- Conn's syndrome.

Table 11.6 Hormones synthesised by the adrenal glands, and the disorders characterised by excess secretion

Region of gland		Hormone secreted	Disorders characterised by excess secretion
Adrenal cortex	Zona glomerulosa	Aldosterone	Primary hyperaldosteronism Conn's syndrome
	Zona fasciculata	Cortisol	Cushing's syndrome
	Zona reticularis	Adrenal androgens	Virilism
Adrenal medulla		Adrenaline (epinephrine) and noradrenaline (norepinephrine)	Phaeochromocytoma

Box 11.3 Causes of Cushing's syndrome

ACTH-dependent
Ectopic ACTH secretion – 15%
Cushing's 'disease' (ACTH-secreting pituitary tumour) – 65%

ACTH-independent
Adrenocortical adenoma – 10%
Adrenocortical carcinoma – 10%
Iatrogenic steroid therapy – variable but should never be forgotten

Conn's syndrome is the more common syndrome, usually caused by a single, small yellow tumour of the adrenal cortex and nearly always benign. This is best treated surgically. Clinical features are vague or absent. Patients complain of lethargy, muscle weakness and thirst. Clinical examination is normal apart from hypertension. Blood tests show hypokalaemia, elevated aldosterone and low renin. Diagnosis is confirmed and the differentiation between Conn's syndrome and adrenal hyperplasia is achieved by CT scan localisation or isotope scanning. Occasionally adrenal venous sampling to measure aldosterone concentrations is necessary to localise a tumour. Adenomas are cured by unilateral adrenalectomy, either open or laparoscopic. Hypokalaemia and hypertension must be corrected medically before surgery. Bilateral adrenal hyperplasia is best treated medically.

Cushing's syndrome

This affects patients between 20 and 40 years of age, and is more common in women. Causes of Cushing's syndrome are shown in Box 11.3. Clinical

Table 11.7 Methods to distinguish between ACTH-dependent and ACTH-independent disorders

	Cushing's disease (pituitary tumour)	Adrenal tumour	Ectopic ACTH secretion
Plasma ACTH	Normal to elevated	Undetectable	Very high
High-dose dexamethasone suppression test	Suppression	No suppression	No suppression

Box 11.4 Phaeochromocytoma, the '10% tumour'

10% are bilateral
10% are familial (e.g. MEN-II, see p. 193)
10% are malignant
10% are extra-adrenal tumours

features include trunk and facial obesity (moon face), buffalo hump, hirsutism, muscle weakness, osteoporosis and hypertension.

Diagnosis is confirmed by 24-hour urinary free cortisol, which is elevated. Plasma ACTH and high-dose dexamethasone suppression test identify the underlying cause of the abnormal cortisol secretion (Table 11.7).

Adrenal adenomas are localised by CT scanning and treated by unilateral adrenalectomy. Carcinomas are rare and usually advanced at presentation.

Virilising tumours

Overproduction of sex steroid hormones can lead to virilisation (androgen) or feminisation (oestrogen). The cause is usually genetic, resulting in abnormal genitalia and virilisation at birth.

Phaeochromocytoma

This is a catecholamine-secreting tumour of the adrenal medulla or in the paraganglionic tissues adjacent to the sympathetic chain (Box 11.4). Extra-adrenal tumours are more likely to be malignant and can be found anywhere from the pelvis to the base of the skull.

Clinical features include profuse sweating, headaches, palpitations, angina and fear of impending death (angor animi). Hypertension is common. Sudden cardiac death may occur.

Diagnosis is established by 24-hour measurement of the urinary metabolites of adrenaline and noradrenaline (VMA) and metanephrines. CT and isotope scanning localise the tumour.

Phaeochromocytomas are dangerous tumours and successful treatment requires effective medical treatment to control hypertension before surgery. Phenoxybenzamine, a non-selective alpha-blocker, is the agent of choice. Beta-blockade is also necessary (propranolol) after alpha-blockade is effectively established. Once hypertension is controlled, surgical excision of the tumour is indicated.

GASTROINTESTINAL ENDOCRINE TUMOURS

These uncommon tumours cause symptoms due to secreted peptide hormones. Most are malignant apart from insulinomas, which are usually benign.

Insulinoma

Insulinomas form 70% of all pancreatic endocrine tumours. They arise from the beta-islet cells. Seventy-five per cent are benign and small (less than 2 cm in diameter); 10% may be multiple and 10% may be associated with MEN-I. They secrete insulin and cause hypoglycaemic attacks.

Diagnosis is suspected when the attacks are precipitated by fasting. Localisation of the tumours is achieved with CT scan, isotope scanning, angiography and portal venous sampling. Before surgery, diazoxide, which inhibits the release of insulin, is administered to restore the blood sugar to normal. Surgical removal, which may be laparoscopic, is curative.

Gastrinoma

This is the second most common islet-cell tumour. One-third of patients with gastrinomas have MEN-I syndrome; 30% are malignant. Secretion of gastrin stimulates excess production of gastric acid leading to the development of Zollinger–Ellison syndrome (severe peptic ulceration). Patients typically complain of epigastric pain secondary to peptic ulceration. Physical examination may be normal. Diagnosis is achieved by elevated fasting levels of serum gastrin. Preoperative imaging may be difficult. Treatment is medical, including proton pump inhibitors. A well-localised tumour may be removed surgically.

VIPoma

These islet-cell tumours secrete vasoactive intestinal peptide (VIP) producing the Verner–Morrison syndrome of watery diarrhoea, hypokalaemic acidosis and achlorhydria. There is an elevated concentration of VIP in the serum. A combination of CT scan, ultrasound and angiography localises the tumour. The mainstay of treatment is chemotherapy rather than surgery, which is reserved for patients without metastases.

Carcinoid tumours

Carcinoid tumours secrete vasoactive substances (serotonin, bradykinin, prostaglandin, substance P) which may give rise to carcinoid syndrome (flushing, diarrhoea, bronchospasm) when there are hepatic secondaries. Localisation is difficult because tumours are mostly submucosal. Appendicular carcinoid is found in a small percentage of appendices as an incidental finding, often at the tip. If the tumour is greater than 2 cm or there is vascular involvement and invasion of the mesoappendix, a right hemicolectomy is recommended. Contrast-enhanced CT scan, MRI scan and radiolabelled octreotide scan (carcinoid tumours may express receptors for somatostatin) are used to detect secondary spread.

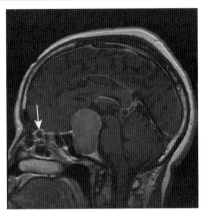

Figure 11.2 MRI scan, sagittal section, showing a large pituitary adenoma. (Courtesy of Dr A. Mehta, with thanks.)

PITUITARY

Pituitary tumours account for 10% of intracranial neoplasms. They are nearly always benign but cause problems due to local expansion (visual field defects due to pressure on the optic chiasma) and consequences of hypersecretion of one of the pituitary hormones (Fig. 11.2).

Prolactinoma

Prolactin-secreting tumours are quite common, and often without clinical significance. Presenting signs in women include delay in the onset of menstruation, period abnormalities, sterility and galactorrhoea. In men, galactorrhoea, decrease in libido and changes in secondary sexual characteristics may occur. Treatment is with bromocriptine (which inhibits the release of prolactin) or surgery.

Acromegaly

Excess growth hormone secretion in adulthood results in acromegaly, the main appearance being overgrowth of the hands and feet and coarse facial features (Fig. 11.3). There are often physiological disturbances including glucose intolerance, osteoporosis and hypertension. Diagnosis is confirmed by elevated plasma growth hormone levels. Treatment is with drugs (octreotide), radiotherapy or surgery.

Cushing's disease

This is a pituitary-dependent adrenocortico-hyperplasia secondary to ACTH secretion by a pituitary adenoma. Patients present with Cushingoid features. Surgical removal gives an 80% chance of cure. Radiotherapy may be used.

MULTIPLE ENDOCRINE NEOPLASIA

There are three familial syndromes of endocrine tumours: known as MEN-I, MEN-IIA and MEN-IIB. The abnormal cells all have the same

Kumar and Clark's Handbook of Medical Management

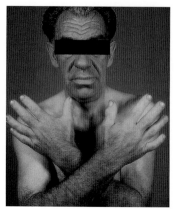

Figure 11.3 Acromegaly. Note coarse facial features resulting from increased growth of connective tissue and cartilage, together with the typical broadening and enlargement of the fingers. (Courtesy of Professor S. R. Bloom, Hammersmith Hospital, London.)

embryological origin, the amine precursor uptake and decarboxylation (APUD) cells.

- **MEN-I**
- Parathyroid hyperplasia
- Pancreatic islet cell hyperplasia (insulinoma, glucagonoma, VIPoma or Zollinger–Ellison syndrome)
- Pituitary adenoma (prolactin or growth hormone)
- Thyroid adenoma.
- **MEN-IIA**
- Medullary carcinoma of the thyroid
- Phaeochromocytoma/Cushing's syndrome
- Hyperparathyroidism.
- **MEN-IIB**
- Medullary carcinoma of the thyroid
- Phaeochromocytoma
- Hyperparathyroidism (rarely)
- Marfanoid features and mucosal neuromas.

Transplant surgery 12

INTRODUCTION AND DEFINITIONS

Advances in surgical technique and immunology have allowed organ transplantation to become routine, limited mainly by shortage of donor organs.

- *Cadaveric donors* who are brainstem dead are the commonest source of organs, often following severe head injury. The procedure for confirming brainstem death requires two senior doctors to perform a series of tests to establish the diagnosis (Box 12.1).
- *Cadaveric non-heart-beating donors* are occasionally used for renal transplants.
- *Live donors* may be related or non-related to the recipient. Living donors are usually first degree relatives of the recipient. Unrelated donors are rare in the developed world, though trading in organs occurs in poor countries.
- *Autograft:* transplantation of an organ from one part of the body to another part of the same individual.
- *Isograft:* transplantation of tissue between genetically identical individuals, i.e. identical twins.
- *Allograft:* transplantation of tissue from an individual of the same species. Most human organ transplants are allografts.
- *Xenograft:* transplantation of tissue from one species to another. This is limited to avascular tissues that have been treated to remove antigens. Porcine heart valves are examples of such grafts. Larger organs are rejected immediately. Using animal organs for human transplants would solve the organ shortage problem but there remain serious difficulties related to rejection and the potential for transfer of infectious diseases from the animal to human population.
- *Orthoptic graft:* the donor organ is transplanted to the same site after removal of the recipient's diseased organ, e.g. liver transplantation.
- *Heterotopic graft:* the organ is grafted to a site remote from the normal anatomic position, e.g. renal transplantation to the iliac fossa.

REJECTION

- *Hyperacute rejection* is caused by preformed circulating antibodies present in the recipient's blood which recognise antigens present on the cells of the donor organ. Rejection begins within hours and immediate loss of the graft ensues.
- *Acute rejection* is cell mediated and usually occurs 5–14 days after transplantation, though sometimes it may take several months.
- *Chronic rejection* involves cell- and antibody-mediated processes and causes graft ischaemia. Deterioration is slow and insidious but inevitably results in graft failure.

Box 12.1 Defining brain-stem death

1. Fixed pupils
2. No corneal reflex
3. Absent oculo-vestibular reflexes
4. No response to supraorbital pressure
5. No cough reflex or gagging response
6. No observed respiratory effort in response to disconnection of the ventilator (such that CO_2 >6 kpa)

Assuming:

no doubt of coma due to irreversible brain damage

no depressant drugs

not hypothermic

no reversible metabolic

endocrine or circulatory cause

no potentially reversible causes of apnoea

(from Academy of Medical Royal Colleges 2008 A Code of Practice for the Diagnosis and Confirmation of Death)

The rejection phenomenon is a consequence of the requirement to distinguish between self and non-self (e.g. infecting organisms) or abnormal self (e.g. tumour cells or cells with intracellular infections). The recognition of foreign and abnormal cells by the immune system allows the elimination and removal of the infection or tumour. Transplanted tissue activates the same process, and prevention of rejection requires suppression of the immune system. Current immunosuppressive therapy is highly effective but, not surprisingly, side effects include a higher susceptibility to infections and incidence of tumours.

MATCHING DONOR TO RECIPIENT

Tissue typing

The molecules that are involved in immune recognition are the major histocompatibility (MHC) antigens. Class I MHC antigens are expressed as integral proteins of the surface membranes of all nucleated cells and platelets. Class II MHC antigens are found on lymphocytes. The genes coding for the MHC proteins are located on the short arm of chromosome 6, termed the human leucocyte antigen (HLA) loci (Table 12.1). Tissue typing identifies which of the HLA-A, -B and -DR alleles are present for a donor or recipient.

ABO blood group compatibility

ABO compatibility requirements are the same as for blood transfusion. Rhesus matching is not required since rhesus factor is only expressed on red blood cells, not on the cells of the transplanted organ.

Direct cross-matching

Direct cross-matching is required in case a recipient has preformed antibodies which may react with donor cells. Such antibodies may result from blood transfusion, pregnancy or viral infections.

Table 12.1 The four HLA loci and their importance in organ transplantation. Modern immunosuppressants have made HLA compatibility less critical

HLA locus	Number of alleles identified/function
HLA-A	20 alleles
HLA-B	30 alleles (less importance for graft outcome)
HLA-C	No apparent role in immune response
HLA-DR	The most important: if donor and recipient match graft prognosis is better

Box 12.2 General complications of immune suppression

Bacterial
  TB
  Listeria monocytogenes
Fungal
  Candida albicans
  Aspergillus
Protozoal
  Pneumocystis carinii
  Cryptosporidium
Viral
  Cytomegalovirus (may be transmitted in the graft)
  Epstein–Barr
  Measles
  Herpes simplex and zoster
Mitotic – benign
  Multiple viral warts
Mitotic – malignant
  Squamous skin carcinomas
  Lymphomas

Extended-range tissue matching

Using plasmapheresis and heightened immunosuppression, it has been possible in recent years to perform ABO incompatible transplants.

IMMUNOSUPPRESSION

Immunosuppressive therapy prevents or reverses rejection of the transplanted organ but at the expense of increased risk of infectious and malignant disease (Box 12.2). Prophylaxis against rejection usually requires different agents to be used in combination. The main immunosuppressive agents, mechanisms of action, doses and side effects are summarised in Table 12.2. Acute rejection crises require high-dose intravenous steroids

Kumar and Clark's Handbook of Medical Management

Table 12.2 Immunosuppressive agents, mechanisms of action and specific side effects

Drug	Mechanism of action	Dose	Specific side effects
Azathioprine	Metabolised in liver to 6-mercaptopurine, a purine antagonist that reduces DNA/RNA synthesis	1–2 mg/kg/day	Myelosuppression Hepatotoxic, cholestatic jaundice Pancreatitis
Ciclosporin	Reduces transcription of gene of IL-2	3–5 mg/kg/day	Nephrotoxic Hepatotoxic Gum hypertrophy Hypertrichosis Neuropathy Tremor
Tacrolimus	Reduces transcription of gene of IL-2	0.05–0.1 mg/kg/day	Diabetogenic Tremor
Sirolimus	Inhibits T-cell proliferation and B-cell differentiation	15 mg loading dose 5 mg maintenance	Interstitial pneumonitis
Prednisolone	Non-specific anti-inflammatory and immune suppression. Anti-macrophage and anti-IL-2 activity	0.1 mg/kg/day	Poor wound healing Growth reduction in children Diabetogenic Hypertension Pancreatitis Osteoporosis Peptic ulceration
MMF (mycophenolate mofetil)	Depresses T- and B-cell proliferation	1–2 g/day	

(methylprednisolone 500 mg three times a day) and occasionally mono-clonal antibody therapy with basiliximab.

ORGAN RETRIEVAL AND MANAGEMENT OF CADAVERIC ORGAN DONORS

Most cadaveric organ donors are head injury patients who have their diagnosis of brainstem death confirmed while they are ventilated on ITU. Brain death leads to hypothermia, coagulopathy, reduced cardiac output and endocrine disturbance. Active intervention is required to ensure the organs are retrieved in as good a condition as possible. This includes the following measures:

- full ITU monitoring
- maintain core temperature >35.5°C
- strict asepsis for ventilatory support; ensure adequate oxygenation and avoid high positive end-expiratory pressure (PEEP) if possible
- adrenaline (epinephrine) is the best inotrope to support blood pressure
- thyroxine infusion
- treatment of diabetes insipidus (replace urine with 5% dextrose and desmopressin)
- maintain good urine output
- blood products as required for coagulopathy.

The retrieval operation is started by the renal/liver team followed by the heart/lung team. The organs are cold-perfused before removal then trans-ported in double plastic bags in crushed ice.

KIDNEY TRANSPLANTATION

Kidney transplantation is indicated for end-stage renal failure. The com-monest causes are:

- chronic glomerulonephritis
- chronic pyelonephritis
- diabetic nephropathy
- hypertensive nephropathy
- polycystic kidney disease
- analgesic nephropathy.

Around 1700 kidney transplants are performed each year in the UK and over 5000 patients are on the transplant waiting list.

Ischaemic time comprises warm ischaemic time (between stopping the circulation through the organ and perfusing it with cold perfusion fluid) and cold ischaemia time, from the moment of cold perfusion to re-establishing blood flow after grafting. The shorter the ischaemia time, the sooner the graft will function after transplantation (Fig 12.1).

Renal transplants are heterotopic. The iliac vessels are exposed via an extraperitoneal approach and the graft placed in the iliac fossa with the renal artery and vein anastomosed to the internal or external iliac artery and vein. The ureter is implanted into the bladder and may be stented. Immune suppression is started immediately together with prophylactic antibiotics. Graft function is monitored postoperatively by measurement of urine output (oliguria is common at first), urea, creatinine and creatinine clearance. Early complications are usually technical and include thrombo-sis of artery or vein, urinary leak and ureteric stenosis. Occlusion of either vessel usually results in graft infarction. Cadaveric graft survival rates are 90% at one year and 50% at 10 years.

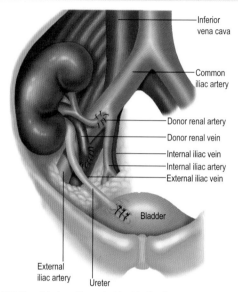

Inferior vena cava

Common iliac artery

Donor renal artery

Donor renal vein

Internal iliac vein

Internal iliac artery

External iliac vein

Bladder

External iliac artery

Ureter

Figure 12.1 Completed renal transplant in right iliac fossa.

Living donors

Great advances have been made in living-related donor surgical technique, minimising the morbidity rate for the (usually healthy) donor. Laparoscopic harvest and even natural orifice transluminal endoscopic surgery (NOTES) harvest has been achieved.

LIVER TRANSPLANTATION

Liver immunology is rather mysterious. Some patients develop spontaneous tolerance to their new liver and immune suppression may be reduced or withdrawn. One-year survival is 70–90% and most one-year survivors are still alive at 5 years.

Indications for liver transplantation are summarised in Box 12.3. Outcome after transplantation for malignant disease is unpredictable and results are poor with high recurrence rates.

Approximately 700 liver transplants are performed each year in the UK. Liver transplantation is orthotopic, and the recipient's hepatectomy is particularly demanding since the patients are always very sick and portal hypertension makes the abdomen hostile. Complex anastomotic work is required for the transplant. Primary graft failure occurs in up to 10% and this is usually fatal.

PANCREAS TRANSPLANTATION

Pancreatic transplantation is indicated for insulin-dependent diabetes and may either be performed alone or together with renal transplantation for

Box 12.3 Indications for liver transplantation

Acute liver failure
    Poisoning, e.g. paracetamol overdose
    Viral hepatitis
Chronic liver failure
    Primary biliary cirrhosis
    – Primary sclerosing cholangitis
    Autoimmune chronic active hepatitis
    Alcoholic cirrhosis
    Cryptogenic cirrhosis
    Anatomic defects including Budd–Chiari syndrome (post-hepatic
        venous obstruction) and biliary atresia
Primary hepatic malignancy
    Restricted to small hepatocellular carcinomas
Genetic defects
    Alpha-1-antitrypsin deficiency
    Wilson's disease (copper storage abnormality)
    Crigler–Najjar syndrome (inability to conjugate bilirubin)

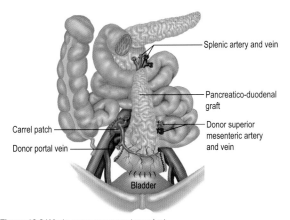

Figure 12.2 Whole organ pancreas transplant.

diabetics with advanced nephropathy. The operation is not widely performed in the UK though it is more popular in North America. There are two techniques: whole organ or segmental graft. The whole organ method has lower complication rates (Fig. 12.2). Results are improving but in the future it is likely that grafting of the pancreas will be replaced by transplantation of islet of Langerhans cells only.

SMALL BOWEL TRANSPLANTATION

Small bowel transplantation is inherently problematic due to the high concentrations of lymphoid tissue in the transplanted bowel (graft versus host reaction) and the colonisation of the graft with intestinal flora. Only limited numbers are performed worldwide per year, with a 2-year survival of about 50%.

HEART AND LUNG TRANSPLANTATION

Heart, lung and heart-lung transplantation are discussed in Chapter 14.

CORNEA

The cornea was the first solid tissue successfully transplanted between humans and it is the most commonly performed transplant. Opaque or distorted cornea from any cause is an indication for grafting. A button of the recipient's cornea is removed and replaced with a corresponding graft from the donor using microscopic sutures. The cornea is avascular and rejection is not usually a problem. In close HLA-matched cases, graft survival is 95% and is expected to last for life.

IMPROVING DONOR RATES

There is significant variation between countries in the numbers of organs made available for transplantation (per head of population). Utilising specialist transplant co-ordinators in each hospital helps, but there has been little appetite in the UK to adopt an opt-out (presumed consent for donation) system.

Vascular and endovascular surgery

ATHEROSCLEROSIS

Atherosclerosis is a disease affecting arteries of all sizes and means literally 'hardening of the arteries'. Large elastic arteries (aorta, iliac, carotid) and medium-sized muscular arteries (coronary, femoral and popliteal) are most commonly affected. The basic lesion of atherosclerosis is a localised fibrofatty plaque in the wall of the artery causing narrowing of the lumen. The plaque is often calcified and contains a core of cholesterol covered with a fibrous cap.

Atherosclerosis is a multifocal condition. A patient with peripheral vascular disease is highly likely to have coronary disease or cerebrovascular disease and vice versa.

The pathogenesis of atherosclerosis is complex and not fully understood. The development of atheromatous lesions is aggravated by risk factors including smoking, hypercholesterolaemia, hypertension and diabetes mellitus (see 'Vascular risk factors and their modification', below). Low-density lipoproteins and monocyte-derived macrophages accumulate in the tunica intima, forming a fatty streak. In certain susceptible arteries, smooth muscle and inflammatory cells are recruited into the intimal fatty streak, promoting the development of the fibrofatty plaque covered by a collagen fibrous cap.

The symptoms caused by atherosclerotic disease depend on the arteries affected. Thus coronary artery disease gives rise to angina and myocardial infarction; cerebrovascular disease leads to strokes and transient ischaemic attacks (TIAs); and peripheral vascular disease results in limb ischaemia. Most deaths and serious morbidity in the Western world are due to these conditions resulting from atherosclerosis.

Atherosclerosis causes symptoms via three mechanisms:

- limitation of blood flow
- embolisation
- thrombosis.

An atheromatous plaque may allow sufficient flow through a vessel to satisfy end-organ demands at rest but cause problems when the flow needs to increase, for example angina on exertion due to stable coronary artery disease. Another example is intermittent claudication (see p. 210). Such symptoms may be unpleasant but not necessarily imminently dangerous.

Embolisation and thrombosis are related in that they both depend on plaque stability. Their consequences are much more serious. The fibrous cap covering an atherosclerotic plaque may be quite smooth and covered by endothelial cells. In an unstable plaque, the cap may fissure or rupture, exposing the highly thrombogenic core of the plaque causing immediate platelet activation and formation of thrombus. A small thrombus may break off and embolise. More major plaque disruption may cause complete thrombosis and occlusion of the artery. In the carotid circulation this is a common cause of TIAs and strokes. In the heart this may cause unstable angina or myocardial infarction. In the peripheral circulation, acute limb ischaemia results.

The beneficial effects of statin therapy for individuals with coronary and peripheral artery disease extend beyond their lipid-lowering properties. In addition to lowering blood cholesterol concentration, statins have plaque-stabilising effects that greatly reduce the likelihood of stroke and myocardial infarction.

Vascular risk factors and their modification

Fixed (non-modifiable) risk factors

These are of limited interest since no-one can alter their age, the population into which they were born or the age at which a parent had a heart attack or stroke.

Vascular disease in any one arterial territory is an important risk factor for adverse events in others. Patients surviving strokes are more likely to die of a heart attack than another stroke. Similarly, intermittent claudication is a major risk factor for stroke and ischaemic heart disease.

Major modifiable risk factors

Smoking, hypertension, hypercholesterolaemia and sedentary lifestyle each increase the risk of acute myocardial infarction. When two or more are present, the risk is multiplied, not added. The benefit of removing a risk factor by lifestyle changes or treatment depends on the background risk set by an individual's fixed risk factors.

- Smoking There is a dose-response relationship between smoking and atherosclerotic disease in all arterial territories. This is complicated by the fact that some individuals may smoke heavily without obvious ill effects, while others are much more susceptible to harm from smoking even a few cigarettes. The excess risk reduces rapidly when an individual stops smoking.
- Hypertension Hypertension is a progressive cardiovascular syndrome which may cause organ damage before blood pressure elevation is substantial. Hypertension cannot therefore be classified solely by strict blood pressure thresholds.

The International Society of Hypertension defines hypertension as systolic pressure over 140 mmHg and diastolic pressure over 90 mmHg. These levels are arbitrary, since the risk of ischaemic heart disease and stroke rises steadily across the whole range of blood pressure and only around one-third of strokes occur in patients with 'hypertension'. The effect of the entire population lowering their blood pressure by only 5 mmHg by lifestyle changes would be dramatic, reducing heart attacks by nearly a quarter and strokes by a third.

- Cholesterol Like hypertension, the definition of hypercholesterolaemia is arbitrary and the risk of vascular disease rises steadily across the whole range of blood cholesterol concentrations. Treating patients with established vascular disease with statins provides protection against heart attack and stroke even for patients with normal cholesterol levels, an effect mediated by stabilisation of atherosclerotic plaque.
- Exercise Regular aerobic exercise confers considerable protection against myocardial infarction. Thirty minutes of moderate activity most days of the week is the current recommendation. Cardiac arrest is five

times more likely during vigorous exercise but individuals who regularly undertake such activity still have only half the risk of fatal heart attack compared to those who remain sedentary.

- **Diabetes** Patients with diabetes are at greatly elevated risk of vascular disease in all territories (cardiac, carotid and peripheral). Good diabetic control improves prognosis.
- **Alcohol** Heavy drinkers tend to have higher blood pressure but those who consume modest quantities of alcohol on a regular basis have lower mortality rates than teetotallers (the J-shaped curve).
- **Homocysteine** The blood level of this amino acid is an independent risk factor for arterial disease and increasing intake of vitamin B_6 and folate effectively reduce homocysteine concentrations. It is not yet clear whether this will be an important way of reducing atherosclerotic disease.

ANEURYSMS

An aneurysm is an abnormal dilatation of a blood vessel. They may either rupture causing bleeding, or thrombose causing distal ischaemia. The two commonest sites for aneurysms are the infrarenal aorta (often in association with iliac aneurysm) and the popliteal artery.

Thoracoabdominal aortic aneurysms (TAAAs)

The aetiology of TAAAs is different from infrarenal AAAs, with medial degeneration and dissection being more common. Patients are often symptomatic with back pain due to compression of surrounding structures. Prognosis for large or symptomatic TAAAs is poor with only about 25% 5-year survival without treatment.

Surgery is high risk, especially for extensive aneurysms. Open repair involves an extensive thoracoabdominal exposure. Spinal cord ischaemia due to damage to intercostal vessels and the artery of Adamkiewicz may cause paraplegia. Manoeuvres such as reimplantation of the larger intercostal vessels, intraoperative hypothermia and CSF drainage may protect the spinal cord from ischaemia.

Endovascular repair is the preferred treatment for aneurysms of the thoracic aorta. Branched and fenestrated stents grafts allow endovascular grafting of complete aneurysms involving visceral branches of the aorta. Hybrid surgical/endovascular procedures are increasingly used for aneurysms of the aortic arch.

Infrarenal abdominal aortic aneurysms

The infrarenal aorta is considered aneurysmal if its diameter exceeds 3 cm. The natural history of AAAs is gradual enlargement until rupture occurs. Ruptured AAA accounts for around the same number of deaths per year as upper GI malignancies. Males are eight times more likely to be affected (1 in 20 men over 65 have an AAA) but females with an aneurysm are more prone to rupture.

The main risk factors are age, male gender, smoking and family history. The aneurysm wall becomes chronically inflamed, elastin and collagen are degraded and vascular smooth muscle cells are lost, leading to weakening and dilatation of the aorta. The risk of rupture rises sharply once the diameter exceeds 6 cm; therefore repair is advised for aneurysms over 5.5 cm in all but very unfit patients.

Most AAAs are asymptomatic until they rupture. Screening programmes reduce deaths due to aneurysms. Many AAAs are detected incidentally during investigation for other problems.

Clinical examination is unreliable for diagnosing and measuring AAAs. Ultrasound is highly sensitive and specific, and is used to diagnose and monitor aneurysm growth. Once an aneurysm has reached 5.5 cm and repair is indicated, CT scanning is vital to define aneurysm anatomy and determine whether endovascular or open repair is appropriate.

Open repair comprises replacement of the aneurysmal aorta with a Dacron graft sutured into place just below the renal arteries (p. 376). Mortality for elective surgery is around 5–10%, higher for less fit patients. Smoking, reduced FEV, impaired renal function and female gender are adverse risk factors.

Endovascular aneurysm repair (EVAR) allows a stent-graft to be delivered inside the aneurysm via the femoral artery, then expanded and fixed in position under fluoroscopic guidance (Fig. 13.1). The whole procedure is performed via small groin incisions, or even percutaneously in some cases. Recovery is quicker than for open repair and less fit patients can be

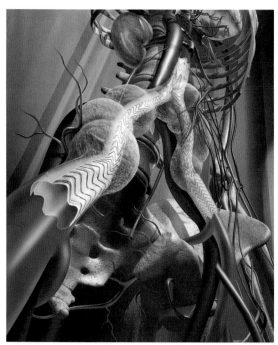

Figure 13.1 Schematic depiction of an endovascular repair of an abdominal aortic aneurysm with a bifurcated stent-graft. (© 2012 W L Gore & Associates, Inc, with permission.)

treated. The mortality for EVAR is less than 2%, one third of that for open repair. Long term complications of EVAR include endoleaks, graft migration, iliac limb occlusion and aneurysm rupture. Long term surveillance with duplex scanning ± CT is required.

Ruptured AAA (p. 96)

The presentation of a ruptured aortic aneurysm is very variable depending on the size and site of the rupture. This commonly leads to diagnostic confusion. Misdiagnoses such as ureteric colic and pancreatitis may lead to delayed diagnosis with disastrous results.

A large leak, especially one which ruptures into the peritoneal cavity, causes a swift death. Other patients have a contained retroperitoneal bleed causing pain of sudden onset which is severe and continuous, in the central abdomen and radiates to the back. The site of pain may be very variable and may be felt only in the back, or one or other flank. The signs of acute haemorrhage; tachycardia, hypotension, vasoconstriction and depressed conscious level, depend on the size of leak. In many patients the initial rupture is contained and tamponaded by the periaortic tissue and posterior peritoneum to the extent that no haemodynamic disturbance occurs, indeed the patient may even be hypertensive during this early stage. The aneurysm may be palpable as a pulsatile expansile mass in the epigastrium, but even a large aneurysm may be difficult to feel, and haematoma surrounding the aorta may mask the aortic pulsation. For these reasons, the abdominal signs of aortic aneurysm rupture are not as clear-cut as might be expected.

Immediate management of suspected ruptured AAA

The diagnosis is made on clinical grounds. Call the duty vascular surgeon and anaesthetist immediately. Give 100% oxygen, put up two large-bore IVs and take blood for FBC, U&E, amylase, clotting and cross-match. Request at least 10 units of blood and inform the haematologist that fresh frozen plasma and platelets are likely to be required urgently. Pass a urinary catheter. Do not give excessive IV fluids to patients who are conscious: a systolic pressure of 80 mmHg is more than adequate. Excessive fluid at this stage only increases bleeding into the abdomen and makes the operation more difficult. Treatment is immediate aneurysm repair and nothing should delay transfer to the operating theatre. Time spent in A&E doing X-rays, ECGs, and central lines may be lethal; these can be done in theatre.

For open repair, the anaesthetic must be induced on the operating table after preparing and draping the abdomen. As soon as the muscle relaxant is given, the abdominal muscles become paralysed and the blood pressure may collapse. It is then a race against time to get a clamp on the aorta above the leak. The rest of the operation proceeds along the same lines as for elective repair.

For emergency endovascular repair, the procedure is performed using local anaesthetic infiltration of the groins for femoral artery exposures.

In stable patients where the diagnosis is not clear, a CT scan is crucial. This confirms or excludes the presence of a ruptured aorta and may also detect pancreatitis or ureteric obstruction, the two main differential diagnoses.

An ultrasound scan is not sufficient to exclude a rupture in patients who have an AAA.

Kumar and Clark's Handbook of Medical Management

Popliteal aneurysms

The popliteal artery is usually considered aneurysmal if its diameter exceeds 1 cm. The risk factors are the same as for AAAs, indeed around 20% of individuals with a popliteal aneurysm also have an AAA, and vice versa. Rupture is rare (under 4%) but embolisation (causing chronic critical limb ischaemia) and thrombosis (causing acute limb ischaemia) are common. Mural thrombus lining the aneurysm sac leads to chronic micro-embolisation over many years causing severe damage to the distal small arteries. When the patient finally presents with critical limb ischaemia the situation may be difficult to salvage since successful bypass requires a patent distal vessel to accept a graft. For this reason popliteal aneurysms greater than 2–3 cm in diameter should be treated with femoropopliteal vein bypass with ligation of the proximal and distal ends of the aneurysm. Such surgery for asymptomatic popliteal aneurysms is very successful with 5-year graft patency of around 80% and limb preservation of over 95%. If treatment is delayed until the aneurysm becomes symptomatic, the outcome is poor, with nearly 20% of limbs requiring amputation.

Endovascular covered stenting is an alternative for patients with no suitable vein for bypass, or who are unfit for surgery.

Other peripheral aneurysms

True aneurysms of the femoral artery are much less common than the popliteal variety. Rupture is rare but symptoms result from local compression or distal ischaemia due to embolisation. Treatment is usually surgical reconstruction.

Visceral artery aneurysms

Aneurysms involving the splenic, hepatic and mesenteric arteries are rare. Splenic aneurysms are four times commoner in females and hepatic aneurysms more frequent in men. Multiple aneurysms in the same patient are usually associated with a connective tissue abnormality such as Ehlers–Danlos syndrome. Rupture is uncommon but may be fatal. Endovascular coil embolisation is the treatment of choice.

Mycotic aneurysms

This is quite different from an infected false aneurysm, where arterial damage is the primary insult and infection supervenes. Mycotic aneurysms result from infection in the vessel wall which weakens, dilates and eventually ruptures. Normal arteries are very resistant to infection so mycotic aneurysms are usually due to a particularly virulent organism or arise in immune compromised patients. The commonest cause of aortic aneurysms used to be syphilis, which affects the aortic arch. Tuberculous aneurysms are seen frequently in Africa, often in association with AIDS.

A mycotic aneurysm typically manifests as a painful, tender pulsatile mass associated with pyrexia. Mycotic aneurysms expand rapidly and rupture is often fatal. Successful treatment depends on accurate antimicrobial therapy and, where possible, avoidance of prosthetic material in any surgical reconstruction.

False aneurysms

False aneurysms occur where an artery has been damaged. Such aneurysms comprise a cavity of blood in continuity with the artery lumen

Table 13.1 The La Fontaine classification for lower limb ischaemia	
Asymptomatic	I
Intermittent claudication	II
Rest pain	III
Ulceration/gangrene	IV

surrounded by haematoma and connective tissue. Trauma, surgery or infection are the commonest causes. A frequent example is the femoral artery which has been punctured for an angiogram but fails to seal. False aneurysms may also occur at the site of an old vascular anastomosis, especially if prosthetic material was used or if it has become infected. Some splenic and gastroduodenal artery aneurysms are false aneurysms caused by erosion of the artery wall by proteolytic enzymes following pancreatitis.

Treatment depends on the site and symptoms. Duplex-guided compression is successful in inducing thrombosis in many angiogram-related femoral false aneurysms. Thrombin injection may achieve the same result, albeit with a risk of distal embolisation. More complex false aneurysms may require surgery, or endovascular treatment with a covered stent.

LOWER LIMB ISCHAEMIA

Classification of chronic lower limb ischaemia, as described by La Fontaine, is shown in Table 13.1.

Causes of lower limb ischaemia

Atherosclerosis accounts for the vast majority of lower limb ischaemia in the West. Presentation of limb ischaemia in a younger adult should prompt a search for causes of accelerated atherosclerosis and consideration of less common causes of lower limb ischaemia. These include:

- aortic dissection
- aneurysms (see p. 208)
- accelerated atherosclerosis (hyperlipidaemia, hyperhomocysteinaemia, AIDS)
- Buerger's disease (common in male smokers in the Middle/Far East)
- popliteal entrapment (artery passes medially to medial head of gastrocnemius causing compression; seen in athletes and may progress to permanent arterial damage if untreated)
- fibromuscular dysplasia (most commonly affects carotid and renal arteries but can narrow the iliac arteries in young adults)
- cystic adventitial disease (popliteal artery develops ganglion-like cysts that may connect to the knee joint)
- persistent sciatic artery (associated with atresia of the ileofemoral vessels).

Investigation of lower limb ischaemia

This may include:

- ankle-brachial pressure index (ABPI)
- duplex ultrasound

Kumar and Clark's Handbook of Medical Management

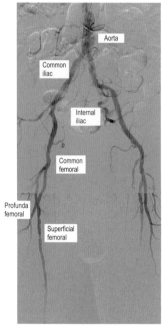

Figure 13.2 Digital Subtraction Angiogram (Aortogram) highlighting the major arteries from the aorta to the knee. Left SFA (by convention to the right of the picture) is occluded.

- angiography (Fig. 13.2)
- CT
- magnetic resonance angiography
- intravascular ultrasound.

Intermittent claudication

Intermittent claudication (IC) is the tight cramp-like pain felt typically in the calf muscle on walking when the blood supply to the lower limb is limited (derived from the Latin, *claudere,* to limp). The severity of the claudication is defined by the distance walked before onset of the pain. On resting or slowing down, the pain passes off within a few minutes. Walking uphill, carrying a heavy bag or rushing all shorten the claudication distance.

Although unpleasant, IC is a relatively benign condition as far as the leg is concerned. Most patients either stay the same or improve and only a small minority (5%) progress to critical limb ischaemia (Fig. 13.3). Diabetics and patients who continue to smoke have a worse prognosis.

The main differential diagnosis is spinal claudication due to congestion of the spinal canal. The pain of spinal claudication resembles IC but the

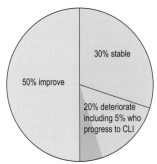

Figure 13.3 Pie chart of intermittent claudication prognosis.

onset is variable; patients have good days and bad days. This is never so with vascular IC, which is very consistent. The pain of spinal claudication extends beyond the calf muscle up the back of the thigh and round onto the shin. There is often a history of back problems and straight leg raising may be limited.

A diagnosis of IC is supported by absent peripheral pulses and reduced ABPIs, typically 60–79% of normal. Non-invasive duplex imaging localises the culprit arterial flow-limiting lesions and guides treatment.

Risk factor modification
In many respects the true significance of IC is not the symptom but the risk of death from other aspects of vascular disease. Claudicants have a mortality around three times that of age-matched controls, mainly due to coronary heart disease, strokes and aneurysms. Attention to vascular risk factors including smoking, hypertension, antiplatelet and statin therapy (see p. 204) is therefore of paramount importance.

Exercise
Many patients can cure their IC by walking as much as possible. 'Walking through the pain', i.e. continuing to walk as long as possible after the pain starts, encourages collateral blood vessels to open up. Patients effectively do their own bypass. Simply advising patients to walk achieves limited benefit but supervised exercised programmes are highly effective.

Drugs
There is no practical drug therapy for IC though cilostazol helps some patients and may have beneficial effects after angioplasty.

Angioplasty
Angioplasty is most effective for stenoses or short occlusions in the aorto-iliac segment. Femoropopliteal disease can also be treated but the risks are higher and any benefit less durable.

Surgery
Bypass surgery for IC is becoming uncommon. The value of exercise therapy and the effectiveness of angioplasty for iliac lesions have greatly reduced the number of patients who end up requiring operations for claudication. The crucial thing to bear in mind when contemplating surgery (or even angioplasty) for claudication is that however unpleasant the IC, claudicants have a high cardiovascular mortality, and in most cases

Kumar and Clark's Handbook of Medical Management

the legs will remain stable or improve if left alone. This must be weighed against the consequences of complications following intervention that could lead to loss of life or limb. In selected patients, however, surgery is highly effective and durable. This is particularly so for occlusions and stenoses of the common femoral artery which is easily accessible surgically and not readily treated with angioplasty. Here a localised endarterectomy may be the best treatment.

Critical lower limb ischaemia

Critical leg ischaemia (CLI) is ischaemia that endangers all or part of the limb and is usually defined as persistently recurring rest pain for more than 2 weeks, or ulceration or gangrene of the foot. The ankle pressure should be lower than 50 mmHg.

In the UK around 20 000 patients per year develop CLI (40 per 100 000) and this is increasing as the population becomes more elderly.

Twenty-five per cent of CLI patients are dead within a year and only half survive more than 5 years, mainly due to deaths from myocardial infarction and stroke. Unlike claudication, therefore, treatment aims are relatively short term and focus on quality of life rather than long term durability of any procedure.

The pain of CLI is felt in the toes and forefoot and is typically worse at night when cardiac output drops. Patients wake up in the early hours with severe pain, relieved by hanging the leg out of the bed allowing blood to flow down to the foot. Some patients take to sleeping in a chair. Many patients get up and walk around in the night, which stimulates flow and reduces pain. During the day the patient may suffer short distance claudication. This pattern of symptoms – calf claudication by day and rest pain in the toes at night – is strongly suggestive of CLI.

It is rare to have rest pain in the presence of palpable pedal pulses unless the problem is due to microembolisation. Pedal and usually the popliteal pulses are absent. There may be ulceration of the foot or frank gangrene of the toes. The leg may become swollen if the patient has to hang it down all the time to ease the pain. Accumulation of metabolites may make the foot look surprisingly red but it will go white if elevated for a few minutes (Buerger's test).

Investigation of limb ischaemia is considered on page 210. Endovascular therapy is usually first-line treatment. Many of these patients die of other problems before the benefits of angioplasty have worn off. The durability of angioplasty is not as good as surgery but the effects may be sufficient to heal the limb and convert rest pain to claudication. Moreover, occlusion of the angioplastied site frequently does NOT result in clinical deterioration and an attempt at angioplasty seems not to prejudice subsequent surgical intervention if required.

In both endovascular and surgical treatment, the strategy is to treat the most proximal flow-limiting lesions first. Thus iliac and above-knee stenoses should be treated before more distal problems.

Acute limb ischaemia

This is described on page 96.

The diabetic foot

Diabetics are prone to ulceration and infection of the foot which may progress to tissue necrosis requiring amputation. This is due to a

Table 13.2 Wagner classification of diabetic foot ulcers

Grade 0	No ulcer on a high risk foot
Grade 1	Superficial ulcer
Grade 2	Deep ulcer penetrating to ligaments/muscle but not bone and no abscess formation
Grade 3	Deep ulcer with cellulitis or abscess, often with bone infection
Grade 4	Localised gangrene
Grade 5	Extensive gangrene

Table 13.3 Texas classification of diabetic foot ulcers

		A	B	C	D
Grade I	Superficial	No infection, no ischaemia	Infected, no ischaemia	Ischaemic, not infected	Infection and ischaemia
Grade II	Penetrates to capsule/tendon	No infection, no ischaemia	Infected, no ischaemia	Ischaemic, not infected	Infection and ischaemia
Grade III	Bone involvement or deep abscess	No infection, no ischaemia	Infected, no ischaemia	Ischaemic, not infected	Infection and ischaemia

combination of vascular disease and neuropathy. Diabetic foot ulcers are classified using the Wagner (Table 13.2) or Texas systems (Table 13.3).

Sensory neuropathy robs the diabetic foot of the protective mechanism of pain, allowing ulceration to develop in response to minor trauma or rubbing.

Autonomic neuropathy reduces sweating and opens arteriovenous shunts in the foot. The diabetic foot is typically warm, and may have strong pedal pulses and dry, cracked skin. The skin fissuring allows entry of bacteria, causing localised infection.

Motor neuropathy causes wasting of the small intrinsic muscles of the foot with collapse of the longitudinal and transverse arches. Abnormal pressure areas then develop which progress to ulceration.

Atherosclerosis in diabetics develops at a much younger age and is more extensive and distal. It is not uncommon for a diabetic to have a critically ischaemic foot in the presence of a normal popliteal pulse due to occlusion of the crural arteries. In addition to disease of the major arteries, the capillary basement membranes thicken, impairing oxygen diffusion to the tissues of the foot.

Management

Management is aimed at prevention by careful foot care. Good diabetic control helps reduce the severity of foot complications. There is no specific treatment for neuropathy. Localised sepsis should be treated with debridement and drainage in the usual way. Plain X-rays may show evidence of osteomyelitis and MRI is an accurate way of defining the extent of sepsis in the foot. Ischaemia, if present, should be corrected.

A multidisciplinary team approach including a diabetologist, vascular surgeon, radiologist, podiatrist and infectious disease specialist improves outcomes and reduces major amputations.

AMPUTATIONS

There is only one indication for a major amputation and that is to save the life of the patient. Amputation is a last resort in a patient with non-salvageable critical limb ischaemia or extensive gangrene/necrosis as a result of tissue infection. In this situation, without amputation, the gangrene/infection will progress, causing death. The most frequently performed major amputations are below-knee amputation (transtibial) and above-knee amputation (trans-femoral). The procedures have a high morbidity and mortality, not least because patients requiring such operations are very sick to start with. Surgical technique is important to obtain a well-shaped stump that heals without complication.

Rehabilitation takes several weeks but, with modern prostheses, a good proportion of patients will achieve a satisfactory degree of independence. The level of function and independence achieved depends greatly on the patient's general health and strength, co-morbidities and social support.

CAROTID ARTERY DISEASE

A high proportion of strokes result from embolisation from diseased carotid arteries. The origin of the internal carotid artery is prone to localised atheromatous plaque formation. Platelet thrombi form on the surface of the rough plaque then break off and embolise to the brain. This may give rise to different symptoms depending on how large the embolus is and which part of the brain it ends up in.

The goal of carotid surgery is to prevent strokes. A stroke is defined (by the WHO) as rapidly developing signs of focal (or global, i.e. coma) disturbance of cerebral function lasting more than 24 hours (unless interrupted by death), with no apparent cause other than a vascular origin. 'Strokes' lasting less than 24 hours are referred to as transient ischaemic attacks (TIAs).

There are two main types of stroke: ischaemic (due to cardiac or other emboli, intracerebral thrombosis) and haemorrhagic (subarachnoid haemorrhage, intracerebral haemorrhage). In the West, 80% of strokes are ischaemic.

Carotid embolisation

Embolism from the carotid artery may manifest in several ways.
- *Asymptomatic.* CT and MRI scanning often reveal evidence of multiple small brain infarctions with no history of preceding symptoms.
- *Amaurosis fugax.* Small emboli which pass through the retinal artery cause the characteristic symptom of a greying out of the vision in the eye on the *same* side as the source of the embolus. Patients often describe

it as a curtain coming down. The vision returns to normal within a few minutes.

- A *transient ischaemic attack* (TIA). These resolve within 24 hours by definition.
- *Strokes* result from embolisation of branches of the middle cerebral artery and cause neurological deficit on the *contralateral* side to the embolising artery. Strokes lasting less than 3 weeks are said to be 'transient strokes'. Persistent deficits after 3 weeks are 'established strokes' and subsequent recovery may be good, moderate or poor.

These clinical distinctions are important since prognosis after carotid surgery is related to the presenting symptom.

Any patient presenting with symptoms attributable to carotid artery embolisation should have a carotid duplex scan. This identifies whether the internal carotid artery is diseased and, if so, what degree of narrowing (stenosis) is present. The percentage of stenosis is the best predictor currently available of likelihood of subsequent major (fatal or disabling) stroke.

A patient who presents with amaurosis fugax, TIA or stroke, associated with a stenosis of the relevant internal carotid artery greater than 70%, has a risk of major stroke in the following 18 months. Correcting vascular risk factors (stopping smoking, treating hypertension, instigating antiplatelet and statin therapy) go some way to reduce this risk but carotid endarterectomy is highly effective at reducing subsequent stroke risk down to normal levels.

Carotid endarterectomy

Carotid endarterectomy involves exposing the carotid bifurcation, opening the artery and carefully removing the atheromatous plaque, leaving a smooth non-thrombogenic luminal surface. The artery is usually closed with a patch to avoid narrowing. A shunt may be used during the operation to preserve cerebral blood flow while the artery is open but this is not always necessary if the circle of Willis is complete. The operation is increasingly performed under local anaesthetic so the patient remains conscious throughout. Carotid endarterectomy has a risk of death and stroke of around 2%, which is much less than the natural history of the condition left untreated. The other main complication is damage to the hypoglossal (XII) nerve, which crosses the internal carotid artery at the upper limit of the dissection.

Symptomatic carotid artery stenosis should be corrected as soon as possible after the symptom, ideally within 48 hours. This is because the risk of major stroke is greatest immediately after the TIA or transient stroke and this risk tails off gradually over the following weeks. Even though the operative risk of endarterectomy is slightly higher when operating soon after an acute symptom, more strokes are prevented by early surgery than by waiting, as many patients will stroke in the interim.

The benefits of surgery for severe (>70%) asymptomatic carotid stenosis are much more finely balanced. Improvements in medical therapy, especially use of statins, have reduced the risk of stroke caused by asymptomatic carotid artery stenosis to less than 2% per year. Successful surgery halves this risk, but only patients with a good life expectancy benefit from this modest improvement likelihood of stroke.

In summary, carotid surgery for symptomatic stenosis should be performed very promptly, and for asymptomatic stenosis very selectively.

Carotid artery stenting (CAS) is a less invasive method of correcting carotid artery stenosis. It is associated with a higher risk of stroke but a lower risk of heart attack. The results of carotid artery endarterectomy are superior to stenting for most patients in most centres.

VENOUS DISEASE

Varicose veins

Varicose veins are dilated tortuous superficial veins occurring usually in the lower limb. They are common and run in families (female to male ratio 3:1).

Anatomy

In health there are two venous systems in the lower limb: the deep and superficial veins. The deep veins run alongside the arteries and are contained within the fascial compartments. Muscular activity compresses the deep veins, driving blood up into the abdomen (the so-called muscle pump). Reflux is prevented by valves ensuring blood flows upwards towards the heart.

The superficial veins are just beneath the skin in the subcutaneous fat. There are two main superficial veins, the long and short saphenous veins, which drain into the deep system via the saphenofemoral and saphenopopliteal junctions. Valves in the veins and at the junctions ensure that blood flows from superficial to deep. There are also a number of perforating veins connecting the superficial and deep systems and again blood flows from superficial to deep.

The commonest cause of varicose veins is the development of incompetence of the valves at the saphenofemoral or popliteal junctions. This allows blood to reflux from the deep system into the superficial system causing dilatation and tortuosity of the saphenous tributaries.

Symptoms

Characteristic discomfort due to varicose veins is an aching sensation exacerbated by standing for long periods and eased by elevating the leg. This may be associated with a sensation or actual appearance of swelling of the leg. Varicose veins may be painless but cause considerable distress due to their appearance. Chronic venous hypertension causes skin changes including venous flares and brown pigmentation (lipodermatosclerosis) which may itch and irritate and progress to ulceration.

Signs

Varicose veins invariably crop up in clinical surgical examinations and it is worthwhile practising to become slick in examining them.

Ask the patient to stand up to allow the veins to fill. Ask about family history of varicose veins and past DVT. Inspect for:

- great or small saphenous distribution?
- associated skin changes/ulceration?

Palpate:

- groin for cough impulse or saphenovarix
- using the tap test: gently feel the lower varicosities while tapping on the proximal saphenous vein. The impulse is transmitted readily down the incompetent trunk
- using the tourniquet (Trendelenburg) test. A popular ritual in clinical examinations but rarely performed by vascular surgeons who use handheld Doppler and duplex scanning to determine the sites of reflux.

- **Hand-held Doppler** Hand-held Doppler readily confirms saphenofemoral and saphenopopliteal incompetence.
- **Tests** Colour duplex imaging has revolutionised venous assessment, and other tests (venography, plethysmography) are rarely needed.

Treatment (see also 'Leg ulceration', below)

Treatment for varicose veins has changed from surgical operating-theatre based therapy to a range of minimally invasive procedures which may be performed under local anaesthetic, so-called office-based vein treatment carried out in an outpatient clinic.

Treatment options include:

- high saphenous ligation (crossectomy) and stripping (traditional treatment, usually performed under general anaesthetic)
- foam sclerotherapy
- radiofrequency ablation (RFA)
- endovenous laser therapy (EVLT)
- mechano-chemo-ablation ('Clarivein')
- phlebectomy
- perforator vein ablation/ligation.

Patients often require a combination of these treatments. Treatment is usually in two components. The first is to deal with the underlying incompetent vein which is causing the varicose vein. This is usually the great and small saphenous vein which may be effectively closed by an endothermal method (RFA or EVLT). The surface varicoscities are then removed by phlebectomy or sclerotherapy.

Chronic venous insufficiency

Untreated varicose veins, deep venous incompetence secondary to DVT or deep venous obstruction may cause the post-thrombotic syndrome (PTS). This unpleasant condition causes pain, limb swelling, chronic skin changes and ultimately ulceration. Treatment is usually non-surgical in the form of compression bandaging or compression stockings. Rarely the deep veins can be reconstructed but the results are limited.

LYMPHOEDEMA

Lymphoedema is limb swelling resulting from failure of the lymphatic system to transport tissue fluid via lymphatic vessels and lymph nodes. The affected limb becomes progressively more swollen, heavy and uncomfortable. As the swelling worsens, skin complications of ulceration, hyperkeratosis and fissuring develop. The limb is prone to recurrent attacks of cellulitis, which exacerbates the swelling further.

The causes of lymphoedema are shown in Table 13.4. There are three types of primary lymphoedema, determined by age of onset.

The main differential diagnosis is chronic venous insufficiency, which can usually be excluded with duplex scanning. Isotope lymphography demonstrates sluggish lymphatic flow in lymphoedema and may indicate the site of the hold-up.

The results of surgical attempts to correct lymphatic obstruction are poor. Treatment is supportive in the form of compression stockings and skin care. Attacks of cellulitis require prolonged antibiotic therapy (e.g. phenoxymethylpenicillin 500 mg four times a day for one month) and elevation during the acute early stage of the infection.

Table 13.4 Causes of lymphoedema

Primary	Congenital (symptoms appear as an infant)	Familial (Milroy's disease) Non-familial
	Praecox (adolescence)	Familial and non-familial types
	Tarda (over 35 years)	Often associated with obesity
Secondary	Infection (commonest cause worldwide but not in the West)	Filariasis (causes elephantiasis)
	Cancer	Malignant obstruction of lymph nodes by metastases
	Surgery/Radiotherapy	Especially to axilla for treatment of breast cancer

Various debulking procedures have been designed to reduce limb swelling (e.g. Homan's and Charles' operations). Liposuction techniques may also help in some cases.

LEG ULCERATION

Causes

Leg ulcers are mainly due to:
- venous insufficiency
- arterial insufficiency
- neuropathy (impaired sensation).

There are other less common causes but the vast majority of leg ulcers seen in vascular clinics (and surgical clinical examinations) are due to one or a combination of these three problems. The 'mixed' ulcers (i.e. due to more than one factor) are the most difficult to heal and most likely to recur.

In a clinical examination situation, e.g. a short case, you can score marks efficiently by asking four questions and examining four features as you inspect the ulcer's characteristics.

Ask:
1. 'Do you smoke?'
2. 'Are you diabetic?'
3. 'Are you on tablets for blood pressure or cholesterol?' This takes care of the commonest vascular risk factors. Most importantly, find out whether there is pain suggestive of arterial ischaemia, which typically causes pain in bed at night which is relieved by hanging the leg down.
4. 'Is the ulcer painful, and does your leg feel more comfortable with it up or hanging down?'

Legs with chronic venous insufficiency feel better up on a stool or in bed. Legs with chronic arterial insufficiency feel more comfortable hanging down. This is a *very* discriminating question when trying to tease out whether the arterial or venous aspect is dominant.

Examine:
1. The ulcer site. Ulcers due to arterial insufficiency tend to be on the tips of the digits. Those due to impaired sensation are on bony prominences.

Venous ulcers are characteristically in the 'gaiter' distribution above the ankles.
2. Pedal pulses.
3. Varicose veins.
4. Sensation.

These manoeuvres will allow you to decide whether an ulcer is mainly arterial, venous or neuropathic, or whether a rarer cause should be considered (e.g. ulcerating tumour, infection, vasculitis).

VASCULAR MALFORMATIONS

The definition and classification of vascular anomalies is confusing. There are two main types, which are histologically different.

Haemangiomas

Haemangiomas in skin affect infants and enlarge by marked endothelial hyperplasia to cause disfiguring lesions. Fortunately, they almost always regress completely without treatment. The term haemangioma is often used incorrectly to include vascular malformations.

Vascular malformations

Vascular malformations are congenital abnormalities of blood vessels which have normal endothelial cell turnover but abnormal structure. They may be subdivided into high-flow (due to multiple arteriovenous fistulas), and low-flow. Low-flow lesions are subdivided further into:

- capillary
- venous
- lymphatic
- mixed.

Vascular malformations are present at birth though they may grow markedly in response to puberty, pregnancy, trauma or a misguided attempt at excision.

Symptoms and signs vary widely. A dermal component may be easily apparent but this may represent only a small part of a much larger abnormality. Some lesions are painful. Others cause extreme deformity. High-flow lesions may have a bruit. Lymphatic malformations may weep; dermal vesicles ulcerate and become infected.

The differential diagnosis includes soft tissue tumours and it is vital not to confuse a malignant soft tissue tumour with a benign vascular malformation. Arteriovenous fistulas resulting from trauma may mimic a high-flow malformation.

Hand-held Doppler may help detect arteriovenous shunting. Colour duplex ultrasound easily distinguishes high- and low-flow lesions and may demonstrate the anatomical extent of the malformation.

Plain X-rays will demonstrate associated bony deformity or overgrowth. CT scanning is useful but has been superseded by MRI.

Angiography is only indicated in those lesions being considered for active treatment.

Cure by surgical excision is usually impossible. Most lesions are best left alone. Non-operative measures such as compression stockings for lower limb lesions are often highly effective. Embolisation and surgery are reserved for particularly symptomatic malformations.

Cardiothoracic surgery 14

ISCHAEMIC HEART DISEASE

Epidemiology and aetiology

Ischaemic heart disease (IHD) includes all the consequences of narrowing or occlusion of the coronary arteries by atherosclerosis. These include angina, myocardial infarction and heart failure, arrhythmias and mitral valve incompetence. Myocardial infarction is the commonest cause of death in the UK. The risk factors and pathogenesis of atherosclerosis are the same as for peripheral vascular disease, discussed on page 203. The heart is supplied by the right and left coronary arteries. The left coronary artery is the bigger vessel and has a main stem 1 cm in length which divides into the left anterior descending artery and the circumflex artery (Fig. 14.1).

Clinical features

The manifestations of coronary artery disease vary depending on which vessels are affected and are summarised in Box 14.1.

Investigation

- CXR
- ECG
- Stress (exercise) ECG
- Echocardiography
- Stress echocardiography (exercise or dobutamine)
- Cardiac isotope scanning
- Coronary angiography.

Coronary angiography is the definitive investigation for patients suspected of having ischaemic heart disease. Non-invasive techniques such as MRA are likely to replace diagnostic coronary angiography in the future.

Treatment

Risk factor modification and medical therapy

The modification of vascular risk factors is discussed in Chapter 13 on page 204. Medical therapy is aimed at reducing myocardial oxygen demand, but more severe disease requires coronary artery intervention by either angioplasty/stenting or coronary artery bypass grafting (CABG).

Percutaneous transluminal coronary angioplasty and stenting

Coronary angiography is performed by passing a catheter via the femoral artery into the proximal aorta and into each of the two coronary ostia. Contrast is injected and images of the coronary vessels obtained.

Left main stem disease is significant narrowing of the first part of the left coronary artery before it divides into the anterior descending and circumflex artery. Triple vessel disease is narrowing of the right coronary

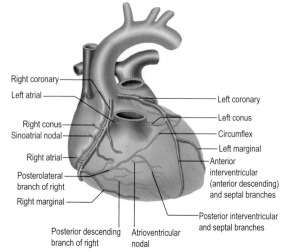

Right coronary

Left atrial

Right conus

Sinoatrial nodal

Right atrial

Posterolateral branch of right

Right marginal

Left coronary

Left conus

Circumflex

Left marginal

Anterior interventricular (anterior descending) and septal branches

Posterior interventricular and septal branches

Posterior descending branch of right

Atrioventricular nodal

Figure 14.1 Anatomy of the coronary arteries.

Box 14.1 Clinical manifestations of coronary artery disease

Angina
Acute coronary syndrome
Myocardial infarction
Mitral valve incompetence (due to papillary muscle infarction)
Arrhythmias secondary to ischaemia of the atrioventricular node (atrial fibrillation) or conduction pathways (heart block)
Ventricular aneurysm
Heart failure

---

artery, anterior descending and circumflex arteries. Single vessel disease is narrowing of one of these, excluding the main stem.

Significant stenoses may be dilated by balloon angioplasty. Combining this with stenting reduces the need for subsequent re-interventions. Drug eluting stents are available which reduce smooth muscle proliferation in the vessel wall and reduce in-stent restenosis.

Coronary artery bypass grafting (CABG)

Coronary artery bypass graft is one of the most commonly performed major operations. Most are performed using cardiopulmonary bypass with hypothermia (Fig. 14.2).

Most operations are carried out through a median sternotomy incision using cardiopulmonary bypass. Mini-thoracotomy and endoscope operations are becoming more widely used. Some procedures are performed on

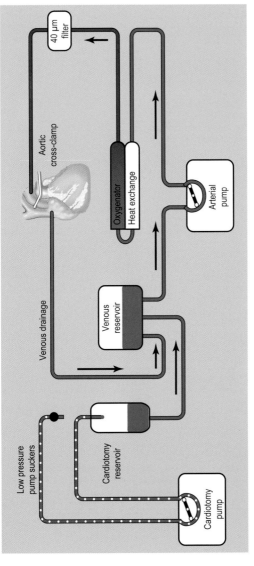

Figure 14.2 Cardiopulmonary bypass.

> **Box 14.2** Indications for coronary artery bypass surgery
>
> Failure of medical therapy with chronic stable angina
> Unstable angina
> Left main stem disease
> Symptomatic three-vessel disease
> Post-infarct angina
> Acute myocardial infarction with cardiogenic shock
> Failed PTCA
> Reoperation for recurrent symptoms
> Congenital anomalies, e.g. anomalous origin of any coronary artery
> Kawasaki disease
> Coronary disease concomitant with other cardiac procedures

---

the beating heart without bypass (off-pump surgery). The internal thoracic artery is the first choice conduit, followed by the long saphenous vein or radial artery. First elective operations have a mortality of 0.5–2.5%, rising to as high as 20% for revision or emergency procedures.

The results for angina are excellent, with 85% of patients relieved of symptoms without medication; a further 5% are improved but require anti-anginal drug therapy.

Other procedures that may be carried out at the time of CABG include:
- left ventricular aneurysm excision (mortality 5%)
- mitral valve repair/replacement (mortality 15%)
- ablation of ventricular arrhythmic focus (mortality 30%)
- ventricular septal rupture (mortality 30%).

Complications include:
- death
- stroke (risk raised if carotid arteries stenosed)
- myocardial infarction
- limb ischaemia/compartment syndrome (especially if intra-aortic balloon pump used perioperatively)
- pneumonia
- wound problems from saphenous vein harvest
- intrathoracic bleeding
- graft occlusion with recurrence of angina/infarction
- arrhythmias.
- Stenting versus CABG for ischaemic heart disease Indications for coronary bypass surgery are summarised in Box 14.2.

Large clinical trials have shown that PTCA and stenting are effective in treating angina, with lower morbidity than surgery. However, the re-intervention rate is higher. CABG achieves better long-term survival, and is more effective in patients with triple vessel disease (Fig. 14.3).

This is a subject of intense international debate.

Experimental therapies for ischaemic heart disease

Percutaneous autologous muscle transplantation is an innovative technique that allows striated muscle taken from the thigh to be cultured then transplanted via percutaneous catheter to the myocardium. The effectiveness is not yet established.

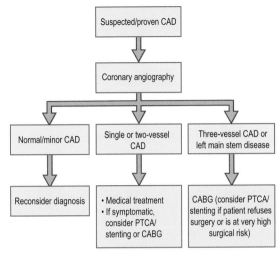

Figure 14.3 An algorithm for the management of patients with suspected coronary artery disease (CAD). This pathway is changing as stent technology improves.

VALVULAR HEART DISEASE

Infective/subacute infective endocarditis

This is a common condition which mainly affects aortic and mitral valves, and tricuspid in intravenous drug users. There is often an underlying valve abnormality (Table 14.1). The common organisms responsible are indicated in Table 14.2.

Rheumatic heart disease

Rheumatic fever in childhood may lead to progressive valve damage (mitral or aortic) in later life. This is an autoimmune reaction stimulated by infection by group A haemolytic *Streptococcus*.

Degenerative

Age-related aortic valve stenosis is the commonest degenerative problem. Marfan's syndrome and ankylosing spondylitis are both associated with aortic valve incompetence.

Clinical features

Haemodynamic symptoms

- Low cardiac output – fatigue, lethargy, shortness of breath on exertion
- Aortic stenosis – syncope and angina
- Pulmonary congestion – any combination of stenosis or regurgitation of the left-sided heart valves causes breathlessness on exertion, cough, frothy sputum and haemoptysis

Table 14.1 Abnormalities associated with infective endocarditis

Site	Abnormality
Aortic valve	Congenital bicuspid valve Degenerative valve disease Rheumatic disease
Mitral valve	Rheumatic disease
	Prolapsing valve
Any prosthetic valve	Adherent thrombus
Congenital cardiac abnormalities	Patent ductus arteriosus Septal defect

Table 14.2 Organisms involved in infective endocarditis

Bacterium	Antecedents	Pathological features
Streptococcus viridans	Dental extraction Other instrumentation: GI endoscopy, cystoscopy, bronchoscopy	Often congenital abnormality of valve
Enterococcus	Prostatic disease Pelvic surgery	Older patients
Staphylococcus aureus	Intravenous prostheses Drug addicts	Acute ulcerative disease Abscess formation
Streptococcus epidermidis	Intravenous prostheses Drug addicts Artificial heart valves	Low-grade disease
Fungal infection	Immunosuppression	Indolent disease

- Right heart failure – fatigue, headache, right upper quadrant pain from liver congestion, ascites, ankle swelling.

Infective symptoms

Fevers, rigors, sweats, malaise, weight loss and splinter haemorrhage may be seen where there is underlying valve infection. Embolism of vegetations may cause stroke or limb ischaemia.

Physical signs of valvular disease

General examination reveals many signs of heart disease, especially right heart failure (cyanosis, pitting ankle oedema, liver enlargement). If the JVP is high, it may be necessary to sit the patient up more than the usual 45° (Table 14.3). Thrills, displacement of the apex and sternal lifting may be detected on examination of the precordium. Auscultation should proceed methodically over the aortic, pulmonary, tricuspid and mitral valve areas, listening for the heart sounds and any murmurs.

Table 14.3 Features of physical examination of peripheral circulation in heart disease

Feature	Findings	Significance
Fingers and hands	Cool Capillary pulsation Splinter haemorrhages Clubbing	Low cardiac output Aortic regurgitation Bacterial endocarditis Cyanotic heart disease
Arm pulse	Low amplitude High amplitude Jerking Double pulse	Low cardiac output Aortic regurgitation Aortopulmonary shunt CO_2 retention Cardiomyopathy Mixed aortic stenosis/ aortic regurgitation
Carotid pulse	Slow rising; low amplitude Bouncing full Head nods Systolic murmur Systolic thrill	Aortic stenosis Aortic regurgitation Aortic regurgitation Referred from aortic stenosis Carotid artery stenosis Carotid artery stenosis
Neck veins	High jugular pressure (JVP)	Congestive heart failure Right ventricular failure Tricuspid regurgitation Tamponade (JVP rises on inspiration) Constrictive pericarditis

Investigations

- Blood tests – ESR, Hb, CRP, blood cultures
- ECG – left ventricular hypertrophy often seen in aortic valve disease, atrial fibrillation in mitral valve stenosis
- CXR
- Echocardiography (transthoracic or transoesophageal) – the most widely used and useful method for investigating valve function
- Angiography – allows measurement of pressure gradients and assessment of coexisting coronary artery disease.

Treatment

Indications for surgery include:

- pressure gradients >50 mmHg across aortic valve, or >10 mmHg across mitral valve
- mitral valve area <1.3 cm^2
- ventricular decompensation (dilating left or right ventricle shown by serial CXRs or echocardiography)
- increasing symptoms of lung congestion or heart failure
- valve infection.

The operative options and their relative merits are indicated in Table 14.4.

Table 14.4 Indications and advantages and disadvantages of different heart valve operations

Technique	Indication	Advantages	Disadvantages
Mechanical valve replacement	Under age 65	Durable Good haemodynamics Low incidence of infection Low incidence of reoperation	Requires lifelong anticoagulation with warfarin Anticoagulant complications (Low) risk of thromboembolic complications
Xenograft	Over 65 Females of childbearing age	Anticoagulation only required for 3 months	Poor durability 30% reoperation rate at 10 years Unsuitable for children Increased infection risk
Homograft	Complex anatomy Indications outstrip supply	No anticoagulation needed	Limited availability Prone to fungal infection Lasts <20 years
Valve reconstruction	Persistent regurgitation of mitral or tricuspid valves treated previously by valvotomy	Suitable for complex and recurrent problems Low infection risk Improved ventricular function Anticoagulation not required	Technically demanding High incidence of early complications

> **Box 14.3** Congenital heart disorders
>
> **Common**
> Ventricular septal defect
> Atrial septal defect
> Pulmonary valve stenosis
> Patent ductus arteriosus
> Aortic coarctation
> Fallot's tetralogy (ventricular septal defect, right ventricular outflow obstruction, over-riding aorta, right ventricular hypertrophy)
>
> **Rare**
> Pulmonary artery atresia
> Tricuspid valve stenosis
> Atrioventricular canal
> Left heart hypoplasia
> Single ventricle
>   Congenital valve disorders are best treated by repair rather than replacement to allow for growth.

TRANSCATHETER AORTIC VALVE IMPLANTATION (TAVI)

TAVI is an endovascular alternative to aortic valve replacement. A replacement aortic valve is deployed via a sheath inserted through the common femoral artery. At present the technique is used chiefly in patients considered unfit for standard surgical aortic valve replacement.

CONGENITAL HEART DISEASE

Congenital heart defects affect around 1 in 100 live births and result in 40 operations per million population per year in the UK. The commonest lesion is a ventricular septal defect (Box 14.3). The causes are multifactorial and include rubella (persistent ductus arteriosus and pulmonary valve stenosis), maternal alcohol abuse (septal defects), maternal drug and radiation treatment and genetic and chromosomal abnormalities (e.g. Down's syndrome).

CARDIOMYOPATHY

Hypertrophic cardiomyopathy (HCM)
The commonest cardiomyopathy, half are of genetic origin, the rest unknown.

Dilated or congestive cardiomyopathy
This may be primary or secondary to amyloidosis, alcoholism, sarcoidosis, systemic lupus erythematosus or thyrotoxicosis.

Restrictive cardiomyopathies
The most common cause is amyloid.

Management
Early disease is managed medically, with cardiac transplantation for severe symptoms and cardiac failure.

CARDIAC TRANSPLANTATION

Retrieval, tissue typing, transplantation ethics and immune suppression

These topics are all discussed in Chapter 12, pages 196–199.

Indications

Over 3500 heart transplants are performed worldwide each year. The results of heart transplants are now so good that the indications have broadened. Indications include:

- severe cardiomyopathy
- severe ischaemic heart disease, unsuitable for coronary revascularisation or after failed CABGs
- inoperable ventricular aneurysm
- severe valve disease
- severe congenital cardiac abnormalities.

Operation

The recipient's heart is removed, leaving atrial cuffs in situ, to which the donor atria are then sutured. The pulmonary artery and aortic anastomosis are then completed. See Table 14.5 for prognosis.

Heart-lung and single lung transplantation

Heart-lung grafting is indicated for severe pulmonary hypertension, end-stage cystic fibrosis and severe congenital cardiac abnormality. Sometimes a 'domino' procedure is performed, where a patient with a normal heart but diseased lungs (usually cystic fibrosis) receives a heart-lung graft and donates their heart to a second recipient.

Single lung transplantation is used for young patients with severe emphysema. Results are poor (usually due to chronic lung infection), but improving (Table 14.6).

CARCINOMA OF THE BRONCHUS

Epidemiology, aetiology and pathology

Lung cancer is the commonest cancer in the UK and causes over 20 000 deaths per year. The incidence is rising in females. Risk factors are smoking

Table 14.5 Survival for UK cardiac transplant patients

1 year	72%
3 years	67%
5 years	62%

Table 14.6 Survival after single lung transplantation

1 year	62%
3 years	46%
5 years	38%

Kumar and Clark's Handbook of Medical Management

(especially total number of cigarettes smoked and age on starting smoking) and asbestos exposure. Types of pathology are:

- 60% squamous
- 15% adenocarcinoma
- 20% small cell carcinoma (oat cell)
- 5% bronchoalveolar.

Tumour (local) symptoms are:

- cough
- haemoptysis
- chest pain
- shortness of breath
- dysphagia
- arm symptoms (pain/numbness) from brachial plexus invasion (Pancoast's tumour)
- hoarse voice (recurrent laryngeal nerve invasion)
- superior vena cava obstruction.

Metastatic symptoms include:

- bone pain
- pathological fractures
- cerebral metastases.

Some lung cancers secrete antidiuretic hormone (ADH) causing the syndrome of inappropriate secretion of ADH (SIADH).

General features of cancer are superimposed:

- weight loss
- anaemia
- fatigue
- arteriovenous thromboembolism due to hypercoagulable state of malignancy.

Diagnosis

Investigations aim to establish a tissue diagnosis and assess the stage of the tumour. Biopsy is crucial not only to establish a tissue diagnosis, but to distinguish small cell carcinoma from the other varieties, since behaviour is so different:

- CXR
- CT or MRI of the thorax
- PET scan
- bronchoscopy
- mediastinoscopy
- bone scan
- liver ultrasound
- brain CT/MRI if cerebral metastases suspected.

Spread is by:

- direct spread to local tissues
- lymphatic spread to axillary and cervical nodes
- transcoelomic spread across the pleural cavity
- blood-borne metastases, especially to bone, liver and brain.

Treatment

Operable tumours may be resected. Metastatic spread may be inhibited by early ligation of the pulmonary vein. More advanced tumours may respond to chemo- or radiotherapy. Palliative therapy is often the most common option for symptom control in advanced cases.

Prognosis

For operable primary lung cancers treated by resection, the 5-year survival is only 45%. The prognosis for squamous cancers is slightly better, early tumours having a 50% 5-year survival, but only 2% of patients with more advanced cancers survive 5 years. Small cell tumours are usually lethal but do initially respond well to chemo.

BENIGN LUNG TUMOURS

Hamartomas and carcinoid tumours are the most frequent benign lung tumours and they are rare compared to carcinoma. Usually showing well-circumscribed nodules on CXR, the distinction between benign lesions and early cancers can be difficult. Features suggestive of benign tumours include:

- slow growth (compare with previous chest films)
- calcification
- well-circumscribed edge (in contrast, cancers show spiky projections as they invade).

CT-guided biopsy may confirm the diagnosis but small lesions are difficult to target and resection is sometimes performed for suspicious lesions which turn out to be benign. Thoracoscopic resection is possible in some cases.

'SURGICAL' LUNG INFECTIONS

Bronchiectasis

Bronchiectasis is gross dilatation of the terminal bronchioles caused by chronic infection, sometimes following measles or tuberculosis. Haemoptysis and excessive sputum production are unpleasant. Antibiotics and chest physiotherapy are the mainstays of treatment, but localised highly symptomatic bronchiectasis responds well to surgery.

Tuberculosis

Antibiotics have rendered obsolete many of the operations performed in the past for TB. Remaining indications include:

- persistent bronchopleural fistula
- major haemoptysis
- gross lung destruction or large lung cavities/abscesses resistant to antibiotic penetration.

These interventions for advanced complicated TB carry a high risk of complications.

PNEUMOTHORAX

Aetiology

Traumatic pneumothorax is discussed on page 63. Spontaneous pneumothorax has three main causes:

- rupture of pleural bleb (commoner in asthmatic patients)
- cystic lung disease – alpha-1-antitrypsin deficiency in the young; emphysema in the elderly
- opportunist infections in immune deficiency (e.g. *Pneumocystis carinii*).

Pathology

As air enters the pleural cavity the lung collapses. With both spontaneous and traumatic pneumothorax, if air continues to leak out of the lung with each breath, since there is no route for it to escape, the pressure in the pleural cavity increases, causing a tension pneumothorax (see p. 63).

Clinical features

There is pleuritic pain associated with breathlessness. Signs of simple pneumothorax are minimal unless the pneumothorax is large (>25%). They are:

- reduced movements of respiration
- hyper-resonant percussion note
- absent breath sounds.

Management

- Observation (for small (<20%) pneumothoraces)
- Needle aspiration and daily X-ray until resolution
- Chest drain.

Table 14.7 Indications for diagnostic and therapeutic thoracoscopy

Diagnostic	
Problem	Possible diagnosis
Pleural effusions	Malignancy, tuberculosis, lymphoma
Pleural nodules/thickening	Mesothelioma, tuberculosis, malignancy, fibromas
Diffuse parenchymal lung disease	Sarcoid, lymphoma, HIV-related conditions, opportunistic infections, granulomas
Staging of lung cancer	Mediastinal and hilar node sampling
Lung nodules	Primary or secondary tumours, granulomas, including tuberculosis
Therapeutic	
Indication	Procedure
Empyema	Drainage and breakdown loculi
Recurrent pneumothorax	Pleurectomy or pleural abrasion (talc) Stapling of apical bullae
Pericardial effusion	Creation of pericardial to pleural window
Malignant effusion	Pleurectomy or talc or tetracycline pleurodesis
Lung masses	Resection as wedge or lobectomy

Recurrent pneumothorax may require chemical pleurodesis (instillation of a sclerosant into the pleural cavity to stick visceral and parietal pleura together) or surgical pleurectomy.

MEDIASTINOSCOPY AND THORACOSCOPY

Indications for diagnostic and therapeutic chest endoscopic procedures are summarised in Table 14.7.

Hernia 15

DEFINITIONS

A hernia is a protrusion of a viscus or other structure beyond the normal coverings of the cavity in which it is contained, or between two adjacent cavities, e.g. abdomen and thorax. Hernias most frequently occur in the inguinal, femoral and umbilical regions and are classified into congenital or acquired. The commonest congenital hernia is found in infants where a patent processus vaginalis occurs, giving rise to an inguinal hernia. Acquired hernias may be primary, occurring at natural weak points, e.g. femoral hernias or umbilical hernias, or secondary at sites of surgical incisions (incisional hernias).

Predisposing factors include increased intra-cavity pressure due to heavy lifting, chronic cough, straining to pass urine or faeces, abdominal distension or the presence of ascites or tumour. A weakened abdominal wall occurs with abnormal collagen, metabolism, age, malnutrition, or damage or paralysis of motor nerves.

A hernia consists of a sac, its coverings and contents. The sac is composed of a mouth, neck, body and fundus. The coverings of hernia refer to the layers which are attenuated as the hernia emerges, consisting of skin, subcutaneous fat, aponeurosis, muscle, fascia and endothelial lining. The contents of the hernia may vary, but are most usually the small bowel or greater omentum.

Any abdominal hernia regardless of site may be reducible, irreducible, incarcerated, strangulated or obstructed.

- **Reducible hernia** The contents can be returned to the abdomen but the sac persists.
- **Irreducible hernia** The contents cannot be returned due to a narrow neck with or without adhesions forming between the contents and the sac.
- **Incarcerated hernia** This describes a hernia that is irreducible but not strangulated.
- **Strangulated hernia** The contents of a hernia become stuck in the sac, impeding the blood supply. Initially the venous return is occluded causing further engorgement of the contents until eventually the arterial flow is also compromised. This leads to ischaemic necrosis of the contents of the sac. If the sac only contains omentum, the necrosis is sterile. If bowel is involved, gangrenous intestine occurs which may result in fatal peritonitis. A strangulated hernia is therefore a surgical emergency.
- **Obstructed hernia** Bowel stuck in a hernia may obstruct, causing intestinal obstruction. Abdominal hernia is a common cause of small bowel obstruction (see pp. 85 and 87-88).

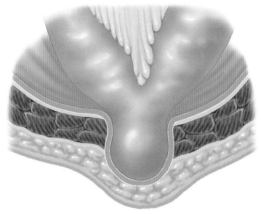

Figure 15.1 Richter's hernia. Part of the bowel wall has strangulated in the hernia but the lumen of the bowel is not obstructed. This is most commonly seen in strangulated femoral hernias.

Special types of hernia

Sliding hernia (en glissade)

An extraperitoneal structure forms part of the wall of the sac (5% of all inguinal indirect hernias). The caecum and ascending colon are involved on the right side, and the sigmoid or descending colon on the left side. Occasionally a portion of the bladder may slide into a direct hernia.

Richter's hernia

A portion of the circumference of the small intestine is trapped, which may become ischaemic but without the development of intestinal obstruction (Fig. 15.1).

CLINICAL FEATURES

Symptoms

- A lump which varies in size which may disappear when lying down
- Pain – ache or symptoms of complication including intestinal obstruction or strangulation.

Signs

The patient should be examined in the supine and erect positions. The area of the swelling is palpated to determine its reducibility and whether an expansile cough impulse is present. A hernia is more likely to be reducible with the patient supine. Control of the hernia by direct pressure over the point at which reduction occurs locates the neck of the sac. Other hernial sites should be examined (bilateral groin hernias are common).

A strangulated hernia is painful, tender and irreducible. The surrounding tissues may be inflamed. Signs of small bowel obstruction may be present.

A general physical examination must be carried out to search for predisposing causes, e.g. benign prostatic hyperplasia or chronic cough.

INVESTIGATIONS

Clinical examination is the gold standard but herniography, ultrasound, CT scan (especially if the patient is obese) and laparoscopy are occasionally used.

PRINCIPLES OF MANAGEMENT

The natural history of a hernia is of progressive enlargement and the risks of complications, i.e. irreducibility and strangulation, increase with time. Most hernias should therefore be operated on. A hernia may be repaired under general anaesthetic, regional block or local anaesthetic. Surgical appliances (trusses) are not advised, due to the increased likelihood of incarceration or strangulation caused by irritation and scar tissue formation at the site of the truss. Most elective operations are now done as a day case or short stay. Groin hernias are now often repaired via the laparoscopic approach (usually bilateral or recurrent).

LAPAROSCOPIC HERNIA SURGERY

In the UK, the National Institute for Health and Clinical Excellence (NICE) has made recommendation that laparoscopic surgery is one of the treatment options for the repair of inguinal hernia, as long as the patient is fully informed of all the risks and benefits of open and laparoscopic surgery either by TAPP (trans-abdominal pre-peritoneal) or TEP (total extra-peritoneal) approaches, to enable them to choose between the procedures.

Surgical techniques

Herniotomy, the removal of the sac and closure of its neck, is all that is required for infant inguinal hernia and is the first step in nearly all hernia repairs.

Herniorrhaphy involves restoration of normal anatomy, increasing the strength of the abdominal wall and constructing a barrier to recurrence. The most commonly used procedure is the insertion of a prosthetic mesh. Patients with obstruction and strangulation need general preoperative resuscitation prior to surgical exploration. Non-operative treatment may be considered in infants.

Outcome

For elective repair, the overall mortality is less than 0.5%. For emergency operations it is 5%. Mortality is dependent on the age of the patient and whether or not the contents of the sac are gangrenous.

Postoperative morbidity

Particular, persistent wound pain occurs in up to 11% of patients. Cutaneous anaesthesia is also common following hernia repair. Recurrent hernia with the use of a mesh is now less than 1%.

SPECIFIC SITES OF ABDOMINAL HERNIAS

Inguinal hernia

Inguinal hernias account for 80% of all abdominal hernias. They are most common in infants and the elderly. Inguinal hernias are twenty times more common in men than women and occur more frequently on the right side.

An *indirect inguinal hernia* passes through the internal ring, lateral to the inferior epigastric artery, along the canal to emerge at the external ring above the pubic crest and tubercle. Its coverings are attenuated layers of the cord. An indirect hernia may extend into the scrotum.

A *direct inguinal hernia* bulges through the posterior wall of the canal, medial to the inferior epigastric artery and is therefore not covered by layers of the cord. Direct hernias cannot extend into the scrotum.

A *pantaloon hernia* is a combination of the two.

Indirect hernias are usually derived from a remnant of the processus vaginalis which does not close. It is therefore more common in infancy. Sixty per cent occur on the right side and they are twenty times more common in men than women. Direct hernias are acquired lesions and usually a condition of later life. The differences between an indirect and direct inguinal hernia are shown in Table 15.1.

A key feature in distinguishing between an inguinal and a femoral hernia is the pubic tubercle, which may be found by feeling laterally along the pubic crest on the upper border of the symphysis pubis or by following the adductor longus tendon from the medial side of the thigh to its origin from the body of the pubis. The tubercle is directly above this. A reducible indirect inguinal hernia can be completely controlled with a fingertip firmly placed over the internal ring at the midpoint of the inguinal ligament. Differential diagnosis includes a femoral hernia, hydrocele, hydrocele of the cord or canal of Nuck, undescended testis, lipoma of the cord or epididymal cyst.

General principles of hernia repair have been given above. Postoerative complications include urinary retention in the male, scrotal haematoma or

Table 15.1 Differences between indirect and direct inguinal hernia

	Indirect	Direct
Patient's age	Any age but usually young	Older
Cause	May be congenital	Acquired
Bilateral	20%	50%
Protrusion on coughing	Oblique	Straight
Appearance on standing	Does not reach full size immediately	Reaches full size immediately
Reduction on lying down	May not reduce immediately	Reduces immediately
Descent into scrotum	Common	Rare
Occlusion of internal ring	Controls	Does not control
Neck of sac	Narrow	Wide
Strangulation	Common	Rare
Relation to inferior epigastric vessels	Lateral	Medial

damage to the ilioinguinal nerve, causing an area of anaesthesia, or continued postoperative groin pain. Recurrent inguinal hernias should be repaired to avoid the same complications that occur with primary hernias. Note the possibility of orchidectomy or testicular damage, which may occur with open repair due to damage of the testicular artery. Damage to the vas deferens is also possible.

Femoral hernia

The differential diagnosis of a femoral hernia is shown in Table 15.2. Femoral hernias account for 7% of all hernias and are four times more common in women than men (although inguinal hernias are still more common in women than femoral). They are most common in late middle age and are rare in children. Bilateral hernias occur in 20%. The femoral canal is bounded by the inguinal ligament (anteriorly), the lacunar part of the inguinal ligament (medially) and the pectineal part of the inguinal ligament (posteriorly). This narrow femoral ring produces considerable risk of incarceration of any hernia. The narrow canal makes femoral hernia the one most likely to result in a Richter's hernia.

Clinical features

The patient is typically a middle-aged or elderly woman, complaining of a low lump in the groin; 20% present with strangulation. Cough impulses are difficult to detect. The femoral hernia is always below and lateral to the pubic tubercle, distinguishing it from an inguinal hernia. Small bowel obstruction may classically present in a strangulated femoral hernia and the hernia may easily be missed on clinical examination if the diagnosis is not thought about.

All femoral hernias should be repaired by direct incision over the hernia and closure of the femoral canal or occasionally from above in patients with obstruction or strangulation.

Table 15.2 Inguinal swellings which may resemble a femoral hernia

Condition	Findings
Inguinal hernia	Swelling is above and medial to the pubic tubercle
Saphena varix	Compressible Palpable thrill on coughing
Enlarged lymph node	Usually multiple Not fixed on deep aspect and therefore more mobile Seek cause – infection, tumour, lymphoma
Lipoma	Soft but not reducible
Femoral artery aneurysm	Expanding pulsation Bruit
Psoas abscess	Fluctuant Lateral to femoral artery Associated swelling in the iliac fossa
Ectopic testis	Empty scrotum

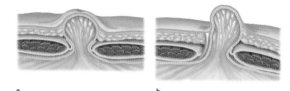

Figure 15.2 (a) Umbilical and (b) para-umbilical hernia.

Umbilical hernia

Two types of hernia occur:
- true umbilical hernia: a protrusion through the umbilical scar
- para-umbilical hernia: usually at the superior aspect between the umbilical vein and upper margin of the umbilical ring.

Typically, umbilical hernias are found in obese, middle-aged patients. Women are five times more likely to develop this than men. The neck of the hernia is narrow. The contents are usually omentum but small bowel or transverse colon may enter the sac if the hernia is large. These hernias are at great risk of strangulation. There may be an underlying cause of ascites or symptoms of local pain and swelling at the navel.

Management

In true umbilical hernias, an underlying cause should be sought and dealt with. Para-umbilical hernias, if symptomatic, require treatment (Figs 15.2 and 15.3). A strangulated umbilical hernia needs urgent exploration.

Epigastric hernia

Three-quarters of these are asymptomatic, found incidentally on examination, but may present with local pain or ill-defined pain which may mimic peptic ulceration. The swelling is palpable in the midline and is often tender and irreducible. Patients who present with upper abdominal symptoms should also be investigated for peptic ulcer, gallbladder or pancreatic disease before symptoms are attributed to the hernia. Surgically, the herniated fat is excised and, if a sac is present, the contents are reduced and the sac excised. The fascial defect is closed by suture ± mesh.

Incisional hernia

An incisional hernia occurs through the wound of a previous operation (1% of all abdominal incisions).

Aetiology

Incisional hernias may be caused by preoperative, operative or postoperative factors.

Preoperative factors

- Age – the tissues do not heal well in elderly people
- Malnutrition
- Sepsis
- Uraemia
- Jaundice
- Obesity

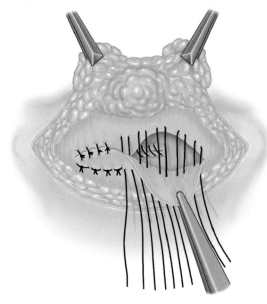

Figure 15.3 Repair of a para-umbilical hernia.

- Diabetes
- Steroids
- Peritonitis.

Operative factors
- Type of incision – vertical incisions are more prone to hernia than transverse
- Technique and materials used
- Type of operation
- Drains.

Postoperative factors
- Wound infection
- Abdominal distension
- Coughing.

Pathological features
Most incisional hernias occur within a year of operation and, once formed, inexorably enlarge. They may be wide or narrow-necked. Incarceration and strangulation may occur. The overlying skin may become thin and atrophic and the patient may complain of local discomfort. Small symptomatic hernias should be repaired, along with asymptomatic hernias, to prevent the risk of intestinal obstruction or skin ulceration. The outcomes of surgery are variable. Larger defects require mesh repair. Many cases are now repaired laparoscopically.

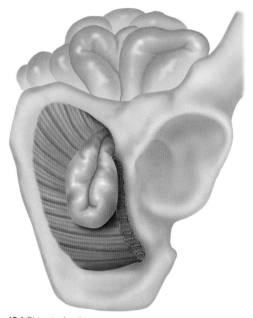

Figure 15.4 Obturator hernia.

Spigelian hernia

This is an interparietal hernia in the line of the linea semilunaris which may present with local pain, worse on straining, or a lump at the lateral margin of the rectus sheath. Strangulation or obstruction may occur. Clinical signs may be difficult to determine and imaging has been found to be useful.

Obturator hernia

This is mostly seen in frail, elderly women (Fig. 15.4). Richter's strangulation is common. Fifty per cent of patients complain of pain along the upper medial side of the thigh with episodes of previous obstructive-like symptoms. Signs are rare and the diagnosis is most often made at laparotomy for small bowel obstruction.

Lumbar hernia

Lumbar hernias may be congenital or acquired, primarily or secondarily as a result of a surgical incision. Most present with a bulge or lump in the flank, associated with discomfort, with a cough impulse and a reducible mass. The contents are most often small or large bowel. Twenty per cent become incarcerated, 10% strangulated. Differential diagnosis includes lipoma, soft tissue tumour, haematoma, tuberculous cold abscess, renal tumour. Hernias are repaired by direct closure of the defect. Large hernias require a mesh prosthesis.

UROLOGICAL SYMPTOMS

Pain

Renal pain is typically a dull ache felt in the flank.

Ureteric pain due to a stone or clot passing down the ureter is a severe colicky pain starting in the loin radiating to the iliac fossa and into the testis/vulva.

Bladder inflammation causes suprapubic pain.

Haematuria

Haematuria is often a sign of malignancy in the urinary tract and requires thorough investigation. Painful haematuria is commonly due to bladder infection; painless haematuria usually signifies cancer. Common causes of haematuria are shown in Box 16.1.

Lower urinary tract symptoms (LUTS)

These symptoms are often divided into irritative and obstructive urinary symptoms. Obstructive symptoms due to bladder outflow obstruction include urinary frequency, incomplete voiding, nocturia, poor stream and terminal dribbling. These are often associated with irritative symptoms of urgency and urge incontinence.

Dysuria

Dysuria (painful voiding) is usually due to urinary infection.

UROLOGICAL SIGNS

Renal masses may be palpable in the flank. A distended bladder is palpable and dull to percussion. The external genitalia are easily examined. The prostate gland is palpable via digital rectal examination. The normal prostate is soft to firm, has a well-defined median sulcus and is non-tender. A malignant prostate is enlarged, hard and irregular.

INVESTIGATIONS

- Urine examination by microscopy, culture, sensitivities, cytology
- Blood tests – urea, electrolytes, creatinine, calcium, alkaline phosphatase (ALP), prostate specific antigen (PSA)
- Plain X-ray – shows abnormal calcification in the urinary tract (Fig. 16.1). 90% of stones are visible.

Intravenous urogram (IVU)

Intravenous contrast is excreted by the kidneys, outlining the anatomy of the urinary tract. Information on structure and function is obtained

Box 16.1 Common causes of haematuria

Systemic
Anticoagulants
Sickle cell disease
Infective endocarditis (emboli)
Henoch-Schönlein purpura
Cyclophosphamide
Non-steroidal anti-inflammatory agents

Nephrological
Mesangial IgA disease
Glomerulonephritis
Renal infarcts
Urinary infection
Tuberculosis
Polycystic disease

Urological
Carcinoma of kidney
Urothelial tumours
Stones
Schistosomiasis
Benign prostatic hypertrophy
Trauma
Infection

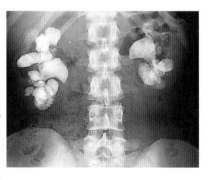

Figure 16.1 Plain film of the abdomen with bilateral stag-horn calculi.

(Fig. 16.2). IVU is used less than in the past – ultrasound and CT are now more common (see Box 16.2).

URINARY TRACT INFECTIONS

Pyelonephritis

The commonest cause is ascending Gram-negative bacterial infection from the bladder. Clinical features include symptoms of high fever, rigors, vomiting, loin pain, and urinary frequency, dysuria and haematuria. The loin is tender but other signs are minimal.

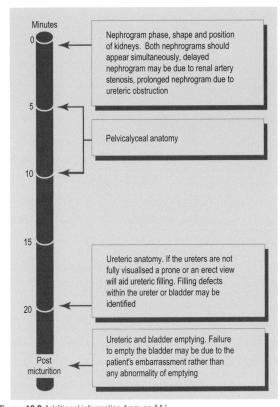

Minutes

0 — Nephrogram phase, shape and position of kidneys. Both nephrograms should appear simultaneously, delayed nephrogram may be due to renal artery stenosis, prolonged nephrogram due to ureteric obstruction

5 — Pelvicalyceal anatomy

10 —

15 —

Ureteric anatomy. If the ureters are not fully visualised a prone or an erect view will aid ureteric filling. Filling defects within the ureter or bladder may be identified

20 —

Ureteric and bladder emptying. Failure to empty the bladder may be due to the patient's embarrassment rather than any abnormality of emptying

Post micturition

Figure 16.2 Additional information from an IVU.

Box 16.2 Imaging modalities useful in urological disease

Ultrasound
Plain AXR
IVU
Retrograde ureterography
Antegrade pyelography
Micturating cystourethrography
Angiography
CT (increasingly used as a first-line investigation)
MRI
Isotope studies

Investigation

Urinalysis and culture (urine contains blood, leucocytes and organisms) are essential to achieve diagnosis. Imaging is necessary to look for renal stones and to exclude ureteric obstruction. Ultrasound and IVU are usually adequate. An obstructed infected kidney may be permanently damaged in under 24 hours and therefore needs emergency treatment.

Treatment

Antibiotics should be started as soon as urine and blood samples have been obtained for culture. Severe cases require IV treatment, e.g. cefuroxime ± gentamicin, converting to oral therapy when the infection is controlled. If the kidney is obstructed it must be decompressed immediately (by ureteric stenting or percutaneous nephrostomy).

Acute cystitis

Bacteria easily ascend the female urethra, which is only 5 cm long. In men, bacterial cystitis is usually associated with bladder outflow obstruction, stones or tumours. Symptoms include urinary frequency, dysuria, suprapubic pain and haematuria. The suprapubic area may be tender and pyrexia is common.

Investigation

Urinalysis and culture as above. Males with cystitis and females with recurrent attacks require cystoscopy to exclude an underlying bladder abnormality, as does any patient with haematuria.

Treatment

Treatment is by rest, hydration and antibiotics with follow-up urine culture after treatment. In females *Candida* often follows antibiotic treatment and should be checked for (with high vaginal swab) and treated if detected.

Interstitial cystitis

This condition is characterised by recurrent irritative urinary symptoms (frequency, dysuria, urgency) but sterile urine cultures. Severe forms may require surgery.

Tuberculosis of the bladder

Recurrent and chronic lower urinary tract symptoms may be due to TB infection of the bladder, which is not detected with routine urine culture. Early morning urine specimens are required, which must be examined specifically for acid and alcohol fast bacilli (AAFB).

Schistosomiasis (bilharziasis)

The parasite *Schistosoma haematobium* is endemic in Africa and the Middle East and causes severe chronic bladder inflammation and fibrosis which may lead to malignant change.

Prostatitis

Acute bacterial prostatitis is most commonly caused by *E. coli, S. aureus, N. gonorrhoeae* or *Chlamydia,* and diabetics are more frequently affected. Symptoms include malaise, fever, rigors with dysuria and frequency. Pain is felt in the lower abdomen and perineum. On examination the prostate is very tender. Chronic prostatitis is often difficult to eradicate.

Investigation and treatment

This involves urine microscopy, culture and sensitivity (MC&S) followed by appropriate antibiotics. Tetracycline, erythromycin and ciprofloxacin are useful if *Chlamydia* is suspected.

Epididymo-orchitis (see also Ch. 5)

In boys, viral infection may be the cause. The main difficulty in this age group is distinguishing infection from testicular torsion. In young males a sexually transmitted infection (e.g. *Chlamydia*) is usually responsible. In older men the infection is a consequence of urinary infection resulting from chronic bladder outflow obstruction. Symptoms include rapid onset of testicular pain, fevers and sometimes vomiting. The testicle becomes very swollen and exquisitely tender.

Investigation

Midstream urine (MSU) should be examined and cultured. In boys, scrotal exploration may be indicated as it is the only completely reliable way to exclude torsion. In younger men the main differential diagnosis is testicular cancer and scrotal ultrasound is required after treatment of the acute episode, to exclude an underlying tumour.

Treatment

Treatment is by rest, analgesics and antibiotics. Abscess formation may require surgical drainage.

Urinary infection in children

Urinary tract infection (UTI) in children is important since it may indicate an underlying congenital abnormality, for example vesicoureteric reflux, which may cause longterm renal damage if untreated. The clinical features of UTI in young children may be very non-specific and include vomiting, distress, weight loss and fever. Any child with a proven UTI should be thoroughly investigated to exclude a significant anatomical abnormality.

Urological trauma

This is discussed in Chapter 4.

UPPER URINARY TRACT – KIDNEYS AND URETERS

Congenital abnormalities

The most commonly encountered anatomical abnormalities of the kidneys and ureters are listed in Box 16.3.

Nephroblastoma (Wilms tumour)

This is the second commonest cause of death in infants. Peak incidence is 2 years. It is a highly malignant undifferentiated embryonic tumour which metastasises throughout the body. Presentation is non-specific with failure to thrive, sometimes with an abdominal mass and haematuria. Treatment requires radical nephrectomy and adjuvant chemotherapy. Small localised tumours have an 80% 5-year survival but this falls to zero if there are metastases in solid organs.

Adenocarcinoma

Aetiology and pathology

This tumour is commonest in men in late middle age and often causes paraneoplastic syndromes (Table 16.1). These cancers are usually well

> **Box 16.3** Congenital renal and ureteric abnormalities
>
> Horseshoe and pelvic kidney
> Cysts
> Congenital pelviureteric junction (PUJ) obstruction
> Ureteric duplication
> Megaureter
> Vesicoureteric reflux

Table 16.1 Paraneoplastic syndromes in renal cell adenocarcinoma

Event	Cause
Raised ESR	Changes in plasma proteins
Anaemia	Depressed erythropoiesis and haemolysis
Polycythaemia	Erythropoietin secretion
Hypercalcaemia	Tumour secretion of parathormone-like substance
Raised alkaline phosphatase concentration	Secretion from the tumour
Pyrexia	Circulating pyrogens
Hypertension	Secretion of renin
Amyloid deposition	Unknown
Peripheral neuropathy and myopathy	Unknown

encapsulated and contain areas of haemorrhage and necrosis. Spread is by local infiltration and blood-borne metastases. The tumour may grow into the renal veins and vena cava.

Clinical features

The tumour may present with symptoms due to the tumour, due to metastases or due to symptoms resulting from secretion from malignant tissue (see Table 6.3, p. 108). Symptoms include:

● aching loin pain
● 'clot colic', resembling renal colic but due to passage of a clot down a ureter
● haematuria
● paraneoplastic syndromes (see Table 16.1)
● pathological fracture (renal cancers are one of the five cancers that commonly metastasise to bone; the others are lung, breast, prostate and thyroid).

The triad of loin pain, loin mass and haematuria is only seen in advanced tumours. Early renal cancers may have no signs at all, often found by chance during a CT scan requested for other reasons.

Investigation

- Urinalysis
- Blood tests (including tests for the common paraneoplastic syndromes)
- CXR (lung metastases)
- Ultrasound, CT, IVU and sometimes angiography are all useful in delineating tumour anatomy.

Treatment

The only curative treatment is radical nephrectomy (this can be done laparoscopically). Embolisation of the renal artery may lessen symptoms in patients unsuitable for surgery. Radiotherapy to the primary tumour is ineffective, but may help pain from bone metastases. Chemotherapy and hormonal treatments are ineffective.

Prognosis

Five-year survival is nearly 70% for early (T1) tumours, falling to almost zero for cancers presenting with metastases.

Carcinoma of the renal pelvis

Ten per cent of all renal tumours arise in the renal pelvis; 90% are transitional cell carcinomas (TCCs), 10% squamous. Many TCCs are associated with tumours elsewhere in the urinary tract. Management requires surgical excision. TCCs have a good prognosis but squamous cell carcinomas have a poor outcome.

Stone disease

Urinary stones are common. Most are due to conditions causing high urinary calcium concentrations, or due to infections (e.g. *Proteus* spp.) which split urea to form ammonia, rendering the urine alkaline.

Symptoms depend on the size and position of the stone, and whether there is associated urinary infection. The classic presentation is of ureteric colic (Fig. 5.7, p. 94) (also commonly called renal colic) due to the passage of a stone along a ureter. Severe colicky pain (said to be as bad as labour pain) is felt in the loin, radiating to the groin and into the scrotum or labia. Vomiting is common. The loin may be tender but physical signs may be absent. Urine dipstix is usually positive for blood. Evidence of infection (dysuria, constant loin pain between colicky exacerbations, fever, loin tenderness) should be taken very seriously since an obstructed infected kidney may be irreparably damaged in less than 24 hours if not decompressed.

The differential diagnosis is important (Box 16.4). In particular, in individuals over 50, especially those who have never previously had urinary stones, ruptured aortic aneurysm must be considered and excluded.

Diagnosis is by intravenous urogram (IVU). CT or ultrasound may also be used.

Most stones pass spontaneously, and analgesia is all that is required. Large (>0.5 mm) obstructing stones in the upper ureter are more likely to need treatment (Box 16.5).

A patient who has formed one renal stone has a 20% chance of developing another. Recurrence may be reduced by ensuring a high fluid intake to ensure more dilute urine. Underlying metabolic abnormality must be excluded (check U&E, calcium, uric acid and ALP, and do 24-hour urine collection for calcium, uric acid and citrate).

Kumar and Clark's Handbook of Medical Management

> **Box 16.4** Differential diagnosis of ureteric (renal) colic
>
> Appendicitis   Pyelonephritis
> Cholecystitis   Ruptured abdominal aortic
> Diverticulitis   aneurysm

> **Box 16.5** Treatment modalities for urinary stones
>
> Extracorporeal shockwave lithotripsy (ESWL)
> Percutaneous nephrolithotomy
> Cystoscopy and ureteroscopy
> Ureteric stenting
> Laparoscopic ureterotomy
> Open surgical removal (rarely required)

Retroperitoneal fibrosis (chronic periaortitis)

This rather peculiar condition causes thick, plaque-like fibrosis in the retroperitoneum, encasing and obstructing the ureters. Onset is slow and insidious. The condition may be associated with inflammatory forms of abdominal aortic aneurysm (and endovascular aneurysm repair is often preferred as treatment to the AAA). Treatment requires relief of ureteric obstruction (usually with stents) and steroids which cause the fibrosis to regress. Surgical exploration of the ureters is sometimes required (ureterolysis).

Urinary diversion

Temporary

A kidney may be drained by a catheter passed percutaneously into the renal pelvis under X-ray control, to allow urine to drain externally (percutaneous nephrostomy).

Permanent

Permanent urinary diversion is most frequently performed by an ileal conduit, where the ureters are drained into an isolated segment of ileum (Fig. 16.3).

LOWER URINARY TRACT

Bladder cancer

Benign bladder tumours are rare. Most bladder tumours are malignant growths arising from the transitional cell epithelium lining the urinary tract. Predisposing factors are male sex (5:1), smoking, chemical industry (rubber/dyes/pesticides) and schistosomiasis (squamous tumours).

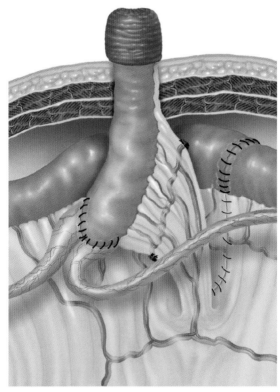

Figure 16.3 An ileal conduit.

Clinical features
Painless haematuria is the commonest presentation. Irritative urinary symptoms and recurrent infection may also occur. Physical signs are minimal unless the disease is advanced.

Investigations
- Urine MC&S
- Urine cytology
- U&E (bladder tumours may obstruct the ureters and cause renal impairment)
- Cystoscopy (the definitive investigation, allows biopsy)
- IVU (CT scan to assess upper urinary tract)
- CXR (to look for lung metastases).

Advanced tumours invading bladder muscle require CT/MRI for local staging. The TNM classification is used, summarised in Table 16.2.

Table 16.2 Local staging of bladder cancer that is no longer superficial

Stage	Findings
T2	Superficial muscle is involved
T3A	Deep bladder muscle is involved
T3B	Extending beyond muscle but bladder still mobile
T4A	Adjacent structures involved
T4B	Fixed to pelvic wall
M0	No distant metastases
M1	Distant metastases

Table 16.3 Survival in bladder cancer

Stage	Grade	5-year survival (%)
pTiS		75
pT1A	1	95
pT1B	1	72
pT1	3	39
pT2		45
pT3		39
pT4		5

Treatment

Superficial tumours require transurethral resection and intravesical chemotherapy, with regular flexible cystoscopic follow-up. More advanced cancers require cystectomy or radical radiotherapy. Prognosis is summarised in Table 16.3.

Urinary retention

This is described on page 93-95.

The prostate gland

Benign prostate hyperplasia (BPH)

This is a normal consequence of ageing and occurs in 75% of men by the age of 70. One-fifth of all men require treatment for the condition during their lifetime. The cause is unknown.

Presentation may be due to:

- obstructive urinary symptoms (hesitancy, poor stream, terminal dribbling, frequency and nocturia); incomplete voiding may cause UTI
- acute urinary retention (p. 93)
- chronic urinary retention (p. 95).

Conservative treatment includes alpha-adrenergic blocking agents, finasteride and thermotherapy. Once retention has occurred, prostatectomy is required, usually via transurethral resection. Complications include bleeding, sepsis, transurethral resection (TUR) syndrome (hyponatraemia due to bladder irrigant entering the bloodstream), retrograde ejaculation, urethral stricture, impotence and incontinence.

Prostatitis (see p. 246)

Prostate cancer

This is the commonest cancer in men, with over 27 000 new diagnoses per year in the UK. The difficulty with prostate cancer is distinguishing between those that will progress and those that are harmless. Autopsy studies on men who have died of unrelated causes demonstrate that half of all men aged 70–79 years and two-thirds of those aged 80–89 have unsuspected prostate cancer. Only around 1 in 200 of men with prostate cancer will die of it. Nonetheless prostate cancer is the fourth most common cause of cancer death in males. This confusion makes screening for prostate cancer problematic, since many cases detected would never have caused any symptoms, or shortened life, if left alone.

- Aetiology and pathology The cause is unknown, age is the only predisposing factor. The tumour is an adenocarcinoma and spreads by local infiltration, lymphatic spread to iliac and paraaortic nodes, and blood-borne spread to bone, where it causes sclerotic (rather than lytic) metastases.
- Clinical features
- LUTS (see p. 243)
- Perineal pain from local infiltration
- Bone pain from metastases
- Renal failure, from bilateral ureteric obstruction.

A malignant prostate feels hard, knobbly and irregular on rectal examination.

- Investigation
- U&E
- PSA
- ALP (raised with bone metastases).

PSA is secreted into blood by both normal and malignant prostate tissue. An elevated PSA may be due to a large benign gland, prostate cancer, prostate inflammation and catheterisation of the bladder. Many men with a mildly raised PSA do not have cancer; equally many men with cancer do not have markedly raised PSAs. This limits the value of PSA as a screening test. However, it is useful in monitoring progression of established disease and monitoring of treatment.

Abdominal ultrasound detects hydronephrosis due to ureteric obstruction. Trans-rectal ultrasound and biopsy establishes histological diagnosis.

Bone scanning (Fig. 16.4) may show bone metastases and MRI scanning complements EUA to establish staging, which is by the TNM classification (Table 16.4).

- Treatment Options include:
- conservative management (watchful waiting)
- radical prostatectomy for suspected early ('organ-confined') concern; may be open or laparoscopic approaches
- external beam radiotherapy
- brachytherapy (radioactive implants placed inside the prostate)
- hormone therapy (LHRH analogues and antiandrogens).

Localised prostate cancer is potentially curable with radical treatment or combinations of these treatments. Asymptomatic, localised,

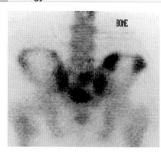

Figure 16.4 Bone scan showing hot spots due to metastatic carcinoma of the prostate.

Table 16.4 Staging of prostate cancer	
Stage	**Findings**
T1a	An incidental finding of tumour with low biological potential for aggressive behaviour in a prostate removed for clinically benign disease
T1b	An incidental finding of a tumour with potentially biological aggressive behaviour found in a prostate removed for clinically benign disease (high-grade or diffuse)
T1c	Tumour identified because of an elevated serum prostate-specific antigen
T2a	Tumour involving half a lobe or less
T2b	More than half a lobe but not both
T2c	Both lobes
T3	Tumour extends through capsule and may involve seminal vesicle
T4	Tumour fixed invasive of adjacent structures other than seminal vesicle

well-differentiated disease may require no treatment at all. Metastatic disease may remain remarkably well controlled for long periods with hormone treatment.

● **Prognosis** Localised disease treated radically has 55% 10-year survival, while metastatic disease at presentation has 25% 5-year survival.

Penis and male urethra

Urethral stricture
Urethral strictures may be congenital, or the result of trauma or infections. They result in obstructive urinary symptoms. Treatment is by urethral dilatation, endoscopic ureterotomy or surgical urethroplasty.

Phimosis
The foreskin does not normally retract until after the age of 2–3 years. Inability to retract after this is the result of too tight a foreskin (phimosis), which is usually due to recurrent infections (balanitis) causing fibrosis. Treatment is by circumcision.

Paraphimosis

If a phimosis is pulled back over the glans (e.g. during intercourse or catheterisation) this causes congestion and swelling of the glans penis as venous return from the glans is occluded. The glans becomes increasingly swollen and painful. Reduction may require local or general anaesthesia. Sometimes a dorsal slit to divide the constricting band, or circumcision, may be required.

Peyronie's disease

Fibrous thickening of the corpora cavernosa causes bending of the erect penis. Treatment requires wedge excision of the affected tissue, which shortens but straightens the penis.

Priapism

Priapism is persistent painful erection of the penis. The causes include idiopathic, iatrogenic (drugs used to enhance potency), sickle cell anaemia and leukaemia. Infarction of the penis may result if treatment is delayed. Aspiration of the corpora cavernosa is required; injection of phenylephrine into the corpus cavernosum may be required if that is not successful.

Testes and scrotum

Undescended testes

Undescended testes occur in 30% of premature infants and 3% of full term boys. By one year only 1% have failed to descend into the scrotum and spontaneous descent is rare after this age. The complications of undescended testes are listed in Box 16.6. Treatment is by orchidopexy between 1 and 2 years of age.

Testicular torsion

This is described on page 92.

Testicular cancer

Testicular cancer accounts for only 1–2% of malignancy in males but is the commonest solid tumour in males aged 20–35. The cause is unknown, but maldescended testes have a much higher incidence of malignant change. Types of testicular tumours are summarised in Box 16.7. For clinical features see Table 16.5.

- **Investigation** Tumour markers aid diagnosis and allow monitoring of effectiveness of treatment (Table 16.6). Ultrasound is helpful in defining the nature of the lesion. CT of the chest and abdomen is required for staging (Table 16.7).
- **Treatment** Orchidectomy for cancer is performed via an inguinal incision. Biopsy through the scrotum is not done because of the risk of seeding of tumour to the scrotal skin. Adjuvant chemotherapy and pelvic/para-aortic radiotherapy may be required.

Box 16.6 Complications of undescended testes

Infertility (fertility may be impaired even after treatment)
Torsion
Trauma
Inguinal hernia
Testicular carcinoma

Box 16.7 Testicular tumours

Seminoma (35% of all testicular cancers, peak incidence age 30–40)
Teratoma (60% of testicular cancers, peak incidence age 20–30)
Mixed (contains seminoma and teratoma, treat as teratoma)
Differentiated teratoma
Intermediate teratoma
Undifferentiated (embryonal) teratoma
Trophoblastic (chorionic) carcinoma

Table 16.5 Clinical features of testicular cancer

Symptoms	Signs
Painless lump in scrotum	Hard lump in body of testis
History of trauma often described	Non-tender
10% of patients had previous orchidopexy	5% of tumours are bilateral
Pain/dragging sensation in scrotum	Gynaecomastia (with choriocarcinoma)
Symptoms due to metastases (e.g. backache, haemoptysis)	

Table 16.6 Tumour markers for testicular cancer 1

Tumour marker	Type of tumour
Alpha-fetoprotein and beta-HCG	Teratomas
Lactate dehydrogenase	Teratomas and seminomas
Placental ALP	Seminomas

Table 16.7 Staging of testicular tumours (Royal Marsden Hospital Staging System)

Stage	Details
Testis	
I	Tumour confined to testis
IM	Rising concentrations of serum markers with no other evidence of metastasis
II	Abdominal node metastasis
A	≤2 cm in diameter
B	2–5 cm in diameter
C	>5 cm in diameter
III	Supradiaphragmatic nodal metastasis
ABC	Node stage as defined in stage II
M	Mediastinal
N	Supraclavicular, cervical or axillary
O	No abdominal node metastasis
IV	Extralymphatic metastasis
Lung	
L1	≤3 metastases
L2	≥3 metastases, all ≤2 cm in diameter
L3	≥3 metastases, one or more of which are ≥2 cm in diameter
H^+, Br^+, Bo^+	Liver, brain or bone metastases

- **Prognosis** All patients with stage I disease should expect cure. For stage II and III disease, 5-year survival is over 80%.

Scrotal swellings

Scrotal swellings can be diagnosed by establishing four features.

- Is the swelling confined to the scrotum?
- Can the testes and epididymis be identified?
- Does the swelling transilluminate?
- Is the swelling tender?

Establishing these properties allows most scrotal swellings to be diagnosed (Table 16.8). Scrotal ultrasound is useful to confirm the clinical diagnosis.

Kumar and Clark's Handbook of Medical Management

Table 16.8 Causes of scrotal swellings

Diagnoses	Confined to the scrotum	Testes and epididymis identified	Translucent	Tender	Comment
Inguinal hernia	No	Yes	No	No	Inguinal hernias extending into the scrotum are not always reducible Strangulated hernias are tender
Infant hydrocele	No	No	Yes	No	Infant hydroceles shrink while the baby sleeps and get bigger when he wakes or cries
Adult hydrocele	Yes	No	Yes	No	See page 92
Testicular torsion Epididymo-orchitis	Yes	No	No	Yes	Pain may make it impossible to define the testicle and epididymis
Epididymal cyst	Yes	Yes	Yes	No	
Testicular tumour	Yes	Yes	No	No	In more advanced tumours, the testicle and epididymis may not be definable
TB epididymis	Yes	Yes	No	No	
Epididymo-orchitis	Yes	Yes	No	Yes	See page 90, 247

Paediatric surgery 17

GENERAL PRINCIPLES OF PAEDIATRIC SURGERY

Newborns and infants present with uncommon surgical disorders, peculiar to their age group. These patients need to be referred to expert centres that are experienced in their special needs. Specialist anaesthetic skills are crucial, sometimes more so than the surgery.

Priorities in care for an infant being transferred to a regional centre include:

- temperature control
- nasogastric intubation
- airway protection
- cardiovascular monitoring
- appropriate intravenous fluids (Table 17.1)

Hypothermia may be controlled by the use of an incubator and warming mattress in the operating theatre and anaesthetic room. The extremities may be wrapped in aluminium foil and the infant nursed in warm cotton wool, exposing only the operating field.

Infection is a constant risk for newborns who need to undergo surgical procedures and broad-spectrum antibiotics, for example benzylpenicillin, metronidazole and aminoglycosides, are given intravenously at the start of all operations. Prolonged antibiotics may be required, particularly for bowel operations, and oral nystatin is given to reduce colonisation by yeasts.

Prenatal ultrasound scanning can identify major anatomical abnormalities, for example anterior abdominal wall defects, diaphragmatic hernia, duodenal atresia and hydronephrosis. Prenatal diagnosis allows the planning of post-delivery care of the baby in a hospital that is equipped to provide specialist services.

The spectrum of disorders seen in mid-pregnancy may be different from that seen in newborns because ultrasound-detected anomalies may be multiple and result in stillbirth. Fetal chromosomes can be checked, echocardiograms performed and scans done for detailed anomaly detection before a prediction of the findings at birth and the prognosis is reached and management planned.

RESPIRATORY DISTRESS

Oesophageal atresia and tracheo-oesophageal fistula

One in 4000 babies has an oesophageal anomaly, most usually a mid-oesophageal atresia with a distal tracheo-oesophageal fistula (Fig. 17.1). Half the infants with oesophageal abnormalities have associated problems, including cardiovascular, renal and skeletal defects.

Clinical features

In the common form with a blind upper oesophagus, the newborn is able to swallow amniotic fluid via the trachea and the fistula into the stomach

Table 17.1 Maintenance fluid requirements in the first week of life

Day	Fluid (mL/kg/24 h)
1, 2	60
3, 4	90
5, 6	120
>7	150

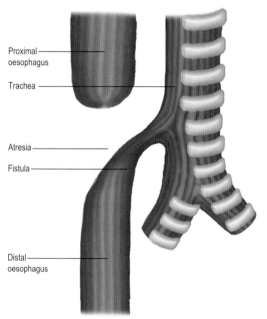

Proximal oesophagus

Trachea

Atresia

Fistula

Distal oesophagus

Figure 17.1 Common variant of oesophageal atresia and tracheo-oesophageal fistula.

but many of the pregnancies are complicated by polyhydramnios. The infant has excessive pharyngeal mucus at birth and, if fed by mouth, a cyanotic episode suggests aspiration into the respiratory tract.

Management

Feeding should be avoided where there is a suspicion of oesophageal atresia. Diagnosis is achieved by the passage of a small nasogastric tube which stops in the midoesophagus. Radiography shows the tube in the proximity of the first or second thoracic body and gas in the stomach confirms the presence of a distal tracheo-oesophageal fistula.

The upper airway is kept clear with suction and hydration is maintained with intravenous fluids. The fistulous opening on the posterior wall of the trachea is repaired via a right thoracotomy and the oesophageal anastomosis is constructed. Staged surgery is sometimes necessary if the gap is too wide to permit primary anastomosis. The outlook is excellent but dysphagia and respiratory complications may continue into adult life.

Diaphragmatic hernia

Diaphragmatic hernia occurs in 1 in 2000 live births, most commonly through a left posterior lateral defect. Agenesis of the hemi-diaphragm can occur, which is more severe. Intestine, stomach and spleen may be found in the pleural cavity and the lung is severely hypoplastic. There is severe respiratory distress and circulatory disability at birth. Diagnosis is confirmed by plain X-ray, which demonstrates lack of small bowel gas in the abdomen with loops of intestine in the pleural cavity and displacement of the mediastinum. Management includes resuscitation, positive pressure ventilation and a nasogastric tube to collapse the stomach. Face-mask assisted respiration is contraindicated. Infants with severe pulmonary hypertension require inotropic support, and intravenous colloids may be required to expand the circulating blood volume. Operative repair is carried out when the neonate is in a stable condition. The contents of the hernia are reduced from the thorax and the diaphragmatic defect repaired. There is a high mortality rate, related to bilateral pulmonary hypoplasia, but the majority of long-term survivors have no long-term problems.

Upper airway obstruction

This may be caused by:
- cystic hygroma: a fluid-filled collection in the neck which may extend to the mediastinum or axilla
- a small jaw (micrognathia), where a hypoplastic mandible causes obstruction of the pharynx by prolapse of the tongue associated with cleft palate. This is the Pierre Robin syndrome
- choanal atresia: a bony membranous obstruction to the nasal passages at the junction of the hard and soft palates. This diagnosis is confirmed by the inability to pass a nasal tube into the pharynx.

NEONATAL INTESTINAL OBSTRUCTION

General clinical features of neonatal intestinal obstruction

The history includes details of maternal illness, for example diabetes mellitus, and medication during pregnancy. A history of intestinal obstruction, Hirschsprung's disease or cystic fibrosis in relatives may be relevant. There is bile-stained vomiting (Box 17.1), failure to pass meconium or stools that change to the characteristic neonatal output, and abdominal distension.

Box 17.1 Bile-stained vomiting

Bile-stained vomiting in a neonate is always a sign of a serious intestinal abnormality and requires emergency specialist paediatric surgical referral.

On examination, a note is made of dysmorphic features, for example Down's syndrome, which is often associated with bowel abnormalities. In the abdomen, dilated loops of bowel may be visible in distal obstruction with bulky, palpable meconium suggestive of meconium ileus. Site and size of the anus should be recorded and the rectum examined. If blood is found, this may be indicative of bowel ischaemia.

Plain abdominal X-rays confirm the presence of dilated loops of bowel and give an idea whether the obstruction is proximal or distal. Free gas means that intestinal perforation has occurred. The presence of small bubbles or intramural gas indicates gangrenous bowel.

Causes of neonatal intestinal obstruction

Duodenal atresia

This is the commonest cause of proximal intestinal obstruction. One-third of the infants have Down's syndrome. The duodenum may be completely obstructed by a short segment of atresia. Partial obstruction may be caused by stenosis or incomplete web situated in the second part of the duodenum at the level of the ampulla of Vater.

- Clinical features Vomiting occurs in the first day of life and is bile-stained. Abdominal X-ray shows the double bubble appearance. The duodenal abnormalities may be corrected surgically.

Volvulus

Volvulus occurs due to mid-gut malrotation and the base of the small bowel mesentery is narrow. The duodenal-jejunal junction is to the right or in the midline and the caecum is mobile on a mesentery and lies close to the midline. Volvulus occurs in the first 4 weeks of life with bile-stained vomiting without distension. Signs of abdominal tenderness and rectal bleeding indicate intestinal ischaemia. Prompt surgical relief is required.

Atresia of the small bowel

This is more common in the ileum but is relatively rare. The cause may be due to a vascular accident in the mesenteric vessels late in fetal development. Features are of intestinal obstruction. Resection of the atresia and anastomosis is possible and the prognosis is good.

Meconium ileus

Tenacious viscid meconium found in 15% of infants with cystic fibrosis obstructs the distal ileum. The terminal small ileum is full of meconium but the colon is empty and appears underdeveloped. Prenatal investigations may reveal cystic fibrosis.

Plain X-ray confirms low small bowel obstruction. Cystic fibrosis is diagnosed by measuring the sodium levels in samples of infants' sweat or one of the specific defect genes found on chromosome 7. Water-soluble barium enema may relieve the obstruction, acting as a cathartic. Fifty per cent of infants require surgery as the condition is often complicated by the presence of atresia, volvulus or perforation.

Hirschsprung's disease

One in 5000 newborns has Hirschsprung's disease. There is a failure of development of the myenteric plexus of ganglion cells controlling para-sympathetic activity in the wall of the large bowel. The aganglionic segment is most usually in the distal sigmoid colon and rectum. A number of abnormal genes have been identified in families and patients with this disease. Most infants present with acute large bowel obstruction at birth or within a few days. Abdominal distension is common. Contrast enema demonstrates proximal dilatation of the ganglionic bowel with a relative narrowing of the aganglionic segment. The diagnosis is confirmed by rectal biopsy which demonstrates lack of ganglion cells in Meissner's plexus.

The obstruction is relieved by stoma. Operative correction occurs a few months later to excise the aganglionic bowel and anastomose normally innervated colon or ileum to the anorectal junction.

Anorectal abnormalities

Examination of the infant's perineum may reveal abnormalities of the anus which may be a skin-covered anus with a narrow anterior ectopic opening to the skin of the perineum or vulva which may be corrected surgically. Absence of the anal canal and distal rectum with or without fistula from the rectum to the urethra or vagina is managed initially with a colostomy. Corrective surgery is delayed until the infant is thriving.

Necrotising enterocolitis

This affects the small or large bowel, occurring in 1 in 1000 infants. The cause is unknown. It is more common in neonates born prematurely. Symptoms include features of sepsis and failure to absorb feeds. Abdominal distension progresses with erythema and tenderness of the abdominal wall or the passage of stool which contains blood. Abdominal X-rays demonstrate dilated loops of bowel. Intramural gas (pneumatosis intestinalis) is diagnostic. Free gas in the peritoneum indicates perforation.

● **Management** Feeding is stopped immediately. Antibiotics are instituted against aerobic and anaerobic bacteria. Resuscitation includes intravenous fluids. Ventilation may be required for respiratory failure. Intensive medical treatment is required prior to laparotomy where any gangrenous bowel is excised and either primary anastomosis or exteriorisation of the bowel is performed. Mortality is high (20%). Longer-term complications include short bowel syndrome or strictures.

ABDOMINAL WALL DEFECTS

The most common abnormalities of the abdominal wall, which are all rare, include:
● exomphalos
● gastroschisis
● exstrophy of the bladder.

Exomphalos

This is a defect with the umbilical cord inserted into a transparent amniotic sac with the vessels spreading out (Fig. 17.2). The sac contains loops of bowel and sometimes liver. There may be associated congenital heart disease or chromosomal abnormalities and neonatal hypoglycaemia. Diagnosis is established by mid-trimester ultrasound scan. Management is primary closure or staged reduction to achieve delayed closure.

Gastroschisis

This is a defect to the right of a normally inserted umbilical cord, with exposure of herniated loops of intestine. The defect is covered with a sterile bag and early operation is recommended to repair the abdominal wall.

Bladder exstrophy

This is more common in boys. There is an anterior opening of the bladder and urethra with absence of tissue of the subumbilical anterior abdominal

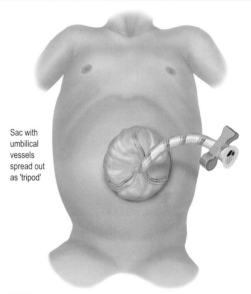

Sac with umbilical vessels spread out as 'tripod'

Figure 17.2 Exomphalos.

Table 17.2 Moist lesions at the umbilicus

Condition	Appearance	Management
Granuloma	Dull and irregular	Cauterisation or surface ligation after excluding an underlying, more serious lesion
Patent vitello-intestinal tract	Red, smooth and leaking digested milk	Specialised investigation and laparotomy for repair
Patent urachus	Leakage of urine	Urological investigation and repair

wall and separation of the pubic bones. Major reconstruction is required in a specialist centre.

Umbilical hernia

There is a higher incidence in Afro-Caribbean children and in patients with Down's syndrome and hypothyroidism. The infant presents with a protrusion that inverts the umbilicus. There is an easily palpable defect of the umbilicus with sharp-edged defect through which usually little more than the omentum protrudes.

Most hernias close spontaneously before the age of 4 years. Persistent umbilical hernias are closed surgically after the first 3 years of life.

Other lesions at the umbilicus are shown in Table 17.2.

Table 17.3 Causes of childhood tumours

Site	Tumour
Upper abdomen crossing midline	Neuroblastoma Ganglioneuroma Lymphoma
Loin	Wilms' tumour (the commonest cause of a solid renal mass in a child)
Pelvis	Urogenital cysts Neuroblastoma arising from pelvic sympathetic ganglia Presacral teratomas Ovarian cysts
Right upper quadrant	Hepatic haemangioma and hepatoblastoma

ABDOMINAL TUMOURS

These may be classified according to site (upper abdomen, loin, pelvis, right hypochondrium). The investigation of all abdominal tumours should include abdominal X-ray and ultrasound scan.

Childhood tumours are summarised in Table 17.3.

Upper abdominal tumours

The commonest tumour is a highly malignant neuroblastoma arising from the adrenal medulla or sympathetic ganglia. These are irregular and cross the midline and spread to lymph nodes, bone marrow, liver and skin. Most tumours are advanced at presentation. Nearly all neuroblastomas produce catecholamines which are metabolised to vanillylmandelic acid (VMA) and homovanillic acid (HVA). Diagnosis is confirmed by measuring urinary catecholamines. CT scan and MRI scan establish the stage of the disease. Treatment includes chemotherapy, surgery and sometimes radiotherapy. Most patients are incurable.

Loin tumours

Tumours arising in the loin are usually of renal origin. These include hydronephrosis, polycystic disease and non-functioning multicystic kidney. The Wilms' tumour is the most common cause of a solid renal mass. This is a malignant nephroblastoma spreading to lymph nodes and via the renal vein to the inferior vena cava and lungs. They are occasionally bilateral. The commonest presentation is a palpable mass in a child of preschool age. Pain indicates haemorrhage or rupture. CT scan stages the disease. Treatment is by radical excision followed by chemotherapy and occasionally radiotherapy. Eighty per cent of patients are cured.

Masses arising from the pelvis

These include urogenital cyst or neoplasia, neuroblastoma, presacral teratomas and ovarian cysts. Urogenital cysts and neoplasms include rhabdomyosarcoma arising from the genitourinary tract. Treatment includes chemotherapy, surgery and radiotherapy. The condition may be cured. Ovarian cysts may be massive with calcification in older girls and are treated by surgical excision. Right upper quadrant tumours include haemangiomas and hepatoblastomas. Presacral teratomas contain elements of the three germ cell layers. The sacrococcygeal region is the commonest site in newborns. Chemotherapy and surgical excision are treatments of choice.

PYLORIC STENOSIS

Hypertrophy of the pyloric circular muscles affects 2–3 per 1000 infants in Europe. The male/female ratio is 5:1. The disorder develops in the first 6 weeks of life. The cause is unknown.

Clinical features

Forceful projectile vomiting develops between the ages of 2 and 6 weeks. The vomit is not bile-stained. There may be signs of weight loss and dehydration. The diagnosis is confirmed by a test feed. The examiner sits to the child's left and palpates the right hypochondrium where the hypertrophied and contracted pyloric pseudotumour is felt as a hard swelling of 2 × 1 cm when the abdomen relaxes. Visible peristalsis from the stomach may occur. If there is clinical uncertainty, imaging with ultrasound may confirm the diagnosis. Complications include metabolic alkalosis with a raised serum bicarbonate and low serum chloride concentration. This is corrected with normal saline with added potassium chloride.

Treatment

Pyloromyotomy (Ramstedt's procedure) is carried out under general anaesthetic and the pyloric muscle is cut longitudinally down to the gastric mucosa. Postoperatively the infant can be re-established on full feeds within 48 hours. The prognosis is good.

INTUSSUSCEPTION

This is an invagination of a segment of bowel into an adjacent segment. The common sites are terminal ileum invaginating into the transverse colon. Two per 1000 infants are affected between the ages of 3 and 12 months. The ratio of boys to girls is 2:1.

Hyperplasia of a Peyer's patch due to infection by a virus is a common cause. The enlarged lymphoid tissue acts as a fixed eccentrically placed bolus in the lumen. The gut is invaginated as it tries to pass the 'lump' distally. The bowel can become strangulated, in which case there are signs of circulatory disturbance. There may be a history of preceding gastroenteritis or upper respiratory tract infection. There may have been a change in diet before the child presents with severe, colicky pain characterised by flexing the hips and facial pallor. Vomiting occurs and, within 24 hours, the passage of rectal blood.

On examination, the infant may be pyrexial and may be collapsed if strangulation has occurred. A sausage-shaped mass may be palpable in the epigastrium or right hypochondrium. Rectal examination confirms rectal bleeding. Many patients may present atypically. Plain abdominal X-rays suggest the diagnosis by the presence of a soft tissue shadow in the region of the transverse colon with empty distal bowel. Intestinal obstruction with a dilated loop of small bowel implies an established obstruction. Ultrasound examination may be helpful.

Management

A contrast barium enema may be therapeutic by reducing the intussusceptive bowel. Otherwise, laparotomy is required after resuscitation. The intussusception is delivered and reduced by manual pressure. Resection is necessary for irreducible intussusceptions or if gangrenous bowel is discovered after reduction. Recurrence may occur in up to 5% of patients.

THE INGUINAL REGION AND MALE GENITALIA

Undescended testes

At the age of 1 year, 1.5% of boys have an undescended testis, most often palpable in the groin – superficial inguinal pouch. However, the testis may lie in the inguinal canal, the abdominal cavity or be absent. It is more common in premature births. Most undescended testes at birth will descend during the first few months of life.

Examination

The cremasteric reflex can be strong in the child, who must therefore be examined in a warm, reassuring atmosphere. The index finger of the left hand passes downwards and immediately over the inguinal canal and may guide the testis towards the scrotum. The infant may be examined in the squatting position, thereby controlling the cremasteric reflex, and the testis may be palpable or persuaded to reach the bottom of the scrotum.

A normal retractile testis does not require intervention but the child should be followed up until the testis drops. An impalpable testis requires laparoscopy to identify the site of the testis, either in the inguinal canal or in the abdomen. If the testicular vessels and the vas are seen to end short of the internal ring, the testis is absent. Once the site has been decided, a surgical decision is made on treatment.

Complications of an undescended testis include reduced fertility, torsion, inguinal hernia and increased risk of malignant change in adult life. Early operation abolishes these risks. If done before the age of 4 years, normal fertility may be achieved by scrotal placement of the testis from the superficial inguinal pouch. The increased risk of malignancy is not altered by orchidopexy. Orchidectomy should be considered for a school-aged boy with a unilateral intraabdominal testis when the contralateral testis is of normal size and position. Orchidopexy should be performed between the ages of 15 months and 4 years. The testis and spermatic cord are dissected free from any hernia and a herniotomy is done. The testis can be mobilised to reach the lower scrotum by being placed in a pouch between scrotal skin and external spermatic fascia (Datos pouch).

Indirect inguinal hernias

This is more common in boys and usually presents in the first year of life. It is more common in premature babies. Irreducibility is common and may result in intestinal obstruction and testicular infarction. The symptoms are usually noticed by the mother who notices a lump in the groin which disappears when the child is at rest. Strangulation may occur, causing pain and distress and features of intestinal obstruction. The swelling is visible and palpable in the medial part of the inguinal region and extends down into the ipsilateral scrotum or labium.

Management

A reducible inguinal hernia is an indication for early elective herniotomy through a small skin crease incision overlying the site of the internal inguinal ring. The hernia sac is isolated and transfixed. Herniorrhaphy is not indicated in this age group. An irreducible inguinal hernia requires analgesia and sedation followed by gentle compression of the lump (taxis), which achieves safe reduction in 90% of patients. Herniotomy is carried out 1–2 days later. A persistent, tender irreducible hernia requires emergency operation.

Hydrocele

The processus vaginalis is usually patent. Hydroceles are common in the first year of life and may resolve spontaneously. Symptoms include the mother reporting an increase in the size of one half of the scrotum. Swelling may fluctuate and transilluminate. If the hydrocele is persistent after the age of 2, an elective operation is recommended to ligate the patent processus vaginalis at the internal inguinal ring. This is similar to a herniotomy.

Torsion of the testis

See page 92.

THE PREPUCE

Circumcision

Removal of the prepuce has been a religious rite for thousands of years. There is no medical indication for this operation, apart from phimosis or a previous episode of paraphimosis.

Phimosis is usually a result of trauma or infection and the flow of urine from the external meatus is obstructed. Marked ballooning occurs on micturition and the tissue around the preputial meatus is white, fibrotic and thickened. The foreskin cannot be retracted.

In paraphimosis the prepuce, which is usually fibrotic, is retracted and trapped in the coronal sulcus of the penile shaft, causing oedema of the glans. If this occurs, oedema is reduced by firm compression and manual reduction is usually possible, sometimes under anaesthetic.

Balanitis is recurrent sub-preputial inflammation with a wide variety of organisms, usually due to lack of cleanliness. Fibrosis may ensue.

Circumcision is usually performed under general anaesthetic and bipolar diathermy is used for haemostasis to prevent testicular vessel thrombosis or corpora cavernosa damage. Absorbable sutures are used and the glans is protected postoperatively by the application of soft paraffin dressing.

Complications of circumcision include bleeding and infection, meatal ulceration and stenosis and, more rarely, a urethral fistula. Removal of too much penile skin leaves the shaft covered by scrotal and abdominal wall skin which may cause sexual problems later in life. Recurrent phimosis can occur if too little inner preputial skin is excised.

Plastic surgery 18

INTRODUCTION

There is no part of the body that is the specific territory of the plastic surgeon; plastic surgeons treat a great variety of problems in many different sites. The development of fibre-optics and microsurgery has also increased the capability of the plastic surgeon to restore form and function. Nevertheless there are several subspecialities:

- oncoplastics
- cranio-facial
- burns
- cosmetic
- hands
- trauma.

SPONTANEOUS WOUND HEALING

This is the natural phenomenon comprising the basic events of blood clotting, fibrin deposition, organisation and collagen synthesis. Many wounds will heal completely without intervention, but the pattern of wound healing may be affected by endocrine, pharmacological and physical manipulation or by the surgery itself. Numerous dressings and topical agents are commercially available that aim to accelerate wound healing although they have not been proven superior – the aim being to provide the optimum environment for re-epithelialisation. The application of negative topical pressure ('vacuum assisted closure' or 'VAC' dressing) has also become increasingly popular.

Vacuum assisted closure

Topical application of negative pressure (see Fig. 18.1) is achieved with:

- suction pump (1)
- tubing
- impermeable film layer (2)
- foam ± interpositional layer (3).

This achieves:

- reduced bacterial load
- reduced exudate
- maintenance of moist environment
- may encourage angiogenesis
- provides protected wound environment (secure dressing).

Disadvantages:

- cumbersome for patient
- noisy
- relatively frequent attention to maintain function
- expensive.

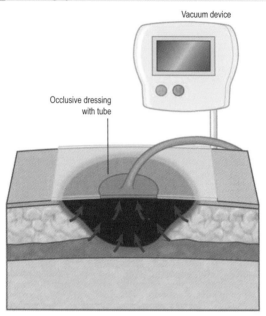

Figure 18.1 Topical application of negative pressure.

DIRECT SURGICAL WOUND CLOSURE

The first choice for wound repair is direct closure by suture, incision of which should be along the same axis line as the local skin creases (Langer lines – see Fig. 23.1, p. 339. Attention to detail is important with minimal handling of the skin edges, meticulous haemostasis and the wound sutured so that the edges are exactly matched but slightly everted. Hopefully hypertrophic scars can be avoided in this way (although true Keloid scarring is unpredictable and often difficult to manage, see Box 18.1)

SKIN GRAFTS

For a wound that cannot be closed directly the logical progression to achieve skin cover is skin grafting. Skin is harvested from elsewhere in the body and may be split or full thickness. The graft is 'free' and its continued survival depends on nutrients from the vascular bed of the wound: therefore drying-out, infection or the presence of necrosis will ensure failure. Split-skin grafts are usually harvested with powered dermatomes cutting the superficial layers of the skin 150–300 μm thick (the epithelial remnants ensure rapid healing of the donor site). Ingrowth of capillary loops is disrupted by any shearing forces so immobilisation of the 'sheet' of donor skin (and of the patient) is crucial, with sutures/staples/glues. 'Meshing' of the skin graft increases the area of cover achievable (Fig. 18.2), although

> **Box 18.1** Keloid scarring
>
> A benign overgrowth of connective tissue at the site of skin injury, beyond the usual confines of the wound (cf. hypertrophic scarring). They are raised, rubbery and nodular and can grow from seemingly innocuous wounds. There is a preponderance among those of African origin. Management is ideally preventative (i.e. avoidance of surgery in those predisposed), ablative (laser, sharp excision – with a >50% chance of recurrence), radiotherapy or intra-lesional steroid therapy.

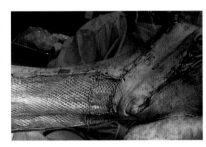

Figure 18.2 Increasing the area of a skin graft by 'meshing'; rotational flap also illustrated.

cosmetically this leaves a cobbled appearance. Smaller wounds may get an improved cosmetic result with a full-thickness graft but consideration also has to be given to colour and texture if the wound is conspicuous (e.g. the face).

FLAPS

For reconstructing a deeper wound (or where skin alone is unlikely to 'take' or leave insufficient cover) the defect can be covered with a flap. This is a 'block' of tissue which retains an attachment to the body known as a pedicle, through which it receives its blood supply and innervation. Until a flap is incorporated within the defect, the pedicle must remain intact for the tissue to survive (a common cause of flap failure) (Fig. 18.3).

Flaps can be classified in three ways:

- the blood supply:
  - random (no named blood vessel)
  - axial (flap based around named blood supply)
- the tissue within the flap:
  - simple (one tissue type, e.g. cutaneous or muscle)
  - composite (fascio-cutaneous – e.g. radial forearm flap; myocutaneous – e.g. transversus rectus abdominis muscle (TRAM) flap)
- the origin of the flap:
  - local (e.g. rotational or advancement flaps)
  - distant (pedicled or free flap).

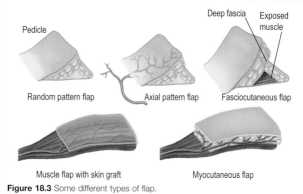

Figure 18.3 Some different types of flap.

Free tissue transfer 'free flaps'

This technique has become possible due to advances in micro-surgery, where blood vessels less than 1 mm can be successfully anastomosed. These free flaps permit sophisticated reconstructions, either for elective (e.g. deep inferior epigastric perforator (DIEP) flap for breast reconstruction) or emergency (e.g. re-attachment of amputated parts) situations. The process involves:

1. Elevation of the flap, isolating it on the vascular pedicle
2. Preparation of the recipient bed and isolation of a healthy recipient vessel
3. Detachment of the flap followed by anastomosis of donor to recipient vessels
4. Inset of flap and closure/coverage of donor site.

OTHER TECHNIQUES

Alternative graft materials

Biological

- Skin:
  - skin substitutes (e.g. composite matrix 'scaffold', allogenic skin).
- Cartilage:
  - costal cartilage or auricular concha.
- Bone:
  - ilium, rib.
- Nerve:
  - sural nerve.
- Tendon:
  - palmaris longus, plantaris.

Inert

- Silicone:
  - breast augmentation.

Tissue expansion

A tissue expander consists of an empty silicone balloon connected to a valved filling tube, implanted subcutaneously adjacent to a defect at an initial operation. After a period of weeks or months, the expander is inflated by serial injections of saline into the balloon, thereby distending the overlying skin. Finally, the expander can be removed and the surplus skin utilised for reconstruction (providing an excellent cosmetic/textural match).

Tissue ablation

Certain conditions affecting the skin can be treated by destroying the specific layer of skin or offending vessel. Dermabrasion is a common treatment for post-acne scarring, and laser is often used to treat vascular lesions such as haemangioma (as well as tattoo ink).

SUBSPECIALISATION ISSUES

Oncoplastics

Resection of some tumours can require multiple disciplines, and the plastic surgeon is a major part of the team, particularly for post-excision reconstruction.

Breast reconstruction

Breast cancer is one of the commonest cancers in women, and unfortunately mastectomy is still often required to achieve local control of the disease. Restoration of an adequately-filled skin envelope requires a combination of surgical techniques including prostheses (± expandable), rotational flaps (latissimus dorsi, TRAM flap) or free flaps (DIEP flap) on the operated breast, and sometimes 'equalising' measures on the contralateral breast, such as mastopexy or reduction mammoplasty, to ensure symmetry.

Trauma

Advances in the management of the multiply-injured patient, particularly in warfare, have allowed the survival of previously non-viable patients. The plastic surgeon is required to:
1. Determine the viability of remaining tissue
2. Debride and clean remaining tissue
3. Undertake reconstruction using the techniques outlined above.

Hand surgery

Post-operative physiotherapy and occupational therapy are vital for a good result which otherwise might result in an irreversibly stiff hand.

Burns

See Chapter 4.

Cranio-facial

Reconstruction of the head and neck demands the highest possible standards and encapsulates all the principles of restoration of form, appearance and function. The procedures undertaken vary from correction of congenital abnormalities (as early as neonatal cleft palate repair) to post-resection reconstruction of complex head and neck tumours.

Decubitus ulcers ('pressure sores')

These remain a depressingly common occurrence in the debilitated and immobilised patient and may represent part of a syndrome of terminal decline. If the patient can become ambulant, the prognosis is good and healing may be augmented by local flap surgery.

Orthopaedics 19

INTRODUCTION

Orthopaedic surgery is a broad speciality concerning management of diseases of the musculoskeletal system. It has become, of necessity, subspecialised; one of the most important subgroupings is between elective and emergency (trauma) work, and also between adult and paediatric care. Small specialist practice areas include bone cancer, hand surgery and spinal surgery.

CLINICAL ASSESSMENT

History

Pain is usually the main symptom, and all the usual features of site, onset, nature, radiation, exacerbating and relieving factors are important. Pain is not always felt at the site of the pathology; for example, hip pain is felt in the groin, or in children, the knee. Spinal root pain may radiate down a limb.

Other key points to ascertain in the history include:

- occupation and right/left handedness
- past trauma (may cause osteoarthritis)
- interference with daily living (e.g. stiff arthritic hip making it difficult to put on shoes or cut toenails)
- requirement for aid (e.g. walking stick or special cutlery)
- severity of pain (night pain may indicate severe arthritis requiring joint replacement).

Examination

This has four components:

- look
- feel
- measure
- move.

Look at the gait (Box 19.1), skin for scars and colour, and the general shape of the joint, swelling, lumps and position. Feel for temperature, tenderness, crepitus, loose bodies, swelling (fluid, soft tissue or bone). Measure limb lengths where appropriate. Move the limb, asking the patient to move it first to determine the range of active movements before ascertaining passive movements.

Check the neurovascular function of the limb by feeling peripheral pulses and assessing power, sensation and reflexes.

Lumps inside muscle are easy to feel when the muscle is relaxed but become immobile and difficult to palpate when the muscle is contracted.

Box 19.1 Abnormal gaits

Antalgic: Painful and with a short stance phase; seen in any condition of the lower leg where the pain is exacerbated by weight-bearing, e.g. osteoarthritis of the hip

Stiff leg: A fused hip or knee joint causes abnormal swing-through when the pelvis has to be rotated to bring the leg through

Trendelenburg: With proximal muscle weakness the pelvis on the opposite side sags during the stance phase – seen in developmental dysplasia of the hip, poliomyelitis and in osteoarthritis of the hip

Short leg: During the stance phase, the short leg results in the pelvis and shoulder on the affected side sagging down

Shuffling: Seen in Parkinson's disease, it has a short swing-through and no real heel strike or toe off

Stamping: The swing-through phase is abnormal with a broad base and high stepping – often caused by peripheral neuropathy with tabes dorsalis

Ataxic: Broad-based with unsteadiness on turning – cerebellar disease, multiple sclerosis or head injury

Foot drop: During swing-through, the foot scuffs on the ground – an L5 root lesion, common peroneal nerve palsy or old poliomyelitis

Scissor: Occurs in children with cerebral palsy with adductor spasm, so the swing-through of one leg is blocked by the other

---

INVESTIGATION

Imaging

Investigations useful in imaging orthopaedic problems are summarised in Table 19.1.

Blood tests

The WBC, ESR and CRP are non-specific markers of inflammation. Rheumatoid factor (an IgM autoantibody) is present in rheumatoid arthritis (80%), Sjogren's syndrome (90%) and systemic lupus erythematosus (50%). Raised uric acid may confirm gout and alkaline phosphatase is elevated in Paget's disease and in the presence of bony metastases. Antistreptolysin (ASO) titres are elevated following streptococcal infection. Protein electrophoresis is abnormal in myeloma.

Aspiration of synovial fluid

WBCs are present in synovial fluid in any reactive arthritis but reach very high concentrations if the joint is infected, and organisms may be identified on the Gram stain or subsequent culture.

Crystals are present in gout and pseudogout.

Table 19.1 Tests used in diagnosing orthopaedic disorders

Test	Indication	Example
Plain X-rays	Excellent definition of most bony and some soft tissue problems	Osteoarthritis: four radiological features are loss of joint space, osteophyte formation, bone cysts and subchondral bone sclerosis
Arthrography	Injection of contrast into a joint space demonstrates capsule abnormalities and loose bodies	Rotator cuff tears of the shoulder
Tomography	Now of limited use, replaced by CT and MRI	Mandible and teeth (orthopantogram)
CT	Detailed information on complex bony lesions	Spine, bone tumours, pelvic fractures, fractures involving joint surfaces
MRI	Provides excellent detail of bone and soft tissue lesions	Spinal cord, knee
Isotope scanning	Technetium-99 labelled biphosphonate is concentrated in areas of increased osteoblastic activity including infected and malignant bone	Prosthetic infection, bone metastases

Arthroscopy

Endoscopic examination of a joint cavity is most commonly performed for the knee, shoulder, elbow, wrist, hip and ankle. In addition to diagnostic examination, therapeutic procedures may also be carried out.

OSTEOARTHRITIS (OA)

OA is the commonest arthritis, and is commoner in women than men. Incidence increases with age and by age 80, 80% of hips show radiological evidence of OA. The disorder is characterised by destruction of the articular cartilage and can affect any synovial joint.

Primary OA is idiopathic and typically affects the hips, knees, spine and distal interphalangeal joints.

Secondary OA has many causes including previous trauma, acquired or developmental abnormalities (e.g. developmental dysplasia of the hip), alcohol, sickle cell anaemia and steroid use.

The main symptoms are progressive pain, stiffness and deformity of the joint. Initially the pain is only during use, then at rest and finally at night. Signs include swelling, crepitus and deformity.

Diagnosis is confirmed by plain X-rays. The four radiological features of OA are loss of joint space, subchondral sclerosis, bone cysts and osteophytes. Severity of symptoms does not always match severity of the X-ray changes.

Damage resulting from arthritis is not reversible and treatment aims to delay progression, relieve symptoms and preserve or restore function.

Non-operative treatment includes:
- pain relief with simple analgesics and NSAIDs
- intra-articular steroid injections
- weight loss
- physiotherapy
- aids (walking stick, special cutlery, etc.).

Operative therapy includes:
- arthroscopic washout
- osteotomy (realignment of joint to allow weight to be borne on a better segment of cartilage)
- arthrodesis (excision of joint surfaces to provide a stiff but painless joint)
- arthroplasty (joint replacement).

RHEUMATOID ARTHRITIS (RA)

This systemic inflammatory disease affects 3% of the female and 1% of the male population. The hands, wrists, elbows, shoulders, neck and feet are particularly vulnerable. The cause is unknown, though an exaggerated immune response to infections has been implicated.

Joint symptoms include pain, stiffness, especially morning stiffness, deformity and progressive loss of function. Systemic symptoms of multiple joint involvement, weight loss, fever, subcutaneous nodules, arteritis and tendon sheath involvement.

The 'rheumatoid hand' has characteristic deformities including swelling of the radial two metacarpophalangeal joints with ulnar deviation of the fingers. Subcutaneous nodules around the wrist and elbow are common, as are scars from previous operations.

> **Box 19.2** Infecting organisms seen in acute osteomyelitis
>
> *Staphylococcus aureus* (85%)
> *Streptococcus pyogenes*
> *Pneumococcus*
> *Haemophilus influenzae*
> *Salmonella* (especially in patients with sickle-cell anaemia)
> *E. coli* (in neonates)
> *Mycobacterium tuberculosis* (usually chronic rather than acute infection)
> *Brucella*

Management is mainly by rheumatologists, with orthopaedic input when surgery is contemplated. Hip joint replacement in RA is problematic as bone quality is poor, infection rates are higher and multiple other joints are usually involved, making rehabilitation difficult.

Rheumatoid involvement of the cervical spine may cause instability of the cervical spine, which necessitates special precautions during general anaesthesia requiring endotracheal intubation.

SEPTIC ARTHRITIS AND OSTEOMYELITIS

Acute osteomyelitis

This is now rare in adults who are not immunocompromised or diabetic. Young children are more commonly affected. The likely culprit organisms are summarised in Box 19.2.

The origin of the infection is not always obvious but it is carried by the blood (haematogenous spread) and lodges in bone capillaries, usually at the metaphysis of a child's long bone. Alternatively, direct infection may occur during an operative fixation of a fracture. An acute inflammatory reaction ensues which may destroy the growth plate and cause major deformity. Untreated, the condition may lead to subperiosteal abscess, suppurative arthritis, chronic osteomyelitis and pathological fracture.

Clinical features

The presentation varies from a mild fever in an unhappy limping child to life-threatening sepsis. The affected area of the limb is painful, red and tender, and swelling may be fluctuant. There may be a recent history of trauma or infection. An infant will keep the limb still (pseudo-paralysis).

Investigation

Plain films may be normal for 10 days. The radiographic signs of osteomyelitis are soft tissue swelling and periosteal elevation. Infected bone appears osteopenic and dead bone is sclerotic. Isotope scanning is a sensitive test.

The ESR, WBC and CRP are all raised and blood cultures identify the infecting organism in about half of cases. Urgent direct aspiration of the infected area provides fluid for culture.

> **Box 19.3** Recognised types of chronic osteomyelitis
>
> Complication of acute osteomyelitis – prevent with prompt treatment of acute infection
> Complication of open compound fracture – prevent by early appropriate treatment of compound fractures
> Infected joint replacement arthroplasty
> Tuberculosis – now less rare, when seen in the spine may lead to vertebral collapse and cord compression (Pott's paraplegia). Immunosuppressed patients at higher risk
> Mycotic infection – long bones and spine
> Syphilis – now rare. Congenital syphilis causes infection of the growth plates
> Brodie's abscess – well-defined walled-off abscess in long bone (usually from acute osteomyelitis)

Treatment

- Splintage of the limb to relieve pain
- High-dose IV antibiotics (after blood cultures have been taken)
- Surgical exploration and drainage for subperiosteal abscess or failure to improve with antibiotics.

Chronic osteomyelitis

This may follow unsuccessful treatment of acute osteomyelitis or an open compound fracture, or may be a consequence of an infected joint replacement. The condition may be complicated by pathological fracture, amyloidosis and malignant change (squamous cell carcinoma in a sinus tract). Well-recognised versions of chronic osteomyelitis are summarised in Box 19.3.

The affected bone may be dormant for long periods with flare-ups of local pain, swelling and purulent discharge. The overlying skin is often densely adherent to the underlying bone and there may be scars and sinuses.

X-rays show grossly abnormal bone with rarefaction and sclerosis. Dead bone (sequestrum) appears as a separate piece of dense, sclerotic bone within a cavity. New bone formation is seen as the involucrum. Isotope bone scan shows increased uptake and CT scanning indicates the exact location of dead bone fragments.

Non-operative treatment with antibiotics is of limited benefit since the affected bone is relatively ischaemic and drugs penetrate poorly. Infrequent flare-ups may be managed with simple dressings. Definitive treatment is surgical and requires excision of all dead bone and infected tissue, lavage and implantation of antibiotic beads.

Septic arthritis

Any joint may be affected but the commonest is the knee. *Staphylococcus aureus, Streptococcus pyogenes* and *Neisseria gonorrhoeae* are the most frequent organisms. The joint is extremely painful and swollen with very limited movement. Plain X-ray is normal but will demonstrate an effusion. WBC, CRP and ESR are raised. Fluid should urgently be aspirated from a joint that is suspected to be infected to allow microscopy and culture. Delayed treatment may cause irreversible damage to the cartilage resulting in osteoarthritis. High-dose antibiotics are required and larger joints should be arthroscopically washed out as an urgent procedure.

TUMOURS OF BONE

Symptoms of bone tumours

Pain is the commonest symptom, usually constant and worse at night. A lump may be felt. Pathological fracture may be the presenting problem and there may also be symptoms from a distant primary tumour.

Signs of bone tumours

Search for a primary tumour. A bony lump may be palpable, which may be tender.

Investigation

Plain X-rays may be diagnostic. Benign lesions have a clear margin with intact cortex. Malignant tumours are less distinct with periosteal disruption and cortical destruction.

Isotope scan distinguishes secondary deposits (usually multiple) from a primary tumour (usually solitary) and detects metastases before symptoms or plain film abnormalities are present.

CT and MRI are both useful for assessing local spread and staging.

Secondary bone tumours

Most bone tumours are metastases; primary bone tumours are relatively uncommon. One-third of patients who die of cancer have bony secondaries. Any bone may be affected but the skull, spine, ribs and pelvis are common sites. Most bony metastases appear osteolytic on plain X-ray apart from prostate secondaries, which are sclerotic. Some breast and prostate secondaries may improve with hormone therapy. NSAIDs and local radiotherapy may alleviate pain. Pathological fractures do not unite spontaneously and require internal fixation.

The five carcinomas which commonly metastasise to bone are:
- breast
- prostate
- lung
- kidney
- thyroid.

Primary bone tumours

Primary bone tumours are not always easily classified as benign or malignant: there is an intermediate group which are locally invasive but do not metastasise. Distinguishing benign from intermediate and more dangerous lesions may be problematic. In contrast to bony metastases, malignant primary bone tumours are rare, with fewer than 500 cases per year in the UK. The characteristics of primary bone tumours are summarised in Table 19.2.

Table 19.2 Characteristics of primary bone tumours

Tumour	Cell of origin	Malignant potential	Clinical features/pathology	Diagnostic features	Treatment and prognosis
Osteoid osteoma	Osteoblast	Benign	Severe pain in long bone of young adult	Rim of sclerosis round a lytic area	Excision or curettage ± bone grafting or internal fixation
Chondroma and osteochondroma	Chondroblast	Benign	Cartilaginous tumours, usually in hands/feet	Sometimes calcify to form exostoses	If symptomatic, as above
Non-ossifying fibroma (bone cyst)	Fibroblast	Benign	Fibrous tissue lesions, more developmental anomaly rather than tumour	Oval defect in cortex	
Haemangioma	Vascular	Benign (but be aware of possibility of haemangiosarcoma)	Vascular malformations (discussed in Ch. 13) may affect bone as well as soft tissues	CT/MRI and angiography	See Chapter 13 (section on vascular malformations)

Table 19.2 Characteristics of primary bone tumours (Continued)

Tumour	Cell of origin	Malignant potential	Clinical features/ pathology	Diagnostic features	Treatment and prognosis
Aneurysmal bone cyst	Vascular	Intermediate (do not metastasise but may recur after treatment)	Blood-filled cavities in spine and long bones	Expansive cyst with thinning cortex	Curettage and grafting Radiotherapy for recurrence
Osteoclastoma (giant cell tumour)	Osteoclast	Intermediate (recurrence common after excision)	Affect long bones near knee in young adults (rare under 20). Pain ± fracture	Multiloculated 'soap bubble' lesion on X-ray	Curettage and grafting. Wide excision ± grafting/ joint replacement for recurrence
Osteosarcoma	Osteoblast	Malignant with blood-borne metastases to lungs	Affects young (10–30), or the elderly with Paget's disease of bone. Long bones near knee are commonest site	Bone destruction, soft tissue mass and bony spicules ('sunray' appearance)	Amputation or radical excision and reconstruction + chemotherapy. 20% 5-year survival

Table 19.2 Characteristics of primary bone tumours (*Continued*)

Tumour	Cell of origin	Malignant potential	Clinical features/pathology	Diagnostic features	Treatment and prognosis
Chondrosarcoma	Chondroblast	Malignant, varies from aggressive anaplastic to low-grade slow-growing tumours	Older patients in flat bones (rib/scapula/pelvis)		Wide excision and reconstruction. Radiotherapy ineffective. Prognosis variable (20–80% 5-year survival) depending on grade of tumour
Fibrosarcoma	Fibroblast	Malignant	Rare, affects 40–60-year-olds at any site		30% 5-year survival
Ewing's sarcoma	Marrow in medullary cavity	Highly malignant	Diaphyses of long bones in young aged 5–20. Causes painful inflamed swelling and pyrexia and may mimic osteomyelitis	'Onion peel' appearance on plain X-ray	Chemotherapy, radical excision and radiotherapy. 35% 5-year survival, improving with new aggressive adjuvant therapy

UPPER LIMB

Shoulder

Symptoms

● Pain:
  ● over the deltoid insertion in impingement problems
  ● anteriorly in arthritis
  ● at the top in acromioclavicular disorders
● Stiffness is common
● Loss of function: difficulty raising hand causes difficulty eating, brushing hair, cleaning teeth, etc. and may be socially embarrassing
● Recurrent dislocation may be the symptom in unstable shoulders
● There is frequently a history of trauma.

Examination

● Look
● Muscle wasting
● Scars
● Shoulder contour: dislocated shoulders lose the rounded contour and the acromion is prominent
● Observe winging of scapula (due to wasted serratus anterior) and ruptured long head of biceps tendon (abnormal biceps contour in flexion).
● Feel
● Skin temperature, tenderness, crepitus on movement.
● Move
● Move through active and passive movements noting painful arcs of movement: pain during mid-elevation suggests subacromial impingement; pain at full elevation is from acromioclavicular disorders.

Investigation

● *Plain X-rays:* demonstrate arthritis and abnormal calcification.
● *Arthrography:* now superseded by MRI but commonly used in the past to demonstrate rotator cuff tears (supraspinatus, infraspinatus, teres minor, subscapularis) by leakage of contrast into the subacromial bursa.
● *CT/MRI:* of increasing value.
● *Arthroscopy:* both diagnostic and therapeutic; it is possible to remove loose bodies, decompress the subacromial space and stabilise the shoulder in recurrent dislocation.

Common problems

● **Acromioclavicular (AC) osteoarthritis and rheumatoid arthritis** AC arthritis causes pain on top of the shoulder aggravated by lifting the arm above the head or across the body. The AC joint may be prominent due to muscle wasting, especially the supraspinatus, and the joint may be tender with crepitus. Passive movement above the shoulder is painful. Excision of the outer end of the clavicle relieves symptoms but causes some weakness.
● **Subacromial impingement** The subacromial bursa and rotator cuff tendons may become trapped between the acromion and the head of the humerus, causing a well-defined painful arc on abduction of the arm. NSAIDs and local steroid injection may help. Arthroscopic excision of the undersurface of the acromion is highly effective and physiotherapy if surgery is not desirable.
● **Rotator cuff tears** These range from minor abrasions of the rotator cuff to complete full-thickness tears. There is usually a history of direct

shoulder trauma or dislocation. Chronic shoulder pain over the deltoid, especially at one point of abduction, is common. There may be muscle wasting, localised tenderness, reduced active but full passive movement. Management may be non-operative (rest followed by progressive rehabilitation) for partial tears and in the elderly, who are prone to stiffness after surgery. Complete tears that fail to settle in the young require surgical repair.

- **Calcific tendinitis** Calcium hydroxyapatite may be deposited in the tendon of supraspinatus. The cause is unknown but the deposit may cause intense pressure with onset of severe pain over a few hours. Inflammation and muscle spasm result in a distressed patient holding the arm very still and septic arthritis may be suspected. Rest, NSAIDs and local anaesthetic injections may help. Surgical incision of the tendon releases the deposit under pressure and relief is immediate.

- **Adhesive capsulitis (frozen shoulder)** The cause of this condition is unknown but there is often a history of minor trauma and the disorder may also complicate myocardial infarction or pneumonia. The shoulder is painful and stiff, and even passive movements are very painful. Frozen shoulder is self-limiting, with the joint returning to normal over 1 to 2 years, so treatment is non-operative. Manipulation under anaesthetic sometimes helps when recovery is slow.

Glenohumeral osteoarthritis and rheumatoid arthritis

OA of the glenohumeral joint is uncommon but disabling; RA is seen more frequently. Treatment may involve:

- non-operative measures: NSAIDs, steroid injections, treatment of the underlying condition in RA
- arthroscopic washout
- arthroplasty
- arthrodesis (salvage procedure after unsuccessful joint replacement).

Elbow

Arthritis of the elbow

The commonest disorders to affect this hinge joint are osteoarthritis and rheumatoid arthritis, OA usually being secondary to trauma. Pain, stiffness, swelling and locking are the main complaints. On examination, ulnar nerve function in the hand must be carefully checked.

Non-operative measures useful in elbow arthritis are:

- analgesia, NSAIDs
- strapping/splinting
- physiotherapy.

Surgical treatments include:

- arthroscopic washout and removal of loose bodies
- ulnar nerve transposition (for ulnar neuritis due to valgus deformity)
- fusion, for severe pain after failure of conservative treatment
- total elbow replacement (for RA)
- arthroscopic synovectomy (for RA)
- excision of radial head.

Tennis elbow

Tennis elbow (lateral epicondylitis) is commonest in middle age and causes pain over the lateral epicondyle radiating down the forearm causing weakening of the grip. NSAIDs, steroid injections and physiotherapy help over 90% to resolve.

Olecranon bursitis

Inflammation of the bursa between the triceps tendon and the olecranon causes pain and swelling. It is usually due to trauma (student's elbow), but occasionally infection is the cause.

The hands

How to examine hands

Be careful shaking hands with a patient with a hand problem as it may be painful. First of all ask the patient to roll up their sleeves above the elbow. Observing this allows inspection of the hands during function and many characteristic abnormalities may be noted. Moreover, there are often clues to the problem further up the arm, for example rheumatoid elbow nodules or synovectomy scars in RA, a patch of psoriasis on the elbow in psoriatic arthropathy, or signs or old trauma around the elbow in an ulnar nerve lesion.

Inspect the hands and note muscle wasting (thenar eminence in median nerve lesions, hypothenar eminence and interosseus muscles in ulnar nerve lesions).

- **Neurological function** Test the median, ulnar and radial nerves.
- Median:
  - abduct the thumb (lift away from the palm)
  - make a circle with the thumb and index finger and test its strength.
- Ulnar:
  - spread the fingers (abduct the little finger)
  - flex little and ring fingers.
- Radial:
  - extend the wrist.

If deficits are detected, look for scars of previous trauma as suggested in Table 19.3.

- **Vascular function** Note the colour and temperature of the skin and whether the veins on the dorsum are filled. Look for digital ulceration. Check capillary refill and feel ulnar and radial pulses.

Allen's test confirms patency of radial and ulnar arteries and may demonstrate impaired perfusion of the digits. While the patient makes a tight

Table 19.3 Sites of causes of neurological deficits in the hand

Abnormality	Possible anatomic site/cause
Median nerve palsy	Carpal tunnel syndrome Operations on antecubital fossa
Ulnar nerve palsy	Operations/trauma near medial epicondyle
Radial nerve palsy	Nerve vulnerable in spiral groove of humerus: look for evidence of arm injury
Combination of more than one nerve	Consider: Brachial plexus injury (birth trauma or motorcycle accident) Spinal root lesion (if sensory loss is dermatomal) Stroke

Kumar and Clark's Handbook of Medical Management

fist, occlude the radial and ulnar arteries by pressure over the vessels at the wrist. On opening the hand, the palm is white. In health, the palm promptly returns to pink when either artery is released.

- **Musculoskeletal function** Look at, feel and move all the joints of the hand and wrist.

Disorders of the hand

- **Arthritis** Osteoarthritis has four characteristic radiological features: loss of joint space, cyst formation, osteophyte formation and bone sclerosis.

- **Dupuytren's contracture** This is a thickening and shortening of the palmar fascia, which becomes adherent to the skin. As it progresses, the ring and little finger develop fixed flexion deformities. Margaret Thatcher had Dupuytren's contracture but it is commoner in men. The cause is unknown and most cases are idiopathic but the condition is associated with alcohol, diabetes, epilepsy (phenytoin) and vibrating tools. Surgical fasciotomy or fasciectomy is required.

- **Carpal tunnel syndrome** Compression of the median nerve in the carpal tunnel is usually idiopathic but specific causes include:
- wrist fracture
- ganglion in the carpal tunnel
- tenosynovitis (tendon sheath swelling) due to rheumatoid arthritis or repetitive strain injury
- oedema due to obesity, pregnancy, diabetes, hypothyroidism, acromegaly and amyloidosis.

The main symptoms are pain and pins and needles in the median nerve sensory distribution, worse at night. The little finger should not be affected. Oddly, there may be an aching pain in the forearm. The hand often looks normal unless the condition is long-standing, when there will be wasting of the thenar eminence. Sensation will be diminished in the median nerve distribution and abduction of the thumb may be weak. Other conditions causing hand symptoms that may mimic carpal tunnel syndrome are cervical spondylosis, thoracic outlet compression syndrome and peripheral neuritis. Nerve conduction studies help confirm the diagnosis.

Carpal tunnel syndrome due to pregnancy resolves soon after delivery. In other cases steroid injections may provide temporary relief but surgical decompression (local or general anaesthetic, open or endoscopic) of the carpal tunnel by dividing the flexor retinaculum is usually highly effective.

- **Ulnar nerve entrapment** This is usually at the elbow due to previous trauma. The patient complains of a weak, clumsy hand. The hypothenar and interosseus muscles may be wasted and ulnar function will be impaired. If the problem is at the elbow, ulnar nerve transposition in front of the medial epicondyle sometimes helps.

- **Trigger finger** Localised thickening of the flexor tendon with associated narrowing of the sheath causes the finger to catch as it is flexed, and straighten suddenly with assistance with a snap. Surgical release of the tendon sheath is the only treatment.

- **Ganglion** Ganglia are tense cysts associated with tendon sheaths or joints. They are commonly found around the wrist and hand. They usually cause no symptoms other than cosmetic, and are best left alone. Recurrence after excision is common.

Box 19.4 The causes of low back pain

Mechanical causes
Lumbar disc prolapse
Spondylosis (degenerate spine)
Spondylolisthesis (slip of one vertebra on another due to disc
  degeneration)
Ligamentous injuries
Spinal canal stenosis

Inflammatory disorders
Arthritis (of facet joints)
Ankylosing spondylitis

Infection
Bacterial discitis
Tuberculosis of the spine (Pott's disease)

Metabolic bone disease
Paget's disease of bone (see p. 293)
Osteoporosis

Tumours of bone (see p. 281-284)
Metastases
Myeloma

Referred pain
Ruptured aortic aneurysm
Pancreatitis
Peptic ulceration
Ureteric colic/pyelonephritis

Spine

Low back pain

- Causes The causes of low back pain are summarised in Box 19.4. Although debilitating, most cases are due to a combination of degeneration and trauma and will settle. Only a small but important minority require surgery, mostly for nerve root decompression to relieve referred pain down the leg (sciatica). A careful history and examination is necessary to make a diagnosis of the cause. Several of the mechanical causes of back pain result in severe muscle spasm, explaining the flare-ups of a chronic problem that many patients experience.
- History Mechanical pain is usually intermittent. Constant pain suggests a more serious (infective or malignant) cause. Pain on coughing and sneezing is commonly due to disc prolapse. A detailed history may narrow the differential diagnosis outlined in Box 19.4.
- Examination Local changes in the back (muscle spasm, local tenderness) may be seen but are not especially helpful in determining the cause. Pain and muscle spasm may alter normal spinal posture; in particular, the lumbar lordosis is often lost. Accurate neurological examination of the lower limbs is critical. Straight leg raising (stretches the sciatic nerve) and the femoral stretch test (with the patient prone, flex the knee and lift the thigh) reproduce nerve root pain.

Kumar and Clark's Handbook of Medical Management

Table 19.4 Comparison of L5 and S1 nerve root compression

L5	S1 (the commonest)
Pins and needles and reduced sensation in L5 dermatome (includes dorsum of foot, hallux and second toe)	Pins and needles and reduced sensation in S1 dermatome (includes lateral thigh and calf and lateral three toes)
Weak extensor hallucis longus	Weak plantarflexion of ankle
Weak dorsiflexion of ankle (tibialis anterior)	Weak eversion of ankle
Wasting of extensor digitorum brevis	Absent/diminished ankle jerk reflex

- **Investigation** MRI scanning is the most useful investigation and has replaced plain films and CT.
- **Treatment** Having excluded the more serious causes, treatment of mechanical low back pain is usually non-operative with a combination of rest, low-impact exercise, analgesia, NSAIDs, manipulation, physiotherapy, and weight loss. There is little consensus across the musculoskeletal disciplines about the most effective therapy for mechanical low back pain. Complementary therapies are widely used. Surgery is effective for referred leg pain due to nerve root compression, but not for most other causes.

Intervertebral disc prolapse

The L5/S1 disc compressing the S1 nerve root is the commonest prolapsed disc. The one above (L4–5 compressing the L5 root) is next. The pain is severe, radiating down the back of the leg (sciatica) into the appropriate dermatome, exacerbated by coughing and sneezing, and straight leg raising. Muscle spasm limits movements. Disturbance of sphincter function is an important symptom indicating a large disc prolapse likely to need surgical treatment. Table 19.4 highlights the signs of the two commonest types of disc prolapse.

Most cases settle with non-operative treatment. Bed rest (once advocated for this condition) is now considered to prolong the problem and patients are advised to try to remain mobile. Analgesics, NSAIDs, muscle relaxants, physiotherapy/manipulation and epidural anaesthesia may all help. Surgery is indicated for persistent cases which fail to resolve, recurrent episodes and large central disc bulges disturbing bladder function.

LOWER LIMB

Osteoarthritis of the hip

History

Hip pain is felt in the groin, thigh or referred to the knee. Pain is worse on walking and at the end of the day, and may disturb sleep. If the hip becomes stiff it becomes difficult to put on shoes and socks and to cut toenails.

Examination

- Look
- Gait: a painful hip results in an antalgic gait (painful limp) progressing to Trendelenburg gait as the hip muscles weaken (the pelvis on the opposite side sags as the bad leg takes the weight).
- Scars and sinuses.
- Hip position: severely arthritic hips are fixed in flexion, internally rotated and adducted.
- Feel
- Crepitus on movement.
- Measure true and apparent limb length. The apparent length is measured from the umbilicus to the medial malleoli with the patient lying flat. True length is measured from the anterior superior iliac spine to the medial malleoli. If the affected limb is fixed in an abnormal position of abduction or adduction, the opposite limb must be placed in a symmetrical position to make the true measurement.
- Move
- Establish active and passive range of movement. The key to hip examination is distinguishing pelvic from hip movement.

Investigation

Plain X-rays are usually sufficient to confirm a clinical diagnosis. ESR is normal and rheumatoid factor is absent; the reverse is true in rheumatoid arthritis.

Management

Non-operative management entails weight loss, physiotherapy, custom-made shoes to adjust for leg length, walking stick and NSAIDs.

Total hip replacement is the definitive surgical treatment. Modern prostheses last 15–20 years. Infection (under 1%) and loosening are the main causes of failure.

The knee

Osteoarthritis of the knee

Pain on walking, later also at rest, is the symptom. Stiffness, swelling and deformity (varus or valgus) develop, and loose bodies may cause locking. Non-operative treatments include analgesia, NSAIDs, physiotherapy, a walking stick and special shoes if leg length is uneven.

Surgical options include arthroscopy (washes out joint and relieves pain for up to a year), osteotomy (realigns the joint surfaces, transferring weight to the healthier side of the knee), knee replacement and arthrodesis. Knee replacement is now the definitive treatment for severe OA.

Knee haemarthrosis

Many acute knee injuries cause bleeding into the joint which causes tense, painful swelling (haemarthrosis). Some will settle with rest and elevation but early arthroscopy allows the blood to be washed out and the precise injury to be diagnosed. The causes of acute knee haemarthrosis are listed in Table 19.5.

Meniscal tears

There are five main types of meniscal problem (Fig. 19.1).

A painful, twisting sporting injury is common when a cracking noise may have been heard followed by pain and knee swelling. The knee may

Table 19.5 Causes of acute haemarthrosis of the knee

Lesion	Percentage
Anterior cruciate ligament rupture	39
Peripheral meniscal tear	26
Collateral ligament injury	13
Capsular tear	9
Osteochondral fracture	7
Posterior cruciate ligament rupture	6

Seventy per cent have more than one lesion, 29% have only one lesion, and in 1% no cause is found.

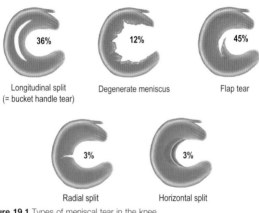

Longitudinal split (= bucket handle tear) 36%

Degenerate meniscus 12%

Flap tear 45%

Radial split 3%

Horizontal split 3%

Figure 19.1 Types of meniscal tear in the knee.

lock or catch if the tear becomes lodged in the joint. Over time the quadriceps wastes.

Mild tears may heal without treatment but persistent symptoms require arthroscopy, which is diagnostic and therapeutic, since the tear may be excised. Physiotherapy is crucial to a successful outcome after surgery. MRI is as accurate as diagnostic arthroscopy.

Anterior cruciate ligament (ACL) injuries

Typically sustained by footballers, these twisting injuries are usually acutely memorable by the victim who hears a loud crack followed by an immediate painful haemarthrosis. The acute symptoms may subside but the knee is left feeling unstable and the footballer has difficulty running round corners.

Examination detects only 70% of ACL ruptures; the remainder require MRI.

Intensive physiotherapy, a knee brace and lifestyle modification may be all that is required. When required, the ACL can be reconstructed using prosthetic or autologous tissue. Early repair is indicated if a fragment of tibia has been avulsed with the tear. Hamstring, or part of the contralateral patellar, can be used for repair.

Posterior cruciate ligament (PCL) injuries

This is less common and may occur when the tibia is forced posteriorly, for example in a head-on car crash. Once the acute injury has settled, the symptoms may be minimal. Walking downstairs exacerbates the sensation of instability. Like ACL injuries, non-operative treatment often suffices but PCL repair is also possible.

Recurrent dislocation of the patella

Full dislocation results from direct trauma to the medial side of the knee, displacing the patella laterally causing severe pain, swelling and a knee locked in flexion. X-rays confirm the diagnosis and may show an associated osteochondral fracture of the lateral femoral condyle.

Ankle and foot

Hallux valgus

Valgus deviation of the metatarsophalangeal joint of the great toe is common, especially in elderly females. The deformity may result in a painful bunion, or osteoarthritis of the joint. A bunion is the painful swelling of the bursa over the prominent head of the first metatarsal. Surgical correction of the deformity (usually by osteotomy) is effective but must be reserved for patients with healthy peripheral circulation.

Paget's disease of bone (osteitis deformans)

This condition affects the elderly; the cause is unknown. The normal turnover of bone is disordered, and healthy bone is gradually replaced by thickened, weak and soft bone. The skull, spine, pelvis and femur are the commonest bones to be affected but sometimes a single bone may be involved (monostosic Paget's disease).

The symptoms are pain and deformity of the affected bone. Pathological fractures may occur. Paget's disease affecting the skull can cause headache and deafness. The diseased bone is very vascular and acts as an arteriovenous fistula and may precipitate high output heart failure. Osteosarcoma complicates <1% of cases of Paget's disease of bone.

Serum calcium is normal but alkaline phosphatase is very high. Isotope bone scan demonstrates increased uptake and plain X-rays show thick, sclerotic bone. Treatment is with bisphosphonate.

Hip disorders in children

Table 19.6 summarises the age ranges for the common hip disorders found in children.

Table 19.6 Age ranges for the common hip disorders found in children

Age	Condition
0–5 years	Developmental dysplasia of the hip (formerly known as congenitally dislocated hip)
5–10 years	Perthes' disease
10–15 years	Slipped upper femoral epiphysis

Kumar and Clark's Handbook of Medical Management

> **Box 19.5** Risk factors for DDH
>
> Female sex
> Family history
>   Affected sibling – 6% chance
>   Affected mother – 12% chance
>   Affected sibling and mother – 35% chance
> First born child
> Breech presentation
> Coexistent talipes
> Any other congenital anomaly
> Oligohydramnios

Developmental dysplasia of the hip (previously called congenitally dislocated hip)

Hip instability at or soon after birth due to an underdeveloped acetabulum and ligamentous laxity is known as developmental dysplasia of the hip (DDH). The incidence is around 1 per 1000 live births and is four times commoner in females; 60% of cases involve the left hip, 20% right and 20% are bilateral (bilateral DDH is particularly difficult to diagnose). Risk factors for DDH are summarised in Box 19.5.

Early diagnosis and treatment yields a 95% cure rate. Delayed diagnosis leads to early osteoarthritis in adulthood requiring joint replacement.

● **Clinical features of DDH** An important part of the postnatal check is examination of the hips. There may be asymmetry of the groin skin creases. Two tests are used: the Barlow test detects an unstable dislocatable hip and the Ortolani test identifies a dislocated but reducible hip. If not diagnosed in infancy, parents notice a waddling (Trendelenburg) gait between the ages of 18 months and 3 years.

● **Investigation for DDH** The most frequently identified radiological signs of DDH are summarised in Figure 19.2. Ultrasound may also be diagnostic especially in the neonate.

● **Management** Diagnosis and treatment at birth result in a normal hip. Delayed detection leads to poor outcome.

Before 6 months a splint is used to hold the hip in abduction and flexion (e.g. Pavlik harness or von Rosen splint). The device is worn until the acetabulum is seen to be developing normally.

After 6 months the hip is dislocated and traction in abduction is required for several weeks to encourage reduction. Surgery may be required to encourage reduction after which further immobilisation in plaster is required.

In older children surgery is needed to reduce the hip and femoral osteotomy may be required. Over the age of 7 years, management is non-operative until osteoarthritis develops in adulthood.

Perthes' disease

This avascular necrosis of the femoral head of unknown cause occurs in 1 in 9000 children, usually in boys (male/female 4:1) aged 5–10. The

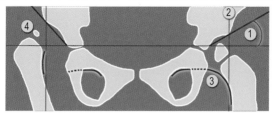

DDH   **Normal**

① Acetabular angle:
should be <30°

③ Shenton's line:
broken on
dislocated side

② Perkins' lines:
ossification centre
should be in inner,
lower quadrant

④ Ossification centre:
smaller on
dislocated side

Figure 19.2 Common radiological features of the dislocated hip.

femoral head collapses and half of cases require joint replacement for secondary osteoarthritis by age 45. Presentation is with limp and ache but few or no signs. X-ray may show an effusion. Management is avoidance of weight-bearing until the pain subsides. If the femoral head subluxes, surgery may be needed.

Slipped upper femoral epiphysis (SUFE)

This is most frequently seen in boys of African descent aged 10–15, usually on the left and bilaterally in 10% of cases. If one side is affected, there is a 1 in 4 chance the other side will also slip.

Hip pain (in groin, thigh or knee) and a limp are the presenting symptoms. A 'frog' lateral X-ray is required since SUFE may be missed on a simple anteroposterior view.

Surgery is always required, either pinning alone or reduction and pinning for more severe slips. Secondary osteoarthritis usually results if the slip progresses beyond 50%.

Irritable hip

This very common condition affecting children aged 2–12 years causes hip pain and a limp. The cause is unknown but postulated to be viral. Irritable hip is self-limiting and benign, but is a diagnosis that can only be made when more serious conditions (Box 19.6) have been excluded.

Blood tests (WBC, CRP, ESR, blood cultures and rheumatoid factor) and X-rays should be normal. Ultrasound may show an effusion, and aspiration allows microscopy and culture of the synovial fluid.

Bed rest is usually advised until the diagnosis is confirmed. Follow-up X-ray at 6 weeks confirms that a more serious pathology (Perthes' disease or SUFE) has not been missed.

Box 19.6 The differential diagnosis of irritable hip in children

Perthes' disease
Slipped upper femoral epiphysis
Osteomyelitis/septic arthritis
Rheumatoid arthritis
Rheumatic fever
Trauma

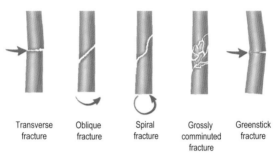

| Transverse fracture | Oblique fracture | Spiral fracture | Grossly comminuted fracture | Greenstick fracture |

Figure 19.3 Classification of fractures. A comminuted fracture is one with more than two bone fragments. Grossly comminuted fractures are usually associated with extensive soft tissue injury. Greenstick fractures occur in children whose bones are more flexible.

FRACTURES

Classification of fractures

A classification of fractures is described in Figure 19.3. A comminuted fracture is one with more than two bone fragments. Grossly comminuted fractures are usually associated with extensive soft tissue injury. Greenstick fractures occur in children whose bones are more flexible.

Every fracture is either closed (= simple) or open (= compound). Closed fractures are not in contact with the exterior. An open or compound fracture communicates to the outside usually via a skin wound, but fractures breaching a mucous membrane (e.g. pelvic fractures and the bladder/rectum or skull fractures involving sinuses) are also considered open fractures.

Fracture healing

Haematoma formation

After a bone fractures, it bleeds into the surrounding tissues forming a variable sized haematoma around the bone ends.

Inflammation: cellular proliferation and organisation

Just like soft tissue damage, bony injury is followed by an acute inflammatory reaction with vasodilatation, increase in local capillary

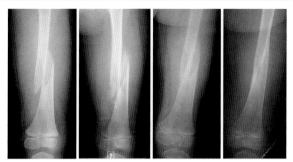

Figure 19.4 Consolidation/remodelling of fracture site (left to right).

permeability and influx of acute inflammatory cells. The haematoma becomes organised into granulation tissue, permeated by new capillary loops and fibroblasts.

Callus formation

Periosteum-derived osteoblasts proliferate and invade the organised haematoma and become calcified to form weak woven bone which envelops the fracture (callus). The callus becomes visible on plain X-ray within 3 weeks (2 weeks in a child).

This phase of early bone formation requires some movement at the bone ends. Completely rigid fixation (e.g. by internal fixation with plates and screws) abolishes callus formation. In this case, bone healing will only occur by direct bone contact.

Callus is progressively replaced by mature (lamellar) bone which immobilises and unites the fracture.

Consolidation and remodelling

After a fracture has united, the new bone is reorganised and the bone regains its original strength (consolidation). The fusiform mass of healing bone takes up to 2 years to return to its normal shape (remodelling, see Fig. 19.4).

Factors predisposing to poor fracture healing

Factors impairing healing of wounds including fractures are listed in Box 2.1, p. 14.

Delayed union

Healing is considered delayed if union has not occurred within 1.5 times the normal time frame.

Non-union

The fracture fails to heal within twice the normal time frame. There are two types of non-union: hypertrophic, due to inadequate immobilisation (the bone ends look like opposing elephants' feet) and atrophic, usually due to poor blood supply (the bone ends look sclerotic). The scaphoid bone is a good example of a bone notorious for non-union. In Figure 19.5 there is a radiological gap between the fragments that can be assumed to be filled with fibrous tissue. There is some, although not much, evidence of sclerosis.

Kumar and Clark's Handbook of Medical Management

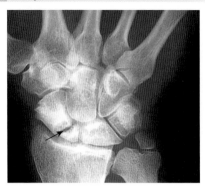

Figure 19.5 Non-union. This fracture of the scaphoid bone has failed to unite.

Mal-union

The fracture unites in a non-anatomical position. The resulting deformity may be of length (shortening), angulation or rotation.

Principles of fracture management

Treatment of fractures requires:
- reduction
- immobilisation
- rehabilitation.

Reduction

Reduction is the term given to restoring a deformity associated with a fracture to a normal anatomical position. Fractures with no deformity are considered undisplaced and do not need reduction. Some displaced fractures may be allowed to heal without compromising function, e.g. fractures of the clavicle and some tibial shaft fractures where up to a 50% transverse displacement is acceptable.

Reduction may be achieved by:
- closed manipulation under anaesthetic
- traction on either skeleton or skin
- open reduction indicated when:
  - closed methods fail
  - the fracture involves a joint and very accurate reduction is required.

Immobilisation

Immobilisation relieves pain and prevents excessive movement at the fracture site which would impair healing. Some fractures, e.g. rib injuries, are held in place by surrounding structures and heal without immobilisation. Other bones require rigid fixation to heal, e.g. scaphoid and shaft of ulna. Methods of fracture immobilisation are summarised in Box 19.7.

Rehabilitation

Rehabilitation should start as soon as the fracture is reduced and immobilised. The injured area should be moved as much as the method of immobilisation permits. The slight movement at the fracture site encourages

Box 19.7 Methods of immobilisation of fractures

External splints
Plaster of Paris
Synthetic resin casts
Cast braces (hinged splints)

Traction (skeletal or skin)
Traction is applied to the distal limb either via a pin through a bone or via adhesive bandages on the skin. This confines the patient to bed for a long period with high risk of complications of chest infections, bed sores, disuse osteoporosis, muscle weakness and deep vein thrombosis

External fixation
The fracture is fixed by a rigid external bridge held in place by pins into the bone above and below the fracture. Mainly used for open (compound) fractures

Internal fixation
Accurate, rigid fixation is achieved by screws, plates and pins, allowing early mobilisation. Indicated for multiple injuries, pathological fractures and fractures involving joints to achieve precise reduction and fixation

Table 19.7 Classification of open fractures

Type of fracture	Surface wound	Description	Infection risk
I	<1 cm	Low-velocity injury, minimal soft tissue damage	Low: under 2%
II	>1 cm	Low-velocity, minimal soft tissue damage	Moderate: under 10%
III	Any size	High-velocity injury with severe soft tissue damage, or grossly contaminated wound (e.g. military or agricultural accident)	Over 10%

callus formation, and the activity prevents joint stiffness, muscle atrophy and disuse osteoporosis.

Open fractures

Open (compound) fractures are surgical emergencies because of risk of infection of the fractured bone. If the bone becomes infected, chronic osteomyelitis results, which may prevent union and even threaten the limb. Open fractures are classified as shown in Table 19.7.

Kumar and Clark's Handbook of Medical Management

Box 19.8 The complications of fractures

Early local
Haemorrhage
Infection
Vascular injury (e.g. spike of bone damaging vessel)
Nerve injury
Compartment syndrome
Delayed union
Non-union

Early general
Deep vein thrombosis
Pulmonary embolism
Fat embolism
Pressure sores
Chest infection
Disuse osteoporosis

Late local
Mal-union
Chronic regional pain syndrome Type 1 (reflex sympathetic dystrophy)
Myositis ossificans
Joint stiffness
Osteoarthritis

Late general
Osteoporosis

Type III fractures are subdivided into:

- IIIa: adequate bone cover possible
- IIIb: wide stripping of periosteum with devascularisation of bone possible
- IIIc: associated vascular injury requiring repair.

Immediate first aid treatment requires a sterile or antiseptic dressing to cover the wound. Antibiotics and tetanus prophylaxis are given early.

Surgical debridement of the wound with reduction and immobilisation as appropriate is required as soon as possible: definitive treatment within 8 hours reduces the infection risk considerably.

Complications of fractures

Fracture complications are divided into early and late, and local and general, and are listed in Box 19.8.

Disorders of the eye 20

CLINICAL ASSESSMENT OF THE EYE

Most eye disorders can be diagnosed by history and examination; special investigations are rarely necessary. Causes of eye symptoms are summarised in Table 20.1.

History

- Pain: onset, duration, relieving and exacerbating factors, periodicity, trauma
- Vision: nature of disturbance, sudden/gradual, partial/total, bilateral/unilateral, change in acuity, visual field loss, double vision
- Redness: onset, presence of discharge
- Tears: excessive tears or dry eyes.

Examination

Equipment needed for a thorough eye examination is a Snellen chart of letters for visual acuity testing, a bright pen torch and an ophthalmoscope.

The important features of eye examination are shown in Table 20.2.

Visual acuity

Visual acuity by the Snellen chart at 6 metres is most commonly used with the subject wearing full refractive correction and bright, ambient illumination.

Pinhole acuity should be measured whenever the acuity with or without refractive correction is worse than 6/9.

Visual fields

The visual fields are assessed by the confrontation method. In addition, hemi-field comparisons may be made along with a kinetic field test using a white hat pin with a 5 mm diameter head.

The rules of interpretation of acuity and field tests are:

- lesions anterior to the chiasma affect one eye only
- lesions at the chiasma usually damage the crossing nasal fibres from each eye to give rise to bitemporal field defects
- lesions posterior to the chiasma damage the temporal fibres from one eye plus the nasal fibres from the other eye, causing a homonymous defect.

Pupils

Abnormal pupillary responses are summarised in Table 20.3. The light reflex (parasympathetic) is intact when a light shone on one eye constricts both pupils at an equal rate and to a similar degree.

Examination of the pupils should occur in both bright and dim light. Observation of the direct and consensual light responses is made when a bright light is shone into one eye. If there is an afferent defect on one side,

Table 20.1 Common symptoms of eye disease

Nature	Type	Causes
Pain	Ocular referred	Uveitis, acute glaucoma Paranasal sinuses Dental
Visual disturbances	Distortion Photophobia Halos Flashing lights Floaters Acute visual loss Chronic visual loss Night blindness	Disease of the macula Uveitis, corneal disease Acute glaucoma Vitreous and retinal disorders, migraines Vitreous and retinal disorders Retinal, vascular and neurological disorders Media opacities, retinal, vascular and neurological disorders Retinal degeneration
Double vision (diplopia)	Monocular Binocular	Cataract, refractive errors Extraocular muscle imbalance
Altered appearance of the eye	Red eye Proptosis	Conjunctivitis, episcleritis, uveitis, acute glaucoma Infection, thyroid eye disease
Lacrimal disturbance	Dry eye Watery eye	Primary lacrimal failure, Sjogren's syndrome Ocular irritation, blocked tear drainage

Table 20.2 Ophthalmic examination

Property examined	Tests and abnormal findings
Visual acuity (normal = 6/6)	At distance At near Pinhole
Visual field	Confrontation Formal perimetry
Ocular motility	Misalignment of visual axis Nystagmus
Pupil responses	Unequal size (anisocoria) Distortion Reaction to light Response to accommodation Afferent pupil defect
Examination of anterior eye by torch	Redness Clarity Depth of anterior chamber
Digital tonometry	Subjective hardness of globe
Fundoscopy	Red reflex Optic disc Macula Retinal vessels

Table 20.3 Abnormal responses of the pupil

Abnormality	Common causes
Dilatation	Third nerve lesion Adie pupil Mydriatic drugs Iris trauma
Constriction	Horner's syndrome Argyll Robertson pupil Drugs: opiates, cholinergic
Failure of accommodation/ convergence	Extrapyramidal disease (parkinsonism) Pineal tumour
Marcus Gunn pupil	Damage to the anterior visual pathway up to the lateral geniculate nucleus

then the stimulus to constriction when the light is shone on the affected side will be reduced. When the torch is swung quickly from one eye to the other, the pupils will dilate when the light is shone on the affected side (paradoxical dilatation).

Eye movements

The ability to move both optic globes is tested by asking the patient to let her eye follow the examiner's finger whilst keeping the head steady.

External eye appearance

Examination of the external eye should include skin lesions, inflammation, the position of the eyelids (ptosis, retraction, entropion or ectropion), proptosis and general facial examination.

Red eye and opacities of the cornea can be seen easily with a torch whilst fluorescein staining reveals areas of the cornea that have been denuded of epithelium (bright yellow fluorescence when viewed with a blue light).

Intraocular pressure

Intraocular pressure is measured using a tonometer.

Fundoscopy

Fundoscopy, using a hand-held direct ophthalmoscope, provides a magnified view of the cornea, aqueous, lens and vitreous. Fundoscopy should be carried out in a darkened room with both pupils dilated using mydriatics, for example tropicamide 1%, and a sympathomimetic (phenylephrine 2.5%). The green/red filters render the blood vessels black and easy to view. Refractive errors in the observer can be dealt with by adjusting the dioptre strength in the ophthalmoscope or by the patient wearing their normal glasses. Features to note are the optic disc, the macula and the retinal vessels.

The optic disc should be sharp and the colour pink. A cup/disc ratio of 0.3 or less is considered normal.

The macula is the area of central vision which lies approximately 1.5 disc diameters temporal to the optic disc. The appearance is a darker hue than the rest of the retina with a central glistening area which is the reflection from the fovea.

The retinal vessels should be inspected for:

- size: arteriolar attenuation (hypertension), venous dilatation (venous obstruction)
- crossing over of the retinal vessels for signs of nipping (hypertension)
- microaneurysms (diabetes).

OPHTHALMIC EMERGENCIES

Box 20.1 lists conditions which should be considered for emergency referral.

THE RED EYE

The features of the dangerous red eye are shown in Box 20.2 and urgent referral to an ophthalmologist is required if these are present.

The presence or absence of pain helps narrow down the possible causes of the red eye (Table 20.4).

THE PAINFUL EYE

It is helpful to elicit if the pain is superficial or deep. Headache associated with visual symptoms occurs in migraine and giant cell arteritis and should not be confused with ocular pain. Common causes include corneal abrasion, keratitis, glaucoma and uveitis.

Corneal abrasions result from trauma, and there is usually a clear history of the injury. Abrasions may be identified with fluorescein 2% stain and cobalt blue light. Treatment is with broad-spectrum antibiotic eye drops four times a day for 5 days and an eye patch if the pain is severe.

Box 20.1 Conditions that require emergency referral to an ophthalmologist

Trauma
    Suspicion of penetrating injury or foreign body
    Blunt injuries or fractures of the orbit
    Damage to either eyelid or tear duct
    Burns
Painful red eyes
Visible corneal lesions
Recent eye surgery
Orbital cellulitis

Box 20.2 Features of the dangerous red eye

Symptoms
Severe pain
Photophobia
Loss of vision
Progression of symptoms

Physical features
Reduced visual acuity
Unilateral
Intense injection
Corneal opacity, epithelial defect
Proptosis
Loss of red reflex

At-risk individual
Neonate
Immunocompromise
Contact lenses

Keratitis is an inflammation of the cornea and may be due to herpes virus infection or bacteria, for example *Neisseria gonorrhoeae*. Predisposing conditions include contact lenses, dry eyes and long-term use of eye drops containing steroids.

Acute anterior uveitis (inflammation of the iris and/or ciliary body) may be associated with systemic disorders, for example HLA B27-positive arthropathies and sarcoidosis. Pain is usually moderate. Redness is most marked around the cornea (Fig. 20.1). Specialist attention is required from an ophthalmologist.

Glaucoma is characterised by optic nerve fibre damage resulting in typical optic disc changes of cupping and visual field loss. Raised intraocular pressure is the key feature. There are many subgroups but acute and chronic glaucoma are the most important. Acute glaucoma is more

Kumar and Clark's Handbook of Medical Management

Table 20.4 Causes of red eye

	Painless	Uncomfortable	Painful
Normal vision	Subconjunctival haemorrhage (may be spontaneous or caused by coughing or minor trauma. Harmless and self limiting, no treatment required)	Blepharitis (acute or chronic inflammation of the eyelid, associated with recurrent styes; treatment is lid hygiene and topical antibiotics)	Anterior uveitis
		Conjunctivitis (usually viral, sometimes bacterial or chlamydial. Discharge is profuse)	Keratitis (peri-peripheral)
		Episcleritis (self-limiting autoimmune mediated inflammation causing discomfort and redness, NSAIDs usually effective)	Scleritis (autoimmune mediated severe inflammation causing severe deep eye pain, often associated with systemic lupus erythematosus, rheumatoid arthritis and vasculitis, ophthalmology referral required)
Impaired vision			Anterior uveitis
			Posterior scleritis (see above, as per scleritis, but redness is less pronounced)
			Keratitis (central)

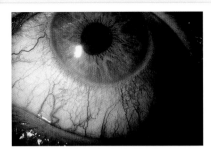

Figure 20.1 Acute anterior uveitis (iritis) with ciliary flush and a fixed, oval pupil.

common with advancing age and causes severe distress, eye pain, blurring of vision and halos around lights. Immediate referral is necessary and urgent treatment to lower the pressure of the eye is required.

OPHTHALMIC INJURIES

Assessment

It is important to determine the force applied, including direction and velocity, the nature of a foreign body and to be suspicious of an undetected injury. Orbital X-ray, CT or ultrasound are used to locate foreign bodies.

Burns

Causes include molten metal, ultraviolet light (welding or sunlamps) and chemicals. Extensive oedema in the eyelids and face after a thermal burn creates difficulty in examination and repeat assessment is necessary. Involvement of the eyelids requires referral to an ophthalmologist for lid repair. Ultraviolet burns are self-limiting and require reassurance that vision will return, along with pain relief. Chemical burns need copious irrigation with saline and urgent referral to an ophthalmologist.

Orbital injuries

Thirty per cent of patients who suffer maxillofacial trauma will sustain an ocular injury, of which 3% are blinding. Orbital and facial fractures require care by both maxillofacial surgeon and ophthalmologist. CT scanning is crucial to assess the injury and plan treatment.

Penetrating injuries

Penetrating injuries may be suspected when there is decreased visual acuity, a soft eye and a distorted iris (tear-drop shaped pupil, Fig. 20.2).

Ocular foreign bodies

Most foreign bodies in the eye are either trapped underneath the upper lid or stuck in the cornea. Removal is possible with the eye well-anaesthetised with topical tetracaine and the instillation of fluorescein to stain any corneal abrasions. A systematic search of the eye is conducted and foreign bodies removed with a sterile cotton bud. A one-week course of topical antibiotic is prescribed postoperatively. Retrieval of intraocular foreign bodies should be carried out by an ophthalmologist.

Kumar and Clark's Handbook of Medical Management

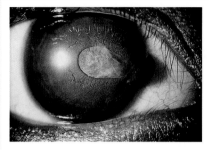

Figure 20.2
Penetrating injury of the cornea with iris prolapse causing pupillary distortion, and secondary cataract.

Table 20.5 Causes of visual loss

Time course	Painful		Painless (white eye)
	Red eye	White eye	
Acute	Trauma	AION – arteritic	CRAO/BRAO CRVO/BRVO AION – non-arteritic
Subacute	Uveitis	Optic neuritis	Wet ARMD Uveitis
	Orbital inflammation		
	Acute glaucoma		
Gradual	Uveitis	Optic nerve compression	Wet ARMD Dry ARMD Cataract Optic nerve compression Uveitis Chronic glaucoma
Transient	Migraine AION – artende		Migraine TIA (amaurosis fugax) Syncope

AION, anterior ischaemic optic neuropathy; ARMD, age-related macular degeneration; BRAO, branch retinal artery occlusions; BRVO, branch retinal vein occlusions; CRAO, central retinal artery occlusions; CRVO, central retinal vein occlusions; TIA, transient ischaemic attack.

VISUAL LOSS

Acute loss of vision

The causes of visual loss are shown in Table 20.5. They may be acute, subacute or gradual, and either partial or total. Unilateral symptoms are

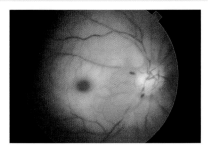

Figure 20.3 Central retinal artery occlusion with 'cherry red spot'.

likely to be from lesions of the eye or optic nerve. Bilateral lesions result from defects proximal to the optic chiasma in the brain.

Retinal artery occlusion

This occurs in the optic nerve, just behind the visible optic nerve head, usually as a result of a thrombosis of atheromatous vessels. Branch retinal artery occlusions are usually embolic, derived from atheroma from the carotid arteries. Emboli may be visualised on fundoscopy as white or yellow particles lodged in the bifurcations of the retinal arterioles. When the central retinal artery is involved, the visual loss is sudden and painless and the deficit profound. At fundoscopy, there is a pale retina with attenuated vessels and a cherry spot at the macula (Fig. 20.3). There is an impaired direct light response. Branch retinal artery occlusion affects vision, depending on the location of the vessel and a visual field defect (scotoma) results.

Retinal vein occlusion

Risk factors include diabetes, hypertension and hyperlipidaemia. Sudden loss of vision of variable severity occurs. Fundoscopy demonstrates dilated veins, haemorrhages and cotton wool spots in the affected area of the retina.

Anterior ischaemic optic neuropathy

This is an infarction of the optic nerve head. Risk factors include hypertension and angina or, in the over-70s, an arteritis usually as a result of temporal arteritis.

Management of acute visual loss

All patients with acute visual loss thought to be vascular in origin should have an urgent ESR and be referred immediately to an ophthalmologist if temporal arteritis is suspected. High doses of systemic steroids are required in this instance to prevent blindness and involvement of the other eye. Temporal artery biopsy may confirm the diagnosis.

If the nature of the visual loss suggests amaurosis fugax (transient clouding over of vision in one eye, typically like a curtain descending) a carotid duplex scan is indicated to look for carotid artery stenosis (see p. 215).

Subacute loss of vision

Optic neuritis

Visual loss develops over a few hours to 2–3 days, associated with ocular pain. Loss of acuity is variable. A swollen optic disc may be seen at fundoscopy. The most common cause is multiple sclerosis with patients in the 20–40-year age group.

Optic nerve compression

The optic nerve may be compressed, resulting in pain, visual loss and diplopia with reduced acuity, loss of colour vision, a relative afferent papillary defect, proptosis and conjunctival chemosis. Aetiologies include Graves' disease, orbital cellulitis, and orbital pseudotumour. In children, an optic nerve glioma should be considered. In adults, meningioma of the optic nerve sheath may also be a cause.

Gradual loss of vision

This is often not noticed by the patient until extensive. Causes include cataracts, macular degeneration, macular oedema and the rarer retinal dystrophies and uveitis.

Cataract

This is an opacity of the lens that interferes with vision. Most are of the idiopathic, senile type. Other causes include trauma, uveitis, diabetes and congenital. It is the most common cause of blindness in many parts of the world. Treatment is by extraction and insertion of a prosthetic intraocular lens when the reduction in vision is sufficient to interfere with lifestyle. Surgery is usually performed as a day case under local anaesthesia.

Macular degeneration

Age-related macular degeneration (AMD) is the most common cause of blindness in the developed world, affecting central vision with a reduction in visual acuity and the formation of a central scotoma. Two types are described: dry and wet. The former is often untreatable but the latter may respond to laser photocoagulation to seal off leaking vessels. Most recently an antibody to vascular endothelial growth factor (VEGF) injected into the eye, has been approved by NICE in cases of 'wet' AMD, halting progression of the disease in up to 90% of patients.

Chronic uveitis

Acute inflammation of the uvea (iritis and iridocyclitis) may present with a red, painful eye, but chronic uveitis may cause visual loss without other symptoms. This may occur in juvenile rheumatoid arthritis (hence children with arthritis must have regular ophthalmic screening). Management of these conditions is difficult and may involve the use of periocular or systemic steroids.

RETINAL DETACHMENT

Retinal detachment is usually spontaneous but may be traumatic. It causes a visual field loss which may be small, and visual acuity is retained unless the macula is involved. If the detachment is small, fundoscopy may be normal. The detachment is seen as an elevated convex area of grey retina which moves with ocular movement and has a wrinkled surface (Fig. 20.4). Treatment aims to oppose the detached retinal and underlying retinal pigment epithelium using laser or cryoprobe.

DISEASES WITH OPHTHALMIC MANIFESTATION

Acquired immune deficiency disease has a number of ophthalmic manifestations due either to a primary effect of HIV on retinal vasculature or

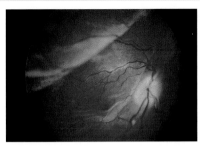

Figure 20.4 Retinal detachment.

to secondary opportunistic infections, for example cytomegalovirus, herpes simplex, staphylococcal and mycobacterial choroiditis. Fungal infections due to *Candida* or *Cryptococcus* may also occur. Toxoplasmosis and Kaposi's sarcoma have also been described.

Rheumatoid arthritis may also be associated with ophthalmic manifestations, as may systemic lupus erythematosus and giant cell arteritis (temporal arteritis). Graves' disease is described in Chapter 11.

Diabetic retinopathy is a leading cause of registration for blindness in the UK, occurring in both type 1 and type 2 diabetes. Visual loss can occur as a result of macular damage, vitreous haemorrhage or retinal detachment. The incidence of retinopathy increases with the duration of the disease and is reduced by good control of blood sugar and blood pressure. Laser treatment is effective in preventing visual loss from retinopathy and all diabetic patients should be screened for this.

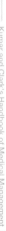

Ear, nose and throat surgery 21

THE EAR

The ear is concerned with hearing and balance, and has three parts: the external, middle and internal ear (Fig. 21.1).

Common symptoms of ear disease include:
- hearing loss (congenital or acquired)
- aural discharge
- otalgia (pain in the ear)
- tinnitus
- vertigo.

Investigations of auditory function

There are three types of hearing loss:
- conductive, due to disorders of the external and middle ear
- sensorineural, due to cochlear and retrocochlear lesions
- mixed conductive and sensorineural.

Tuning fork tests (Table 21.1)
- Rinne test – a vibrating tuning fork is placed near the external auditory meatus testing air conduction and then firmly on the mastoid process testing bone conduction. In a healthy ear, the sound is heard better by the ear (air conduction) than by the mastoid process (bone conduction).
- Weber test – a vibrating tuning fork is placed either on the vertex of the skull or on the forehead. The patient indicates on which side the sound is loudest.

Pure tone audiometry and impedance audiometry, along with electric response audiometry, further refine the investigations (Fig. 21.2).

Diseases of the external ear

Foreign bodies
Skilled personnel should always do extraction of foreign bodies to reduce the danger of forcing the foreign body further into the ear where it may damage the drum and middle ear.

Trauma to the auricle
Haematoma may occur, particularly in boxers and those who take part in contact sports. If blood extravasates between the cartilage and perichondrium, a cauliflower deformity composed of fibrous tissue ensues (classically seen in rugby forwards who damage ears in scrummages).

Otitis externa
- Clinical features There is discharge from the ear and occasional mild pain. In the spreading, necrotising variant, there is systemic disturbance with severe local symptoms which may include the development of a seventh nerve palsy.

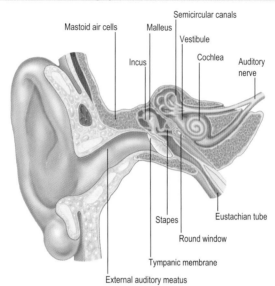

Figure 21.1 The anatomy of the ear.

Table 21.1 Interpretation of tuning fork tests

	Rinne	Weber
Normal	Air conduction better than bone conduction (test positive)	Both sides equal
Conductive deafness	Bone conduction better than air conduction (test negative)	Heard loudest on the affected side
Sensorineural deafness	Air conduction better than bone conduction but both reduced compared to normal (test positive but reduced)	Heard loudest on the good side

- **Management** In the mild type, topical antiseptics and antibiotics are incorporated into eardrops containing steroids. Aural toilet is essential, best done by an ENT surgeon with a microscope and micro-suction equipment. In severe cases, therapy consists of intensive local treatment with excision of dead tissue and administration of systemic antibiotics.

Diseases of the middle ear

Acute otitis media

This is common in young children and rare after 5 years of age. There is usually a history of upper respiratory tract infection. Inflammation of the

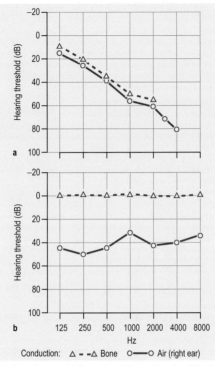

Figure 21.2 An audiogram. (a) Sensorineural loss with reduced hearing levels by both air and bone conduction. (b) Conductive hearing loss with reduced hearing level by air conduction and normal bone conduction.

post-nasal space and adenoids spreads via the Eustachian tube to the middle ear. Oedema in the tube causes blockage. If secondary bacterial infection spreads in the tube, a middle ear abscess results. *Haemophilus influenzae* is isolated in 30% of cases in those under 5 years of age. As pressure builds, rupture of the tympanic membrane occurs in the pars tensa. A small proportion of cases develop complications and there is loss of hearing. Other complications include chronic middle ear effusion, scarring of the tympanic membrane (tympanosclerosis), chronic suppurative otitis media and progression to mastoiditis.

Clinical features are pain and hearing loss. If the drum perforates, a purulent discharge develops with the resolution of pain. There may be malaise and pyrexia. On examination, the drum is reddened and tense. Perforation may be visible. Amoxicillin is the preferred drug for children and is administered for 10 days.

Acute mastoiditis

Mastoiditis is a consequence of preceding otitis media. There may be cellulitis and osteitis in the air spaces, which develop into an abscess. Spread

Kumar and Clark's Handbook of Medical Management

may occur through the temporal bone to cause intracranial complications, for example extradural abscess. Clinical features include pain, fever, aural discharge and hearing loss. There may be an erythematous, swollen mastoid and external canal on examination. Mastoid X-rays may show clouding of the air cells and formation of an abscess with erosion of bone. High-dose IV antibiotics are given. If resolution fails to occur, a cortical mastoidectomy may decompress the inflammatory process, preserving the posterior meatal wall and middle ear ossicles.

Otitis media with effusion (glue ear)

Accumulation of non-purulent fluid is common in children between 2 and 6 years of age. This is most likely caused by low-grade inflammation with partial block of the Eustachian tube. Symptoms include impaired hearing, which may rarely lead to a delay in learning to speak, inattentiveness and recurrent earaches. Many children are diagnosed during routing audiometric screening. Examination demonstrates a lustreless, immobile tympanic membrane with occasional fluid levels.

- **Management** In over 90% of cases, the effusion resolves spontaneously. Unresolved middle ear effusions with hearing loss require an anterior inferior myringotomy, aspiration of the tube and decompression using a grommet. If there is nasal obstruction, the adenoids are curetted.

  Middle ear effusions may occur in adults following an upper respiratory tract infection or allergic or vasomotor rhinitis. Chronic suppurative otitis media often follows acute otitis media which may be divided into tubotympanic suppuration limited to inflammation of the mucosa or atticoantral disease with destruction involving the mastoid bone. The latter may be complicated by cholesteatoma formation (a mass of keratinised squamous epithelium) which initially forms in the developed retraction pocket of a perforated tympanic membrane. Spread may occur, destroying middle ear ossicles and temporal bone causing marked hearing loss or vertigo if the cholesteatoma has eroded the bony wall of the most prominent lateral semicircular canal. CT scan may be helpful to demonstrate the extent of bony erosion. Radical mastoidectomy lays open the mastoid and excises the posterior meatal wall and contents of the tympanic cavity to create a safe cavity. Reconstruction using fascial grafts and artificial ossicles (tympanoplasty) may then be considered. The complications of otitis media are summarised in Box 21.1.

Otosclerosis

This is a localised disease of bone affecting the otic capsule. It is inherited as an autosomal dominant trait with incomplete penetration. New spongy bone develops. If this occurs in the area of the stapes, there may be ankylosis and deafness. There is a strong family history. Both ears are affected in 90% of patients, usually presenting in the second decade. Management includes hearing aids and stapedectomy, which restores the mobility of the ossicular chain.

Diseases of the inner ear

Sensorineural hearing loss

Causes include:

- genetic abnormalities
- maternal infections during pregnancy, for example rubella, cytomegalovirus and syphilis
- perinatal hypoxia

Box 21.1 Complications of otitis media

Intratemporal
Mastoiditis
Labyrinthitis
Facial nerve palsy

Intracranial

Extradural abscess   Temporal lobe abscess
Meningitis   Cerebellar abscess
Lateral sinus thrombosis

- viral and bacterial labyrinthitis
- meningitis
- ototoxic drugs, for example gentamicin, neomycin
- noise-induced hearing loss
- fractures of the temporal bone
- barotrauma to include rupture of the round window.

High audiometric frequencies are usually affected first. Tinnitus is often associated with sensorineural loss. Exposure to high intensity noise causes characteristic bilateral hearing loss on the audiogram.

Management includes hearing aids and air conduction aids consisting of miniature microphone, amplifiers and receivers. Bone conduction aids are used if there is a congenital absence of the pinna and atresia of the canal. Those who do not benefit from hearing aids may benefit from a cochlear implant.

Acoustic neuroma

- Clinical features There is unilateral or marked asymmetric sensorineural hearing loss and tinnitus. The audiogram reveals unilateral sensorineural hearing loss. MRI scan demonstrates the tumour.
- Management The tumour is removed by neurosurgery, hopefully with minimal damage to the facial nerve.

Menière's disease

Distension of the membranous labyrinth caused by endolymphatic hydrops is thought to be the pathological feature of Menière's disease. A characteristic triad of symptoms comprises vertigo, fluctuating sensory loss and tinnitus. Hearing gradually deteriorates over a period of time. Attacks of vertigo are treated with vestibular sedatives, for example diazepam and prochlorperazine. A salt-restricted diet may reduce the frequency of attacks. Decompression of the endolymphatic sac and vestibular neurectomy is indicated if medical treatment fails.

THE NOSE AND PARANASAL SINUSES

Features of nasal and sinus disease

Symptoms include nasal obstruction, mouth breathing, discharge and post-nasal drip. Unilateral discharge in a child probably originates from a foreign body. Bloodstained discharge with unilateral symptoms may be associated with tumour. Copious, watery discharge may suggest CSF rhinorrhoea. Facial pain may also occur, occasionally radiating into the teeth, eyes or ear. There may also be headaches, loss of smell, bleeding and cosmetic nasal deformity.

The anterior part of the nose can be examined using a nasal speculum. Deformities of the septum, mucosal changes, vessels and inferior and middle turbinates can be seen. Polyps, tumours, ulceration and foreign bodies can be identified. The posterior nasal space can be examined through the mouth by introducing a small mirror behind the soft palate.

Investigations of nasal disease:

- X-ray, which may show gross disease
- CT scanning of the sinuses gives precise images demonstrating mucosal swelling, fluid levels or opacities, as well as bony erosion by tumours
- MRI is especially useful for determining tumour infiltration
- Skin prick tests may identify possible allergens
- Smell may be detected by exposure to various bottles containing pungent substances, establishing whether smell is reduced or distorted.

Common conditions

Foreign bodies

Children often insert foreign bodies into the nostril, which may go undetected for some time. They may present with symptoms of unilateral discharge. A radio-opaque body may be seen on plain X-ray, which can then be removed with forceps, or hook; this may require a general anaesthetic.

Fractures of the nose

These may be associated with other fractures of the face, including zygoma, bony orbit and middle third. Symptoms include nasal deformity, obstruction and bleeding. Examination may demonstrate a deviated septum or haematoma. Nasal fractures may be reduced immediately or 7–10 days after the swelling has subsided.

Septal haematoma and abscess may develop between the mucoperichondrial flaps of the septum leading to septal cartilage ischaemia and secondary infection. This may lead to a saddle-type nasal deformity. The haematoma should be incised and drained. Nasal packing should be applied to allow the perichondrium to adhere to the cartilage.

The treatment of deviated nasal septum includes a septoplasty/submucus resection (SMR) where the cartilage is mobilised and the deviated part of the septum is excised.

Epistaxis

Several vessels anastomose in the anterior septum, known as Little's area, a frequent site for anterior nasal bleeding. Causes include:

- trauma
- tumours
- infection with ulceration
- prominent vessels
- atherosclerotic degeneration of greater nasal arteries
- bleeding diatheses
- blood disease
- hereditary telangiectasia.

- **Management** The nose is anaesthetised and decongested with 10% cocaine. The bleeding vessel can be cauterised chemically. If the bleeding point cannot be identified, ribbon gauze impregnated in bismuth iodoform paraffin paste (BIPP) is packed into the anterior nasal cavity. When the bleeding is from the back of the nose, an epistaxis balloon may be introduced through the nose into the post-nasal space and is then drawn forward through the nose and secured. Packs remain for 48 hours. Antibiotics are given. Frequent, repeated haemorrhage may require ligation of the appropriate vessel (e.g. external carotid, maxillary artery, ethmoidal arteries). Modern developments have also allowed embolisation of bleeding vessels by interventional radiologists.

Rhinosinusitis

Mucosal changes in the sinuses are often accompanied by changes in the nasal cavities. The causes are allergy, idiopathic or infective. In allergic rhinitis, inhaled substances including pollens from grass, trees and flowers are responsible for seasonal symptoms. House dust and pet fur cause more perennial symptoms. Acute infective rhinitis occurring secondary to the common cold or viral infections may be complicated by secondary bacterial infection. Common organisms include *Haemophilus influenzae* and *Streptococcus pneumoniae*. Any condition that interferes with mucociliary transport, for example deviated septum, polyps or hypertrophy of the turbinates, may predispose to the development of infective sinusitis. Swollen mucosa blocks the natural ostia and pus reduces the activity of the cilia leading to stasis in the sinuses. In chronic infection, the mucosa may be damaged and granulations may develop.

Symptoms of allergic rhinitis include:
- nasal itching
- sneezing
- profuse, watery discharge
- post-nasal drip.

With infective rhinosinusitis, the symptoms are unilateral, including:
- pain over the affected sinus and around the eye
- headache
- mucopurulent discharge
- nasal obstruction
- loss of smell.

Sinus X-ray and CT scan may reveal opaque sinuses or a fluid level.

Management of allergic rhinitis depends on demonstration of the allergen and advice on how to avoid it. Prophylaxis using sodium cromoglicate and steroid sprays may be effective and is without adverse systemic effects. Occasionally, non-sedating oral histamines may be added. Infective rhinosinusitis is treated with antibiotics and decongestant drops. Surgery may be required to re-establish air flow, including sinus washout, intranasal antrostomy or radical antrostomy (Caldwell–Luc operation).

Complications of infective sinusitis include:
- periorbital cellulitis
- subperiosteal abscess
- blindness
- suppuration of orbital contents
- osteomyelitis
- complications of the frontal bone and maxilla with subsequent sinus formation

- intracranial complications including meningitis, brain abscess and cavernous sinus thrombosis.

Symptoms include:
- diplopia
- restricted eye movement
- reduction of visual acuity
- swollen eyelids proptosis.

Intracranial complications may include:
- headache
- drowsiness
- photophobia.

Cavernous sinus thrombosis occurs rarely and is characterised by proptosis, swelling of the eyelids and ophthalmoplegia. CT scan demonstrates the opaque sinuses, bony defect, abscess formation, displacement of the eye and brain abscess.

Nasal polyps

These are pale grey, pedunculated mucosal tissue masses projecting into the nasal cavity. They originate in the region of the ethmoid. Twenty-five per cent of cases are associated with asthma and possible aspirin sensitivity (8%). Nasal obstruction, loss of smell and sneezing are the common complaints. The lesions may be visible on endonasal examination. Medical management includes topical steroid sprays. In the majority of cases, surgical removal is required, although polyps may recur.

Tumours of the nasal cavity

Benign and malignant tumours in the nasal cavity are rare. Benign tumours include papilloma, which has a tendency to recur, and there is a small risk of malignant change. The tumour is removed using the lateral rhinotomy approach. Osteomas may be an accidental finding on sinus X-ray. They are more common in the frontal area. These may be removed by a fronto-ethmoidectomy. Malignant tumours are squamous cells in origin and present with nasal and eye symptoms. Tumours in the nasal cavity and ethmoids present with nasal and eye symptoms. Maxillary tumours present with dental, orbital and nasal symptoms with facial swelling. Often the first feature is a lymph node in the neck. Treatment is a combination of radiotherapy and surgery. Craniofacial resection may be required when there is an extension of the tumour into the anterior cranial fossa.

SWELLINGS IN THE NECK

Clinical features

Important features include:
- the duration of the swelling
- its size progression
- pain
- other symptoms including hoarseness and dysphagia
- weight loss
- night sweats
- history of chronic exposure to alcohol or tobacco.

On examination, the site and size along with the relationship to other anatomical structures and fixation of the lump including its pulsatility or the presence of a bruit or thrill, tenderness or fluctuation must be noted. A thorough examination of the oral cavity and oropharynx must be made.

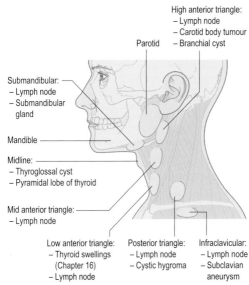

High anterior triangle:
– Lymph node
– Carotid body tumour
– Branchial cyst

Parotid

Submandibular:
– Lymph node
– Submandibular gland

Mandible

Midline:
– Thyroglossal cyst
– Pyramidal lobe of thyroid

Mid anterior triangle:
– Lymph node

Low anterior triangle:
– Thyroid swellings (Chapter 16)
– Lymph node

Posterior triangle:
– Lymph node
– Cystic hygroma

Infraclavicular:
– Lymph node
– Subclavian aneurysm

Figure 21.3 Sites of swelling in the neck and their likely causes.

The nasopharynx and laryngopharynx require indirect examination with a mirror.

Sites of swelling in the neck (Fig. 21.3) may indicate their origin. The most important landmark is the sternocleidomastoid muscle, which divides the neck into anterior and posterior triangles.

● Parotid swellings occur in front of the tragus over the angle of the mandible or below the lobe of the ear. Facial palsy may suggest malignant involvement.
● Submandibular gland swellings may be palpated bimanually via the mouth. They are difficult to distinguish from regional lymphadenopathy.
● Midline submental swellings are commonly a thyroglossal cyst, midline dermal cyst or pyramidal lobe of the thyroid.
● High anterior triangle swellings may be metastatic from the oral cavity but may also include branchial cyst or carotid body tumour.
● Low anterior triangle swellings are related to the thyroid or metastases from primary tumours in the larynx or pharynx.
● Supraclavicular swellings are common on the left side of the neck, caused by disease below the level of the clavicle, for example carcinoma of the lung or stomach.
● Posterior triangle swellings are rarely metastatic but more commonly tuberculosis, toxoplasmosis and lymphoma.

Lymph node enlargement is the commonest cause of a neck lump (see Fig. 21.3). Lymph nodes in the neck should not be biopsied until an ENT surgeon has excluded a primary tumour of the upper aerodigestive tract.

In most cases, multiple cervical masses are accompanied by an acute systemic illness or more chronically may be a presentation produced by tuberculosis. A swelling which is tender and has enlarged over a few days is almost always inflammatory. Lymphomas tend to develop over a period of weeks and are painless. Metastatic nodes may be tender on palpation but rarely cause pain unless there is invasion of surrounding nerves.

Investigation of neck lumps

Fine-needle aspiration (FNA), ultrasound and CT scanning are all useful to determine the cause. Blood tests may help diagnose infection causing lymphadenopathy (e.g. monospot test in glandular fever or HIV antibodies in HIV infection). If FNA suggests squamous carcinoma, an upper aerodigestive tract endoscopy must be done to include examination of the nasopharynx, hypopharynx, larynx and trachea, bronchus and cervical oesophagus. Adenocarcinoma metastases are usually of intra-abdominal or intrathoracic origin. If the cytology suggests lymphoma, incision biopsy may be necessary for further tissue to identify the lymphoma type. If a primary ENT tumour is found at endoscopy, treatment recommended depends on the site and size of the primary and cervical node metastases.

Specific causes of neck swellings

Lymph nodes

The majority of neck swellings are due to lymph node enlargement, most usually due to infection. Making the correct diagnosis and excluding malignancy depends on careful clinical assessment (Box 21.2).

> **Box 21.2** Causes of cervical lymphadenopathy
>
> **Infection**
> Non-specific viral infection
> Tonsillitis
> HIV
> Glandular fever
> Dental infection
> Syphilis
> Toxoplasmosis
> Tuberculosis
> **Lymphoma**
> Hodgkin's
> Non-Hodgkin's
> **Lymph node metastases**
> Squamous tumours of the nasopharynx
> Melanoma or squamous carcinoma of skin of head and neck
> Intra-abdominal and thoracic carcinomas
> **Sarcoidosis**

Lymphoma

The majority of lymphomas in the head and neck are non-Hodgkin's in type. Fine-needle aspiration cytology is insufficient for diagnosis and excision biopsy is required. Even if lymphoma is suspected, a primary ENT tumour must be excluded before excision, since removal of a node which turns out to be a metastasis of a primary cancer of the upper aerodigestive tract may prejudice subsequent treatment. Treatment of lymphomas is by haematologists and oncologists rather than surgical.

Thyroglossal cyst

Presentation occurs during the second or third decade of life. The mass is midline, between the thyroid notch and hyoid bone and moves upwards on protrusion of the tongue. The cyst is removed surgically and the central portion of the hyoid bone may need to be included in the excision.

Branchial cyst

Presentation occurs between the ages of 15 and 35 with a cyst in the upper part of the anterior triangle. It is smooth and mobile. The diagnosis is confirmed by FNA, which produces pale, creamy fluid. Treatment is by excision.

Carotid body tumour (chemodectoma)

Ten per cent are familial, 10% are bilateral and 10% are malignant. The patient presents in adult life with a history of a lump which is ovoid, non-tender and pulsatile. There is mobility in the horizontal but not vertical axis. Auscultation reveals a bruit. CT scan confirms the lesion. Carotid angiography may demonstrate a highly vascular mass. Surgical excision is required, and this is more easily done before the tumour gets too large (>2 cm).

Tumours of the upper aerodigestive tract

Malignant tumours are more common than benign. Squamous cell carcinomas are the most common form followed by lymphomas, salivary gland tumours, melanomas and sarcomas.

Squamous carcinoma

The most important predisposing factors are smoking, high alcohol intake and the presence of pre-malignant conditions. Other factors include chronic irritation, betel nut (common in the Indian subcontinent) and oral syphilis (rare).

Clinical features of upper aerodigestive tract tumours are site specific and may include local problems, for example unilateral nasal obstruction and epistaxis, diplopia, middle ear effusion or loosening of teeth. Local pain and referred otalgia are common. Many lesions are asymptomatic and the presenting symptom is a lump in the neck due to a lymph node metastasis. Hoarseness of the voice occurs in advanced cases. There may also be dysphagia in laryngeal, hypopharyngeal and cervical oesophageal lesions. Investigation depends on the known or likely site of the tumour. The presence of an unexplained hoarse voice for more than 6 weeks is an indication for direct laryngoscopy and biopsy. A diagnosis of functional dysphagia should not be made until both a barium swallow and oesophagoscopy have been shown to be normal.

- **Treatment** A multidisciplinary approach is required, using a combination of surgery and radiotherapy. Eradication of the tumour is a priority but preservation of function, particularly speech and swallowing, is important. Many patients present with advanced tumours and supportive care and analgesia are appropriate. For small tumours (stage T1 and T2), a full course of radiotherapy is the treatment of choice. Recurrences need to be treated by surgery. Large tumours do not respond well to radiotherapy and primary surgery is offered with or without postoperative radiotherapy. The metastatic lymph nodes may be treated at the same time as the primary tumour, either by radiotherapy or surgery. Some primary sites, for example tongue, bone and tonsil, have a high risk of microscopic nodal disease and prophylactic treatment of the ipsilateral neck is undertaken.

Survival rates depend on the size and site of the primary tumour and the presence or absence of metastatic disease. If lymph node metastases have developed, the prognosis for any tumour worsens considerably. The overall 5-year survival rate for all head and neck malignancies is 40%. Reconstruction of the defect after surgery for a large tumour is difficult to achieve and requires plastic surgical techniques including free grafts of split or full thickness, pedicled skin flaps or free flaps with varying results. Restoration of speech is possible by creating a tracheal-oesophageal fistula where a one-way valve is introduced. By occluding the tracheostomy with a finger during exhalation, the patient can divert air through the valve into the pharynx, thus producing speech by the air being set in vibration by the valve.

Diseases of the salivary glands

The three paired salivary glands (the parotid, submandibular and sublingual glands) may be subjected to viral and bacterial infections and neoplasia.

Parotitis

Infection in the parotid or submandibular salivary glands is uncommon but tends to occur in elderly, debilitated patients. In parotitis, the gland swells and becomes acutely tender. A plain X-ray may demonstrate a stone in the duct, which can also occur in the submandibular duct with similar clinical features and the stone identified on X-ray. Parotitis requires excellent mouth care, rehydration and antibiotics. Submandibular sialadenitis is treated in the same way but, if a stone is obvious, excision of the duct and removal of the stone may be required. Care must be taken when removing the duct that damage is not caused to the lingual nerve.

Pleomorphic adenoma

This is the most common benign tumour. If left for many years, it may undergo malignant transformation. The history is of a painless mass, usually in the parotid, which enlarges very slowly over a period of years. Surgical excision is the treatment of choice but requires careful removal to avoid rupture of the capsule (which may lead to tumour seeding and recurrence). A superficial parotidectomy is performed, avoiding injury to the facial nerve. Adenolymphoma (Warthin's tumour) is another common benign tumour of the parotid gland but may occur bilaterally in 10% of cases. Malignant neoplasms of the salivary glands are rare. Mucoepidermoid carcinomas, squamous carcinomas, adenocarcinomas and adenoid cystic carcinomas are the usual histological types. Surgery is the mainstay of removal. If a malignant parotid tumour directly involves the facial nerve, this structure must be sacrificed and continuity re-established using a segment of greater auricular or sural nerve.

Infection of the neck space

Peritonsillar abscess (quinsy)

There is a background history of acute tonsillitis which suddenly progresses with unilateral pain and dysphagia. A fluctuating pyrexia is invariable with the tonsil being displaced downwards and medially on examination. Intravenous antibiotics may be given in the early stages but, if there is a suspicion of pus, the inflammatory mass is incised.

Parapharyngeal abscesses, occurring lateral to the pharyngeal constrictors containing the carotid tree, internal jugular vein and cranial nerves, usually occur as a consequence of dental sepsis. Complications include direct spread to the mediastinum or mucosal oedema and pharyngeal and airway obstruction. Treatment is essential with intravenous antibiotics. A CT scan is obtained to ascertain whether or not there is a collection of pus. If present, this is drained through an incision running down the anterior border of the sternomastoid muscle.

Ludwig's angina

This is a soft tissue infection of the floor of the mouth on both sides of the mylohyoid muscle, usually resulting from dental sepsis. There is gross oedema of the mucosa of the floor of the mouth with upward and posterior displacement of the tongue which may obstruct the airway. Initial treatment with antibiotics and drainage of pus is the treatment of choice but it may be necessary to maintain the airway by nasopharyngeal-tracheal intubation or tracheostomy.

Vocal cord paralysis

This is the consequence of damage to the ipsilateral recurrent laryngeal nerve. Common causes include thyroid surgery, cardiac surgery, carcinoma of the bronchus, thyroid or oesophagus. Diagnosis depends on a detailed search for the cause. Treatment should only be undertaken for those patients who have an identifiable non-reversible cause. Medialisation of the vocal cord is used when one cord is paralysed, which is then moved medially to improve the voice and reduce aspiration, either by the injection of Teflon paste or a piece of thyroid cartilage wedged between it and the thyroid ala. Lateralisation of the vocal cord is used to improve the airway in bilateral palsy. In bilateral paralysis, permanent tracheostomy is usually the best management.

● Tonsillectomy The indications for tonsillectomy are given in Box 21.3.

Box 21.3 Indications for tonsillectomy

Recurrent tonsillitis with more than four attacks per year
Obstructive sleep apnoea with tonsillar hypertrophy in children
Peritonsillar abscess with a past history of recurrent tonsillitis
Persistent sore throat after glandular fever
Unilaterally enlarged tonsil with lymphoma a possibility

Figure 21.4 The two types of tracheostomy.

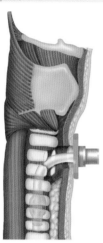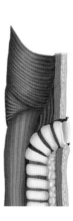

Box 21.4 Indications for tracheostomy

Supralaryngeal obstruction
Ludwig's angina
Severe facial fractures
Glandular fever

Laryngeal obstruction
Epiglottitis
Laryngeal tumour
Bilateral vocal cord palsy

Recurrent aspiration
Coma
Myasthenia gravis
Bulbar or pseudobulbar palsy

Respiratory support
Injury to the chest wall
Seriously ill or injured patients (ARDS)
Prolonged endotracheal intubation (increasingly common indication)

- **Tracheostomy** The two types of open tracheostomy are shown in Figure 21.4, either after a laryngectomy where the divided trachea is brought out and sutured to the skin or more frequently where a side opening is made and a tracheostomy tube is inserted on a temporary, permanent, elective or emergency basis. The indications for tracheostomy are given in Box 21.4. Temporary tracheostomy can be achieved percutaneously and is gaining popularity on intensive care units as it avoids the need for specialist ENT input and can be done at the bedside.

Neurosurgery

Head injuries and spinal trauma topics are covered in Chapter 4.

TUMOURS OF BRAIN, MENINGES AND SPINAL CORD

The commonest brain tumour is metastatic cancer but it is rare for such tumours to present to neurosurgeons unless the primary malignancy is undiagnosed, or the metastasis is solitary and slow growing.

Primary CNS tumours are summarised in Table 22.1.

Clinical features
- Raised intracranial pressure (headache, vomiting, papilloedema)
- Fits (beware late onset epilepsy, tumour must be excluded)
- Neurological deficit.

Diagnosis
Diagnosis is by CT or MRI scanning. Biopsy may be required to determine the type and grade of tumour, and to exclude cerebral abscess which may mimic a tumour.

Treatment
Benign tumours are excised via craniotomy. The options for treatment of malignant tumours are:
- chemotherapy
- conservative treatment (i.e. do nothing).

Prognosis depends on site, type and grade of tumour.

CEREBRAL HAEMORRHAGE

Cerebral haemorrhage is spontaneous bleeding within the cranial cavity. The three types are:
- intracerebral haemorrhage (within the brain substance)
- subarachnoid haemorrhage (within the subarachnoid space)
- subdural haemorrhage (within the subdural space).

Intracerebral haemorrhage

Intracerebral haemorrhage is associated with hypertension or an underlying abnormality such as vascular malformation or aneurysm. Presentation is with sudden onset headache, neurological deficit or coma.

Diagnosis
Diagnosis is as for subarachnoid haemorrhage, below.

Treatment
Cerebellar haematomas should be removed but there is little benefit in evacuating other intracerebral clots.

Table 22.1 Tumours of the central nervous system

Tumour	Origin	Features
Glioma	Derived from supporting tissues of the brain, types include: astrocytoma, oligodendrocytoma, ependymoma	Varying degrees of malignancy depending on cellularity, mitoses, pleomorphism and necrosis
Meningioma	Arise from meninges	Usually benign, rarely recur after removal
Neuroma	Acoustic neuroma (derived from eighth nerve) is commonest	Usually benign
Pituitary	Derived from pituitary gland	Clinical features: Visual disturbance due to pressure on the optic chiasma Metabolic abnormality if the tumour is endocrinologically active
Developmental	Derived from abnormal islands of cells at points of neural tube closure, commonest examples are: craniopharyngioma, colloid cyst of third ventricle, medulloblastoma, choroid plexus papilloma	Variable degree of malignancy

Subarachnoid haemorrhage

Subarachnoid haemorrhage is caused by:
- ruptured aneurysm (70%)
- vascular malformation (10%)
- unknown cause (20%).

Sudden death results in 40% of cases. Sudden onset of headache, neck stiffness and depression of consciousness occur in the remainder. One-third of those who survive the initial bleed die within 6 weeks.

Diagnosis

Diagnosis is by CT/MRI and lumbar puncture.

Treatment

Treatment consists of bed rest, supportive care and treatment of any underlying abnormality (e.g. endovascular coiling or surgical clipping of an aneurysm).

Subdural haematoma

Acute subdural bleeding results from trauma (see Ch. 4). Spontaneous bleeding occurs in cerebral atrophy, especially old age and alcoholism. Onset is gradual and may mimic a tumour.

Diagnosis
Diagnosis is as for subarachnoid haemorrhage, above.

Treatment
Evacuation is required.

HYDROCEPHALUS

Hydrocephalus is enlargement of CSF spaces. CSF is made in the lateral ventricles by the choroid plexuses. It passes into the third ventricle then via the aqueduct into the fourth ventricle and out into the subarachnoid space. It is reabsorbed into the blood by arachnoid granulations over the surface of the cerebral hemispheres.

Non-communicating hydrocephalus

This results from blockage, preventing CSF from reaching the subarachnoid space. Causes include intraventricular haemorrhage, congenital abnormalities and tumours.

Communicating hydrocephalus

There is normal CSF circulation but failure of reabsorption of CSF into the bloodstream. Causes include subarachnoid haemorrhage, head injury and meningitis. Clinical features depend on age and cause (Box 22.1).

Diagnosis
CT or MRI will show enlarged ventricles and may demonstrate the underlying cause.

Treatment
CSF drainage is required.

Box 22.1 Clinical features of hydrocephalus

Infants
Failure to thrive
Large head with tense fontanelle
Failure of up-gaze

Adults
Raised intracranial pressure
Signs associated with the underlying cause (head injury, subarachnoid haemorrhage or meningitis)

Elderly
Confusion
Ataxia
Incontinence

SPINAL DEGENERATIVE DISEASE

Disc prolapse

Prolapse of an intervertebral disc onto a nerve root causes severe pain in the distribution of the nerve dermatome and weakness of the muscles supplied. The L5/S1 disc is the most commonly affected, causing typical sciatica (pain down the back of the buttock, thigh and leg). MRI is the best method of confirming the diagnosis. Most cases resolve with analgesia and various forms of physical therapy. Surgical microdiscectomy is effective for intractable pain or when there is motor weakness.

Cauda equina compression

A large, central disc prolapse may compress the cauda equine causing bilateral sciatica and urinary retention. Surgical decompression is required urgently to prevent permanent sphincter disturbance.

Lumbar canal stenosis: spinal claudication

Age-related spinal degenerative change leads to osteophyte formation and hypertrophied ligaments which may narrow the lumbar spinal canal and impair the blood supply to the cauda equina. This causes pain, numbness and weakness of the legs on walking which is often confused with vascular intermittent claudication (see p. 210). CT or MRI aids diagnosis. Surgical decompression by laminectomy may be required for the most severe cases.

Cervical degenerative disease

Acute disc prolapse may cause pain and weakness in the nerve distribution in the same way as lumbar disc disease. Most settle with analgesia and a cervical collar but some require surgical decompression.

Chronic cervical spine degeneration causing gradual cord compression results in the more insidious myelopathy. Usually the arms are more affected than the legs. The combination of neck pain with upper motor neuron leg signs suggests cervical cord compression.

MRI is the imaging modality of choice, and surgical decompression may be necessary.

PERIPHERAL NERVE LESIONS

Most disorders are due to trauma or entrapment (Table 22.2). Motor and sensory loss result. Nerve conduction studies allow confirmation of the site of the lesion and whether it is complete (i.e. unlikely to recover) or incomplete. Clean traumatic transections of peripheral nerves may be repaired using microsurgical methods. Entrapments can be released by decompression.

INFECTIONS

Brain abscess

This is usually the result of middle ear/sinus infection or immunosuppression. Symptoms and signs are as for a brain tumour plus a swinging fever and localised tenderness if the abscess is in the spinal canal. Brain abscesses require urgent drainage and long-term antibiotic therapy (with the exception of TB, which may be treated with drugs only).

Table 22.2 Features of common peripheral nerve lesions		
Nerve	**Clinical features**	**Causes**
Facial	Facial weakness	Trauma, parotid surgery, acoustic neuroma, Bell's palsy
Radial	Weakness of wrist/finger extension	Fractures of shaft of humerus
Median	Weakness of opposition of thumb, thenar eminence wasting, numbness of lateral three digits	Carpal tunnel syndrome
Ulnar	'Claw hand', wasting of interossei	Entrapment/trauma around elbow (medial epicondyle)
Femoral	Quadriceps weakness	Groin trauma (iatrogenic)
Sciatic	Pain down back of leg, weakness of foot extension and eversion	Lumbar disc prolapse
Common peroneal	Foot drop	Trauma around head of fibula

Meningitis

This is usually due to contiguous bacterial or viral infection but may result from a CSF leak due to a head injury. Symptoms are headache, neck stiffness, photophobia, fever, depression of consciousness and fits. Diagnosis is confirmed by lumbar puncture and treatment is with high-dose antibiotics. CSF leaks usually close spontaneously.

Section 4

Practical skills in surgery

General operative principles 23

This chapter details many aspects of safe surgical practice common to all specialties.

MINIMISATION OF INFECTION

Fundamental to keeping bacterial contamination to a minimum is theatre design and the concept of asepsis (Box 23.1). Operating theatres are divided into zones including the transfer zone, the clean zone, the sterile zone and the disposal zone. The ventilation system of the operating theatre permits temperature control and humidity, air filtration to remove micro-organisms, movement of air from clean to less clean areas and rapid and non-turbulent air change. Twenty to thirty changes per hour is usual. Infection control is achieved by sterilisation of instruments and equipment, skin preparation and draping of the patient, preparation and clothing of the operating team.

Preparation of the patient's skin

Half of all wound infections are caused by bacteria resident on the skin. At the start of the operation, a wide area of skin is cleaned with povidone-iodine or chlorhexidine solution. Excess body hair is most safely removed by clipping rather than shaving as this can cause minor nicks and scratches in the epithelial surface, bringing bacteria to the surface and increasing the incidence of wound infections. The area of the operation is isolated using surgical drapes.

Scrubbing up

This was formerly a ritualised process but it is now known that brisk scrubbing of the skin can cause micro-trauma to the epidermis and increase the bacterial count. An initial scrub of the fingernails at the start of the operating list is all that is required and this should take 3–5 minutes. All jewellery is removed. The fingers, hands and forearms are cleaned using a medicated detergent such as chlorhexidine gluconate (Hibiscrub) or povidone-iodine (Betadine). Gowns and gloves are donned with a closed technique. Newer gown materials such as GoreTex or close-woven polyester have been developed to overcome the problem of permeability to bacteria but these are expensive. Impervious gowns are essential, however, when operating on high-risk patients. All gloves are now talc-free.

Infected and other high-risk patients

'High-risk' patients, i.e. at high risk to the surgeon and operating staff, comprise patients with hepatitis B or C or HIV. Measures to prevent

> **Box 23.1** Infection control
>
> Sterilisation – a process that involves the complete destruction of all microorganisms, including bacterial spores
>
> Disinfection – reduces the number of viable microorganisms but does not necessarily inactivate viruses and bacterial spores
>
> Cleaning – a process that physically removes contamination but does not necessarily destroy microorganisms e.g. hand-washing (see p. 335).

contamination include impervious gowns and drapes, wearing a plastic apron under the operating gown if any contamination is anticipated, double gloving, eye protection, the avoidance of hand-held needles and use of stapling devices for anastomoses to reduce the risk of needle pricks. It should not be forgotten that prions are a potential source of contamination and, where possible, disposable instruments are now used. In addition, operating room discipline, for example passing needles or scalpels between scrub nurse and surgeon in a transit dish to prevent injury through hand to hand passage, and very careful disposal of all contaminated material at the end of the procedure into plastic bags for incineration is essential. Immunisation against hepatitis B should be mandatory for all healthcare workers exposing themselves to these risks.

The common positions for operations are listed in Table 23.1. Careful positioning is important, not only for access to the operating site, but also for prevention of nerve injuries which can occur as a result of traction pressure; for example, the brachial plexus and ulnar nerve, radial nerve and common peroneal nerve may all be damaged by careless positioning of the patient.

WOUND CLOSURE

This can be achieved in a number of ways:

- suturing
- adhesive tape
- staples/glue
- plastic surgery procedures to close defects which cannot be treated with the above methods, e.g. skin grafting, flap transfer (see Chapter 18).

Needles

- Straight needles are hand-held and are typically used to close skin edges in a subcuticular technique
- Curved needles are usually held in a needle holder but very large needles exist for hand-held use. Curved needles can have cutting or round-bodied points. Cutting edges are designed for closing wounds and can penetrate fascial layers. Round-bodied needles are used for

Table 23.1 Common positions for operations

Position	Use
Supine	Suitable for many operations
Prone	Back surgery
Trendelenburg	
Supine, but patient tilted 30–40° head-down	Pelvic organs; small intestine moves out of the way with gravity
Reverse Trendelenburg	
As Trendelenburg but tilt head-up	Upper abdominal organs
Lloyd-Davies	
As Trendelenburg but with legs abducted and hips and knees slightly flexed and legs in rests	Combined procedures involving abdomen and perineum (usually on distal large bowel)
Lithotomy	
Supine, hips and knees fully flexed, feet in stirrups or straps	Access to anal and perianal regions and external genitalia, vagina and uterine cervix, urethra and bladder (endoscopic)
Lateral	
Extension on right or left side with uppermost arm raised above and in front of head. Centre of table may be angled (broken) to improve access	Operations on kidney and in chest
Bowie	
Prone with flexion at hips	Access to perianal area

suturing bowel, vessels and nerves, and are the needles used in micro-surgery. They are designed to push tissues aside instead of cutting through them.

Sutures

There are two types, absorbable and non-absorbable.

Absorbable
- Broken down by the body by hydrolysis
- No foreign material left in wound once absorbed
- Reduced wound infection rate as organisms not trapped in suture material indefinitely
- May be absorbed too quickly before wound has regained tensile strength
- If broken down too quickly in infected wound, may lead to secondary haemorrhage
- Examples include Vicryl, Dexon, PDS.

Kumar and Clark's Handbook of Medical Management

Non-absorbable

- Retains strength for long periods
- Natural (silk, metal) and synthetic (nylon, Prolene, Ethibond) materials are available
- Promotes foreign body reaction and organisms can become trapped around braided suture materials for long periods of time. Infected sutures often have to be removed for infection to clear completely
- Synthetic monofilament sutures are 'slippy' and harder to handle and tie than the natural braided versions. However, they slide through tissues easier than their braided counterparts, causing less local trauma to tissues.

Staples

- Skin – to close wounds quickly
- Intestine – useful for anastomoses in anatomically difficult locations
- Lung – gives an airtight staggered row of staples in lung resection.

Tapes

These are adhesive strips of tape suitable for minor wounds of the skin. They avoid the puncture marks that can be left by sutures. Adhesive strips are particularly suitable for children, who may be anxious about suture removal.

Adhesives

Tissue glues are also suitable for minor skin wounds and are well tolerated by children as local anaesthetic infiltration is avoided. Tissue glue is not suitable for oozing wounds, and mistakes in alignment of the wound edges cannot be easily rectified.

Dressings

- Protect wound from further contamination
- Absorb discharge from the wound
- Enable the application of substances which may help reduce infection and slough.

After 48 hours, sutured wounds can often be left exposed without undue risk of further contamination. Open wounds left to heal by second intention require continued dressings until healed.

Many different substances have been added to dressings in an attempt to accelerate healing or aid debridement. Except in a few specific circumstances, there is little evidence to show that these specialised and often expensive dressings are any better than attentive and thorough surgical and nursing care.

ACCESS AND COMMON INCISIONS

The correct incision must be made to allow adequate access to the operative field. Important considerations for incisions include sound healing and minimal pain during recovery with minimal complications and a satisfactory cosmetic result. Skin incisions, if possible, should follow the skin cleavage lines as described by Langer (Fig. 23.1). Abdominal incisions are shown in Figure 23.2.

The closure of incisions is important and should be meticulous. Many incisions can be closed with a mass closure employing strong, slowly absorbable sutures. Many surgeons prefer to close wounds in layers.

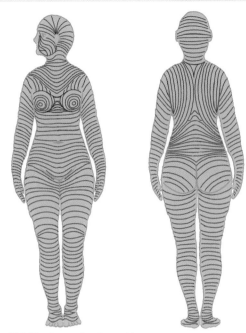

Figure 23.1 Skin cleavage lines (Langer's).

DRAINS

Drains are inserted to evacuate established collections of pus, blood or fluid. They range from simple wicks to low pressure suction applied to tubes. There is controversy concerning their use, with advocates maintaining that drainage of fluid collections removes potential sources of infection, guards against further fluid collections and alerts the surgeon to the presence of leaks or haemorrhage. However, the presence of a drain may increase the chance of infection and can cause damage to nearby structures. In many cases, they are ineffective after a few hours. The different types of drain in common use are shown in Figure 23.3. Most drains in modern surgical practice are closed in nature.

MINIMAL ACCESS SURGERY

The recent proliferation of minimal access surgery techniques has meant that many procedures that were otherwise performed by the open method can now be performed with this technique. The advantages proposed are that the wounds are less painful, surgical tissue trauma is minimised, physiological effects from open operations, for example cooling, excessive handling and drying of internal organs, are avoided. Postoperative

Kumar and Clark's Handbook of Medical Management

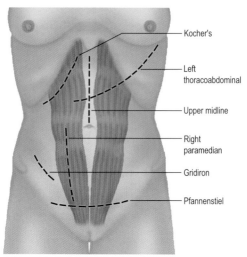

Kocher's

Left
thoracoabdominal

Upper midline

Right
paramedian

Gridiron

Pfannenstiel

Figure 23.2 Types of abdominal incision.

recovery is quicker and there is a reduction in complications related to the wound (dehiscence, incisional hernia and infection). There is also a reduced risk of contact with the patient's blood and postoperative complications such as chest infections and deep vein thrombosis.

Disadvantages of these techniques concern the time that they take to perform, which has a knock-on effect on scheduling and costs, and the special technical expertise necessary to perform them safely. Pneumoperitoneums may compress the diaphragm and lung bases, causing postoperative hypoxia. Not all patients are suitable for this type of procedure and there is a risk of gas embolism although this may be small. Precise control of bleeding is more difficult to achieve but is possible. The extractions of organs may be difficult. Nevertheless, laparoscopic procedures are commonly used for cholecystectomy, oesophageal reflux, gastro-oesophageal malignancy, colonic malignancy, pancreatic malignancy, splenectomy and nephrectomy. Further advances will undoubtedly be made. As part of the informed consent process for any patient undergoing these techniques, it should be emphasised that there is always a risk of converting to an open procedure for technical reasons, anatomical reasons or pathological reasons which the patient must be made to understand.

HAEMOSTASIS

The three main techniques used in stopping haemorrhage are compression, ligation and thermal coagulation. Compression via packing is particularly useful if there is widespread oozing. Ligation may be achieved by the use of haemostats and ligatures, either absorbable or non-absorbable. Ligation may also be achieved by the use of stainless steel clips

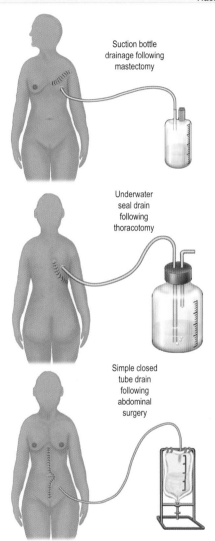

Figure 23.3 Different types of drain.

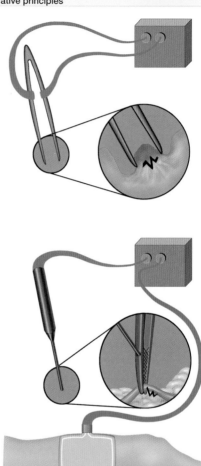

a

b

Figure 23.4 (a) Bipolar diathermy. (b) Unipolar (monopolar) diathermy.

carried on special forceps. Thermal coagulation is achieved by the use of diathermy (Fig. 23.4). The electrical current pathway is either from the point of application through the body of the patient to a large area of contact plate and thence to earth (unipolar) or between two points of the instrument (bipolar). Small blood vessels can be precisely dealt with by either technique. A newer development is the employment of bipolar energy and mechanical compression to reliably seal vessels up to 7 mm in diameter (LigaSure™).

Tourniquets

Many orthopaedic operations on the limb are performed in a bloodless field achieved by the use of a pneumatic tourniquet. Lower pressures are used in patients with little subcutaneous fat and do not exceed 250 mg of mercury for upper limbs and 500 mg of mercury for lower limbs. Reductions in pressures are made for children. The duration of its application must be kept to a minimum by careful planning. One hour is the customary maximum tourniquet time. If the operation is likely to last more than 1½ hours, the tourniquet should be released for 10–15 minutes and bleeding controlled by elevating the limb. Before closing the wound, the tourniquet should be released to ensure that meticulous haemostasis is achieved on completion of the operation. Elevation of the limb for up to 5 days following tourniquet procedures helps to prevent postoperative swelling. Tourniquets should not be used if patients suffer from peripheral vascular disease or sickle cell disease.

FLUOROSCOPY

Many operative procedures require the use of fluoroscopy during the procedure (e.g. an on-table cholangiogram to check arterial patency or to confirm the position of pins and plates in orthopaedics). The same strict safety measures must be taken in terms of protection of the patient and staff with the use of these techniques and thorough understanding of X-rays is mandatory. The patient and staff should be shielded whilst the examinations are being performed. Trained radiographers must control the delivery of the X-rays to the field. Exposure must be the least possible that achieves the desired image. A record must be kept in the patient's notes of the procedure. In the UK, the application of ionising radiation is tightly monitored and subject to regulations set out in The Ionising Radiation (Medical Exposure) Regulations, 2000 (IR(ME)R).

LASERS

The use of laser technology is limited in surgery, although it has a larger place in endoscopic management, for example ablation of gastrointestinal tumours, and in plastic surgery. Precautions must be taken to protect the patient and staff, particularly with respect to prevention of eye damage. The energy generated must be strictly controlled.

Laser treatment for varicose veins is replacing conventional stripping techniques.

Simple practical procedures 24

Most of the following procedures should be within the competence of the junior trainee or senior student. We have selected urinary catheterisation, central venous line insertion, chest drain insertion, venepuncture, blood gas sampling and nasogastric tube insertion, all of which are common day-to-day procedures that can be done on the ward. All procedures require explanation and consent from the patient.

URINARY CATHETERISATION (MALE)

Urinary catheters are made of latex or silicone rubber. A Foley catheter is shown in Figure 24.1. Common sizes for adults are 12–14F and for children 8–10F. The smallest feasible size should be used. You will need:
- catheter
- gloves
- lidocaine gel 0.5%
- antiseptic solution
- pre-prepared catherisation pack
- 10 mL syringe and 10 mL sterile water
- urine drainage bag.

Procedure
- Wash hands and put on gloves
- Arrange everything needed on a sterile tray
- Position the patient flat
- Drape the sterile towels to expose the penis
- Grasp penis with left hand with sterile swab
- Retract the foreskin (if present) and clean glans and urethral opening
- Squeeze lidocaine gel into urethra
- Open catheter, place kidney dish beneath urethral orifice
- Insert catheter with right hand (holding penis with left)
- Peel off plastic wrapping as you go
- Pulling the penis up and then down (Fig. 24.2) will help to traverse the prostatic urethra
- FORCE MUST NOT BE USED
- Insert catheter fully to ensure the balloon is in the bladder
- Check capacity of balloon and after urine is seen inflate 5–10 mL
- Painful? – STOP
- Withdraw catheter to lodge against bladder neck
- Replace foreskin
- Attach drainage apparatus.

Further details of technique may be found in Henry and Thomson, *Clinical Surgery*, 2005, Chapter 11.

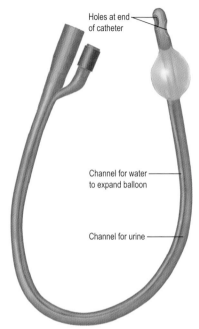

Figure 24.1 A Foley urinary catheter.

CENTRAL VENOUS LINE INSERTION – INTERNAL JUGULAR VEIN

Many patients needing a central venous line insertion are quite unwell and unable to tolerate lying flat. Get everything ready before you put them into this position. The bed must be at 15° head-down tilt at the point of insertion of the needle. There are two methods for the internal jugular vein – high and low. The high method is shown in Figure 24.3. This procedure can result in serious complications (pneumothorax, carotid artery damage, haematoma) and should be done by, or under supervision of, an experienced doctor. It is common to utilise ultrasound to aid placement, as recommended in NICE guidelines, 2002.

Procedure

- If the patient is conscious, infiltrate the skin and proposed route of insertion with local anaesthetic at the level of the thyroid cartilage lateral to the carotid artery
- Open the CVP pack and flush all parts with heparinised saline
- Check the guidewire and practise advancing this
- Flush the needle and syringe to be used for cannulation with heparinised saline

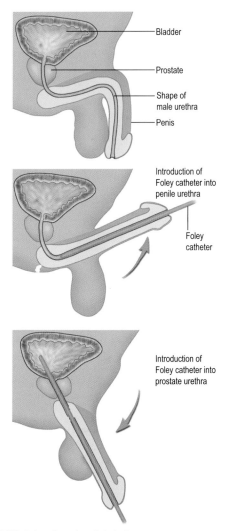

Bladder

Prostate

Shape of
male urethra

Penis

Introduction of
Foley catheter into
penile urethra

Foley
catheter

Introduction of
Foley catheter into
prostate urethra

Figure 24.2 Technique for male catheterisation.

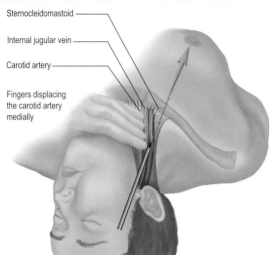

Sternocleidomastoid

Internal jugular vein

Carotid artery

Fingers displacing
the carotid artery
medially

Figure 24.3 The approach used for cannulation of the internal jugular vein.

- Make a small incision at the entry site
- Insert the needle and when deep to skin aspirate as you advance until venous blood is seen in the syringe
- Detach syringe and insert wire and introducer into end of needle
- Never apply force
- When wire is halfway inserted withdraw needle
- Dilate the track with dilator
- Remove dilator and insert central line over the wire, remove wire
- The tip should lie in the superior vena cava
- Aspirate to check free flow of venous blood
- Suture line in place and check CXR to confirm position.

Details of the procedure can be found in Chapter 11 of Henry and Thomson, *Clinical Surgery*, 2005.

INSERTION OF A CHEST DRAIN

Chest drains are inserted for a variety of reasons including pneumothorax, haemothorax, pleural effusion (large) and empyema.

You will need:

- between a 22F and 32F chest drain without the trocar
- 20 mL lidocaine 0.5%
- underwater seal apparatus and bottle
- sterile water
- scalpel
- small and large artery forceps
- heavy silk suture (e.g. silk 0)
- waterproof adhesive tape.

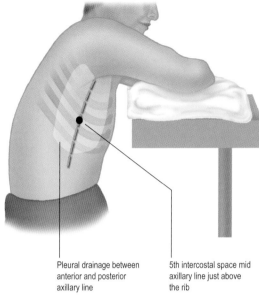

Pleural drainage between anterior and posterior axillary line

5th intercostal space mid axillary line just above the rib

Figure 24.4 The position of a patient during pleural drainage/chest drain.

Procedure

- Position patient as shown in Figure 24.4
- Check physical signs, correct side and CXR
- Mark site of insertion (it is surprisingly easy to lose your bearings once the drapes are on). This will also ensure that you insert the drain at the same site you anaesthetised: the patient will appreciate this
- Prepare skin and drape
- Anaesthetise skin and proposed track down to rib
- Make a 2–3 cm incision at marked site
- Bluntly dissect down to superior border of rib with artery forceps
- Continue to parietal pleura (more local anaesthetic may be needed)
- Puncture pleura, insert finger and sweep any adhesion within pleural space
- Guide drain down track with forceps and finger to pleural cavity
- Advance drain gently into cavity over your finger using Spencer Wells forceps to grasp the tip on the drain (DO NOT USE THE TROCAR THAT COMES WITH THE DRAIN), then attach underwater drainage apparatus
- Close incision and tie to chest drain (Fig. 24.5)
- Insert purse string suture
- Check drain is working
- Secure connection between drain and underwater drainage apparatus

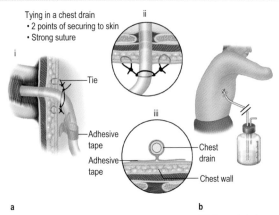

Figure 24.5 (a) Technique for securing of a chest drain. (b) Chest drain in position with underwater drainage.

- Dress and tape drain to chest wall
- Check CXR.

Removal
- Undo dressing, release suture from drain
- Ask patient to take two large breaths and hold (Valsalva)
- Remove drain quickly and tie purse string
- Dress with occlusive dressing
- Concern? Check CXR.

VENOUS ACCESS

Choosing the site

Common sites for cannulation in the body are shown in Figure 24.6. Avoid arteriovenous fistulas, poor venous or lymphatic drainage (see Box 24.1). Avoid the foot if possible. Types of venous cannula are shown in Table 24.1.

You will need:
- clean gloves
- tourniquet
- appropriate needle
- adhesive tape
- 5 mL syringe
- saline flush
- appropriate infusion
- bandage, cotton wool and tape.

Procedure
- Choose the site
- Place tourniquet above site
- Swab area of insertion with alcohol

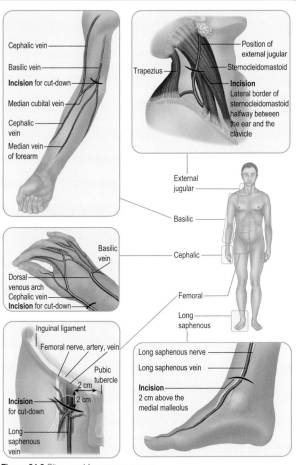

Figure 24.6 Sites used for venous access.

- Advance needle until flashback of blood is seen
- Advance plastic cannula over needle into vein
- Remove tourniquet
- Elevate arm, remove needle, apply fixing dressing
- Connect infusion.

VENOUS CUT-DOWN

This method should only be used if it is not possible to obtain venous access elsewhere (Fig. 24.7).

> **Box 24.1** Aids to location of a vein
>
> Use a sphygmomanometer and inflate it to below diastolic
>   pressure to allow arterial inflow but not venous escape of blood
> Hang the patient's arm over the edge of the bed or couch and tap
>   (not slap) the back of the hand to cause venodilatation
> Immerse the forearm in a bowl of warm water for 2 minutes and
>   place the tourniquet before removing the hand from the bowl
>
> **Additional hint**
>
> In paediatrics or for anxious adults, EMLA cream can be helpful;
> apply over selected veins and cover with an occlusive dressing;
> wipe off after 45–60 minutes. After EMLA cream has been applied,
> veins do not distend as easily

Table 24.1 Types of intravenous cannula

Size	Colour	Use
22G	Blue	Children, small fragile veins
20G	Pink	Low-flow intravenous infusions such as analgesia, sedation
18G	Green	Intravenous fluids and drugs
16G	Yellow	Blood transfusions
14G	Grey	Rapid fluid administration – shock, major trauma and GI bleeding
12G	Brown	Rapid fluid administration – shock, major trauma and GI bleeding

- Prepare skin and drape (e.g. long saphenous vein)
- Infiltrate the area with lidocaine 0.5%
- Make a transverse incision (2.5 cm)
- Bluntly dissect vein from all other structures and free for 2 cm
- Ligate distal end of vein, sling proximal end
- Make a small transverse incision in vein
- Thread 14G (grey) cannula and tie proximally to secure
- Attach infusion
- Close wound and apply dressing.

BLOOD GAS SAMPLING

The vessels of choice are the radial, femoral and brachial in that order. The sites for puncture of the femoral and brachial arteries are shown in Figures 24.8 and 24.9. For radial artery cannulation always check the patency of the ulnar artery first (Allen test).

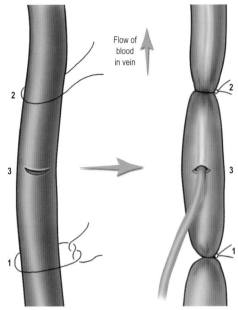

Figure 24.7 Technique for venous cut-down.

You will need:
- 2 mL syringe (often available in a special pack)
- heparin 1000 U/mL
- alcohol swab
- sterile cotton wool/swabs
- syringe cap
- ice.

Procedure

- Draw up 0.5 mL heparin to lubricate whole syringe (prefilled syringes are commonly available)
- Expel completely
- Hold syringe 60–90° to skin, advancing slowly with slight negative pressure
- If syringe fills spontaneously, artery has been entered
- If no filling, artery may have transfixed; withdraw slowly and you may get lucky!
- Obtain 2 mL and cap immediately
- Remove syringe and compress puncture site for 3 minutes (longer if patient anti-coagulated)
- Empty syringe of all bubbles and take immediately for analysis. (Place on ice if not immediately possible.)

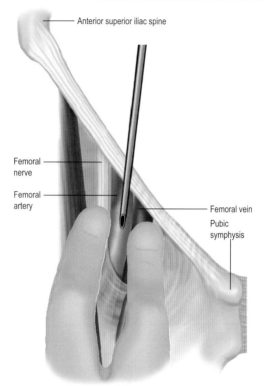

Figure 24.8 The position of the femoral artery in the groin.

INSERTION OF A NASOGASTRIC TUBE

You will need:
- non-sterile gloves
- nasogastric tube 10–16F
- drainage bag
- lubricant
- glass of water.

Procedure

- Inform patient of procedure
- Sit patient upright with chin on chest
- Lubricate tube (preferably cold) and insert into one nostril gently
- Aim backward towards the occiput and advance tube
- Ask patient to swallow when patient feels tube is at back of pharynx

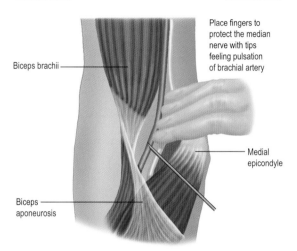

Lateral aspect of
antecubital fossa

Medial aspect of
antecubital fossa

Place fingers to
protect the median
nerve with tips
feeling pulsation
of brachial artery

Biceps brachii

Medial
epicondyle

Biceps
aponeurosis

Figure 24.9 The site for puncture of the brachial artery.

- Give sips of water to aid the above
- If coughing or cyanosis develops, withdraw tube to hypopharynx
- After insertion, check tube is not coiled in back of mouth
- Auscultate below left costal margin and quickly inject air into tube –
  a loud borborygmus confirms position
- Test aspirate with litmus paper for acidity
- Secure nasogastric tube with tape to nose
- Final position is checked by CXR.

Important steps in common operations

Generic checklist for any surgical procedure (as formalised in the WHO surgical checklist, see Chapter 1)

- **Correct patient**
- **Correct surgeon**
- **Correct anaesthetist**
- **Correct assistant**

- Correct diagnosis?
- Correct and complete preoperative tests (e.g. FBC, U&E, ECG)
- ASA grading?
- Correct radiology?
- Group and save/cross-match/clotting
- Hepatitis B, C, HIV status known? MRSA?
- Informed consent
- Type of anaesthetic (general, regional block, local infiltration)
- DVT prophylaxis (stockings, LMWH)
- Site marked clearly by surgeon
- Correct operation?
- Position on table
- Skin preparation (NB allergies)
- Surgeon and staff protection
- Diathermy precautions
- Drapes
- Incision
- Detailed operative notes
- Detailed postoperative instructions to medical and nursing staff.

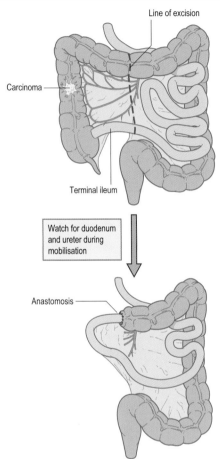

Line of excision

Carcinoma

Terminal ileum

Watch for duodenum
and ureter during
mobilisation

Anastomosis

Figure 25.1 Right hemicolectomy for carcinoma of the right colon.

- Incision (midline, transverse, laparoscopic)
- Preliminary laparotomy, laparoscopy
- Determine operability, stage of disease
- Lateral to medial dissection (open procedure)
- Medial to lateral dissection (laparoscopic)
- Ligation of major vessels
- Radical excision of lymphatic vessels
- Division of terminal ileum, transverse colon
- Ensuring of good blood supply to cut ends
- Anastomosis of ileum to colon (sutures or staples)
- Close mesenteric defect
- Washout with cytocidals (water, Betadine)
- Closure in layers/mass
- No drain
- Return patient in satisfactory condition to recovery unit
- Postoperative instructions.

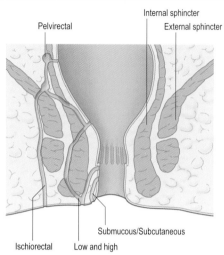

Figure 25.2 Fistula in ano.

- EUA, sigmoidoscopy, proctoscopy and biopsy
- Identify track(s) using probes, dye or H_2O_2
- High or low?
- Relation to internal/external sphincter
- Low – lay open from external to internal opening
- Curettings to histology
- High – consider laying open lower track
- High – consider seton suture (tight/loose)
- Further options: Fibrin glue insertion, Fistula plug, Mucosal advancement flap
- AND SEEK SENIOR HELP IF IN DOUBT.

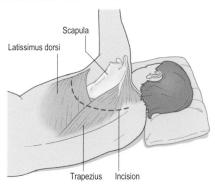

Figure 25.3 Posterolateral thoracotomy.

- Site incision according to operation
- Ribs are not counted until after muscle division
- Upper lobe fourth/fifth interspace, lower lobe sixth/seventh interspace
- Incision from midline skirting scapula to mid-axillary line
- Divide muscles (two layers) – preserve serratus anterior
- Count ribs, divide periosteum and strip with rougine
- Resect 2–3 cm of rib posteriorly
- Warn anaesthetist, open pleura along length
- Insert rib spreader
- Proceed to operation
- Close over two drains (apical and basal)
- Close intercostal layers
- Close muscle layers and skin
- Attach underwater drains and re-expand lung
- Return patient in stable condition to recovery.

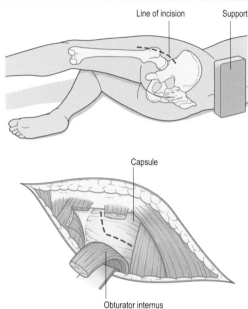

Figure 25.4 Total hip replacement.

- Expose hip joint (anterior/posterolateral)
- Open capsule and dislocate joint
- Remove femoral head at angle corresponding to prosthetic shaft
- Ream the femur with broaches
- Prepare acetabulum by excising all soft tissue
- Enlarge acetabulum to fit cup
- Drill keying holes to provide grip for cement
- Fit acetabular cup
- Insert femoral component into femur
- Reduce the joint
- Close wound in layers with drainage.

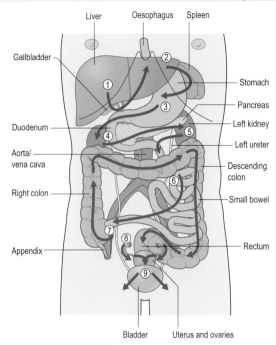

Figure 25.5 General laparotomy.

Identify structures in order as indicated by arrows:
- liver, gallbladder, right kidney
- oesophagus, fundus of stomach, spleen
- body of stomach, duodenum, pancreas, left kidney
- lesser sac, transverse colon
- small bowel, appendix, aorta, ureters
- ascending colon
- descending colon, sigmoid, upper rectum
- uterus, fallopian tubes, ovaries and bladder
- pouch of Douglas.

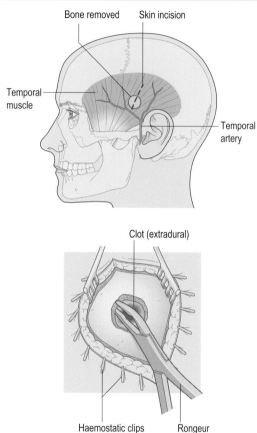

Figure 25.6 Exploratory burr hole for closed cerebral trauma.

- Mark site of pterion burr hole after shaving (3 cm above mid-zygomatic point)
- Incise the scalp and use self-retaining retractor
- Free the pericranium
- Use Hudson brace with perforator
- Move perforator gently to engage outer table and proceed to turn
- Apply firm pressure to the head to prevent lateral movement
- Exchange perforator for burr when inner table has been reached
- Ensure burr hole is vertical
- Stop bleeding from diploe with bone wax
- If extradural haematoma is found, proceed to further burr hole to the limit of the haematoma
- Consider craniectomy
- Remove blood clot carefully, wash with saline
- Secure bleeding point on middle meningeal artery
- Check for subdural haematoma
- Meticulous haemostasis
- Close wounds.

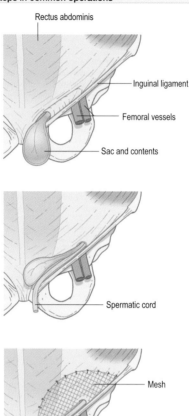

Rectus abdominis

Inguinal ligament

Femoral vessels

Sac and contents

Spermatic cord

Mesh

Figure 25.7 Strangulated inguinal hernia.

- Skin crease incision
- Open external oblique
- Preserve ilioinguinal nerve if possible
- Identify sac and contents, spermatic cord in male
- Carefully separate cord from sac
- Avoid damage to vas and testicular artery
- Open sac; check viability of bowel/omentum
- Resect if necessary
- Reduce contents
- Perform herniotomy
- Attach mesh to transversalis fascia
- Close in layers.

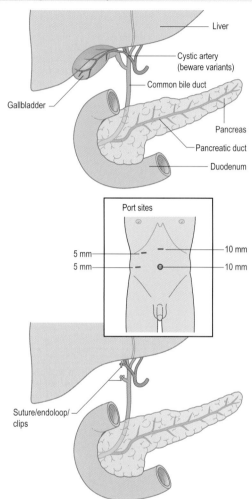

Figure 25.8 Laparoscopic cholecystectomy.

Liver

Cystic artery
(beware variants)

Common bile duct

Gallbladder

Pancreas

Pancreatic duct

Duodenum

Port sites

5 mm

5 mm

10 mm

10 mm

Suture/endoloop/
clips

- Check all instruments, cameras, insufflators, screens etc.
- Preset CO_2 insufflator to 13–15 mm
- Insert first port (Hasson technique/Veress needle)
- Laparoscopy, identify gallbladder, cystic duct and artery
- Beware anatomical variations
- Dissect Calot's triangle, cystic duct and artery
- Operative cholangiogram (if indicated)
- Securely clip artery and duct
- Dissect gallbladder from liver bed (meticulous haemostasis)
- Remove gallbladder via epigastric port using a retrieval bag
- Repeat laparoscopy for damage/bleeding from other sites
- Drain optional
- Check port sites for bleeding
- Close all port site wounds carefully
- Return patient to recovery unit in a stable condition.

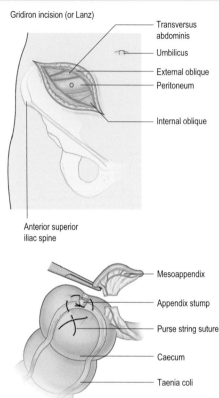

Gridiron incision (or Lanz)

Transversus abdominis

Umbilicus

External oblique

Peritoneum

Internal oblique

Anterior superior iliac spine

Mesoappendix

Appendix stump

Purse string suture

Caecum

Taenia coli

Figure 25.9 Appendicectomy (NB often done laparoscopically).

- Gridiron/Lanz incision
- Identify caecum/appendix
- If normal, examine small bowel for Meckel's, Crohn's disease
- If normal, inspect tubes/ovaries
- Deliver caecum/appendix
- Divide appendicular artery and appendix mesentery
- Clamp base of appendix
- Ligate base, remove appendix for histology
- Purse string to bury stump
- Irrigate pelvis and aspirate if peritonitis
- Close wound in layers – no drain.

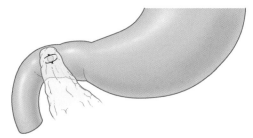

Figure 25.10 Perforated duodenal ulcer.

- Upper midline incision
- Laparotomy
- Identify perforation
- Duodenal? Omental plug (mobilise omentum first)
- Gastric? Excise ulcer, send to pathology, close gastrotomy
- Meticulous lavage with saline
- Drain (optional)
- Close in layers.

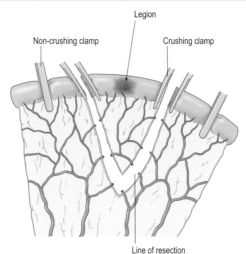

Figure 25.11 Small bowel resection.

- Laparotomy
- Identify pathology (stricture, perforation, tumour, Crohn's)
- Identify arterial arcades
- Resect appropriate segment
- Avoid bowel spillage (use soft bowel clamps) Ensure good vascularity of cut ends
- No tension
- Anastomose ends (extramucosal interrupted using 2-O/3-O Vicryl)
- Start at mesenteric border
- Close mesenteric defect (avoid damaging arcades)
- Lavage with saline
- Close wound
- No drain.

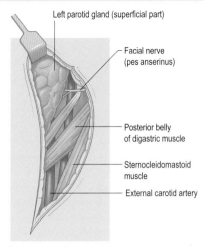

Left parotid gland (superficial part)

Facial nerve
(pes anserinus)

Posterior belly
of digastric muscle

Sternocleidomastoid
muscle

External carotid artery

Figure 25.12 Superficial parotidectomy.

- S-shaped incision behind the ear and down sternomastoid
- Expose the main trunk of the facial nerve
- Reflect the parotid tissue superficial to the facial nerve
- Follow the nerve and branches until parotid border is reached
- Meticulous dissection (ideally with nerve stimulator) Tie the parotid duct
- Remove the gland
- Meticulous haemostasis
- Drain
- Close wound.

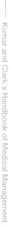

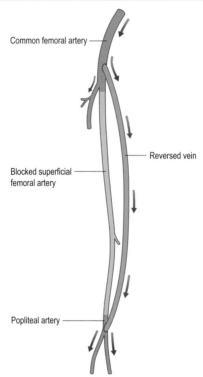

Common femoral artery

Reversed vein

Blocked superficial femoral artery

Popliteal artery

Figure 25.13 Femoropopliteal bypass.

- Expose common, superficial and profunda arteries
- Expose long saphenous vein (LSV) at termination
- Continue down the limb, isolating saphenous vein to knee
- Divide all LSV tributaries and free the vein
- Expose popliteal artery
- Detach the vein at this level and reverse
- Ensure adequate length of vein
- Decide upper and lower levels for anastomosis
- Make subcutaneous tunnel for LSV
- Give heparin
- Anastomose LSV to popliteal artery
- Check forward and back flow
- Anastomose LSV to common/superficial femoral artery
- Check arteriogram and flow
- Close wounds and check pulses.

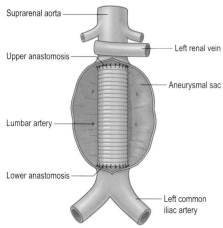

Figure 25.14 Aortic aneurysm repair (straight tube).

- Midline incision
- Reflect root of mesentery to duodenojejunal flexure
- Identify neck of aneurysm and common iliac arteries (limited dissection)
- Give heparin and clamp aorta and common iliacs
- Incise aneurysm and oversew lumbar artery origins
- Oversew middle sacral artery and inferior mesenteric
- Inlay Dacron graft to upper end (beware renal artery origins)
- Test upper anastomosis
- Suture lower end to iliacs or bifurcation
- Check back bleeding and debris is flushed out before releasing clamps
- Close aneurysm sac
- Close wounds.

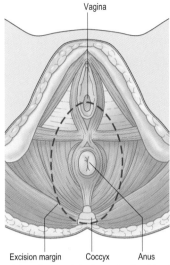

Figure 25.15 Perineal dissection for abdomino-perineal excision (APE).

- Insert purse string around anus
- Incision as shown
- Deepen incision to reach coccyx
- Develop posterior plane to meet abdominal operator
- Deepen lateral dissection to include levators
- Anteriorly in male develop plane between rectum and prostate
- In female posterior wall of vagina may be included in specimen
- Meet perineal operator for lateral ligaments
- Deliver specimen through the perineum
- Ensure meticulous haemostasis
- Close the wound over an abdominal drain
- Deliver the patient in a stable condition to recovery unit.

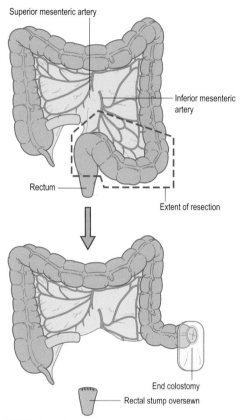

Superior mesenteric artery

Inferior mesenteric artery

Rectum

Extent of resection

End colostomy

Rectal stump oversewn

Figure 25.16 Hartmann's procedure.

- Full laparotomy, determine nature of pathology
- Consider resection and anastomosis with covering ileostomy
- Mobilise left colon to sacral brim
- Identify ureters, preserve spleen
- Ligate inferior mesenteric, preserve left colic artery
- Ligate inferior mesenteric vein
- NB: Radical excision if carcinoma
- Resect specimen (may be very difficult)
- Oversew/staple rectal stump
- Left iliac fossa trephine
- Construct colostomy
- Lavage with cytocidal agent
- Drain to pelvis
- Close wound.

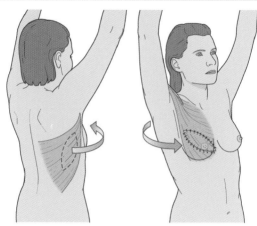

Figure 25.17 Latissimus dorsi flap.

- Mastectomy may be done at the same time
- Preoperative marking of skin paddle (different formats)
- Fashion skin paddle and define margin of latissimus dorsi muscle
- Inferior and medial border of muscle divided
- Dissect the latissimus dorsi from surrounding tissues
- Identify neurovascular bundle (deep surface) (separate axillary incision may be used)
- Transpose paddle to breast pocket.

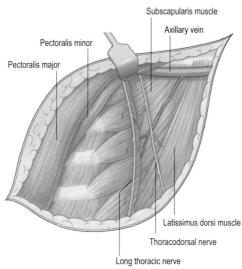

Subscapularis muscle

Axillary vein

Pectoralis minor

Pectoralis major

Latissimus dorsi muscle

Thoracodorsal nerve

Long thoracic nerve

Figure 25.18 Mastectomy and axillary clearance.

- Transverse incision to include nipple
- Fashion skin flaps to incorporate the whole breast
- Avoid buttonhole injury to the skin
- Dissect breast from fascia over pectoralis major
- Meticulous haemostasis
- Irrigate with cytocidal solution
- Open the axilla through a separate incision
- Clean the axillary vessels taking all fat, lymph nodes and fascia
- Lateral thoracic vessels and intercostal brachial nerve are taken
- Avoid damage to brachial plexus and long thoracic nerve of Bell
- All nodes to the apex of the axilla are cleared
- Haemostasis
- Close both wounds over suction drains.

Arterial supply   Venous drainage

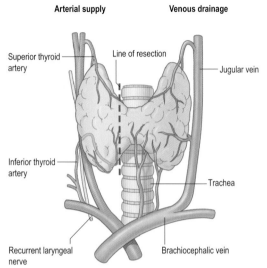

Figure 25.19 Thyroid lobectomy.

- Kocher's incision
- Divide the strap muscles of the neck
- Divide and ligate the middle thyroid veins
- Draw down upper pole and identify superior thyroid vessels
- Ligate superior vessels and draw down upper pole
- Dissect lateral areolar tissue and identify inferior thyroid artery
- Identify recurrent laryngeal nerve (RLN)
- Tie inferior thyroid artery in continuity lateral to the RLN
- Divide inferior thyroid vein
- Mark line of section with haemostats
- Cut isthmus cleanly to trachea and dissect lobe free
- Remove lobe and oversew thyroid remnant to trachea
- Meticulous haemostasis
- Repair strap muscles
- Close wound over a drain.

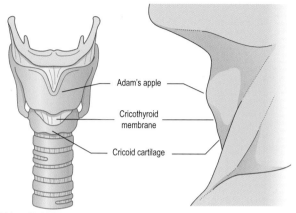

Figure 25.20 Emergency cricothyroidectomy.

For patients with respiratory distress in whom tracheal intubation has failed. It is a temporising measure, maximum duration 72 h (formal tracheostomy if continued surgical airway required) due to the danger of permanent laryngotracheal damage, particularly in children.

- *Very brief* sterilization/drape (e.g. chlorhexidine spray)
- Palpate the cricothyroid membrane (soft area just below the thyroid cartilage and just above the cricoid cartilage)
- Make a 2-cm transverse incision directly over the cricothyroid membrane (stabilising the trachea)
- Palpate the membrane directly and make a further 1-cm incision in the membrane itself
- Insert tracheal tube and secure to the skin (tape/suture)
- Connect to ventilator/ambubag.

Section 5

Self-assessment

QUESTIONS

1. Bone metastases:

(a) occur in less than 5% of patients with malignant disease

(b) 10% of patients with bone metastases develop pathological fractures

(c) breast cancer is commonly a cause of bone metastases in women

(d) are detected by X-ray early in the disease process

(e) osteosclerotic lesions are caused by prostate cancer

2. Osteosarcomas:

(a) affect the epiphyses of long bones

(b) are commonly seen around the knee and proximal humerus

(c) can result in pulmonary metastases

(d) are exclusively a disease of younger people

(e) classical radiology demonstrates a sunburst appearance due to soft tissue involvement

3. Rheumatoid arthritis:

(a) is a disease primarily of the synovium

(b) is associated with the HLA antigens

(c) occurs more often in men

(d) the hands, elbows, knees and cervical spine are the commonest joints involved

(e) extra-articular manifestations occur in 20% of patients

4. **The oesophagus:**

(a) is 25 cm in length

(b) passes behind the left main bronchus in the thorax

(c) is lined by stratified squamous epithelium in the upper two-thirds

(d) is lined by transitional epithelium in the lower third

(e) drains all of its blood into the azygos and hemiazygos veins

5. **The axilla contains:**

(a) the cords of the brachial plexus

(b) the superior thoracic artery

(c) the latissimus dorsi muscle in its medial wall

(d) the thoracodorsal nerve in its posterior wall

(e) the long thoracic nerve in its medial wall

6. **The common bile duct:**

(a) lies in the free edge of the greater omentum

(b) lies posterior to the portal vein

(c) lies to the right of the hepatic artery

(d) may open independent of the pancreatic duct into the duodenum

(e) lies posterior to the first part of the duodenum

7. **The following structures pass beneath the inguinal ligament:**

(a) the tendon of psoas major

(b) the femoral branch of the genitofemoral nerve

(c) the long saphenous vein

(d) the superficial epigastric vein

(e) the superficial femoral artery

8. **Concerning carcinoid tumours:**

(a) the appendix is the commonest primary site

(b) gastric carcinoid tumours produce little 5-hydroxyindoleacetic acid

(c) liver metastases can result in the carcinoid syndrome

(d) octreotide scintigraphy may identify primary and secondary lesions

(e) plasma chromogranin B may be increased

9. **Hashimoto's thyroiditis:**

(a) is an acute suppurative disease of the thyroid

(b) presents as a solitary thyroid nodule

(c) may cause hypothyroidism

(d) anti-thyroglobulin and anti-microsomal antibodies may be increased

(e) increases the risk of thyroid lymphoma

10. **Overwhelming post-splenectomy infection (OPSI):**

(a) is usually due to unencapsulated bacterial infection

(b) is commonly caused by *Streptococcus pneumoniae*

(c) may have a mortality of over 50%

(d) the risk of infection can be reduced with pneumococcal and haemo-philus vaccination

(e) penicillin antibiotic prophylaxis should be considered for all patients

11. **Concerning colonic polyps:**

(a) juvenile rectal polyps are adenomatous in nature

(b) metaplastic polyps are malignant

(c) the risk of malignancy is higher in villous rather than tubular adenomas

(d) villous adenomas occasionally cause hypokalaemia

(e) all patients with untreated familial adenomatous polyposis eventually develop colorectal carcinoma

12. Prostate cancer:

(a) affects 50% or more of men over the age of 80

(b) mostly presents with symptoms of bladder outflow obstruction

(c) a PSA concentration of greater than 10 ng/mL is suggestive of the diagnosis

(d) 80% of tumours are androgen independent

(e) historically orchidectomy treated the disease

13. Hodgkin's lymphoma:

(a) often presents as painless inguinal lymphadenopathy

(b) 50% of patients have splenomegaly

(c) nodular sclerosing type has the best prognosis

(d) stage 3 disease has lymphadenopathy confined to one side of the diaphragm

(e) with modern radiotherapy, stage 1 disease has an excellent 5-year survival

14. A varicocele:

(a) is a dilatation of the testicular artery

(b) is more common on the left

(c) may be associated with a left renal tumour

(d) may be associated with infertility

(e) requires surgery at all times

15. Ultrasound:

(a) can diagnose breast lumps in women aged 35 or older

(b) diagnoses gallstones

(c) diagnoses bone metastases

(d) diagnoses pelvic abscess in a postoperative patient

(e) may detect deep venous thrombosis in any patient with a painful swollen leg

16. Sterilisation of surgical equipment may include the use of:

(a) ethylene oxide

(b) gamma irradiation

(c) autoclave

(d) alcohol

(e) chlorhexidine

17. A postoperative pulmonary embolus:

(a) is always associated with chest pain

(b) is always associated with an abnormal chest X-ray

(c) may be confirmed using a ventilation/perfusion (VQ) scan

(d) may be confirmed on ECG changes

(e) is most commonly seen between 2 and 5 days postoperatively

18. A 5-year-old child is brought to A&E after being hit by a car travelling at 40 mph and sustaining multiple injuries:

(a) the initial priorites for resuscitation are the same as for an adult patient

(b) the correct volume of fluid for initial resuscitation is a bolus of 20 mL/kg

(c) plain X-rays must be avoided because of the risks of ionising radiation

(d) IV access secured via an intraosseous nail cannot be used to transfuse blood

(e) rib fractures indicate a high likelihood of lung contusion and intra-abdominal injury

19. Serum alpha-fetoprotein is increased in:

(a) acute hepatitis

(b) hepatocellular carcinoma

(c) neuroblastoma

(d) teratomas

(e) bladder carcinoma

20. *Clostridium tetani:*

(a) is a Gram-positive rod

(b) is sensitive to penicillin

(c) is widely prevalent in the soil and environment

(d) causes gas gangrene

(e) the toxin acts on the post-synaptic membrane of inhibitory nerve fibres

21. Diathermy:

(a) works by using a direct current

(b) the frequencies used range from 200–400 kHz

(c) the cutting effect is produced using a continuous output

(d) a coagulation effect is produced by using a continuous output

(e) can cause serious burns in patients

22. Ulcerative colitis:

(a) arises in the rectum and spreads proximally

(b) chronic inflammatory polyps occur in 20% of patients

(c) approximately 50% of patients develop total colitis

(d) systemic manifestations include large joint polyarthropathy

(e) overall, 8–10% of patients will develop colonic cancer after 25 years of total colitis

23. Meckel's diverticulum:

(a) occurs in 2% of the population

(b) is found on the antimesenteric border of the small intestine

(c) consists of mucosa without a muscle coat

(d) can present as a gastrointestinal haemorrhage

(e) can cause intestinal obstruction

24. Paget's disease of the bone:

(a) may present with a pathological fracture

(b) causes an increase in serum calcium and phosphate

(c) causes a decrease in serum alkaline phosphatase

(d) malignant change occurs in 10% of patients

(e) the commonest malignant tumour in patients with Paget's disease is a chondrosarcoma

25. The following local factors predispose to poor wound healing:

(a) poor blood supply

(b) localised infection/contamination

(c) previous radiotherapy

(d) haematoma

(e) poor suturing

26. The following systemic factors predispose to anastomotic leakage:

(a) anaemia

(b) dyslexia

(c) jaundice

(d) steroid therapy

(e) severe COPD

27. Prophylactic antibiotic therapy:

(a) works best when the antibiotic is given before the incision is made

(b) requires that the antibiotic be continued until all drains are removed

(c) should always include vancomycin to counter MRSA

(d) is indicated when prosthetic material is being implanted

(e) does not increase incidence of bacterial resistance

28. An abscess:

(a) is a collection of pus

(b) close to the surface causes pain, swelling and erythema

(c) usually requires antibiotics

(d) usually requires drainage

(e) is commoner in left handed medical students

29. Cellulitis:

(a) presents as diffuse reddening of skin and surface tissues

(b) is usually seen with pus formation

(c) does not cause enlargement of local lymph nodes

(d) requires urgent extensive debridement

(e) requires IV antibiotics

30. Necrotising fasciitis:

(a) is colloquially known as the killer superbug

(b) is surprisingly difficult to diagnose in the early stages

(c) causes only mild discomfort

(d) is caused by *Strep. viridans*

(e) requires extensive debridement which may be disfiguring

31. Tuberculosis:

(a) can cause ascites

(b) can cause aneurysms

(c) never occurs in affluent areas

(d) rarely occurs in AIDS

(e) requires radical excision

32. When caring for a severely injured hypotensive patient:

(a) 100% oxygen should not be given

(b) a central line is essential

(c) wide-bore peripheral cannulae are the best IV access

(d) the cervical spine should be immobilised after transfusion

(e) external bleeding should be ignored

33. Hypotension in a severely injured patient:

(a) is always due to hypovolaemic shock

(b) always requires O negative blood

(c) may be due to neurogenic shock

(d) may be due to tension pneumothorax

(e) may be due to cardiac tamponade

34. Shock:

(a) has different causes which require different treatments

(b) always requires 100% oxygen

(c) typically is associated with normal or alkaline blood pH

(d) is sometimes best treated with a cup of tea and a cigarette

(e) may have more than one cause in a single patient

35. Extensive burns:

(a) are more painful when full thickness

(b) are associated with minimal fluid loss

(c) require tetanus prophylaxis

(d) may be associated with airway injury

(e) do not require treatment in a specialist unit

36. Presenting problems of cancer may include:

(a) pain from a bone metastasis

(b) DVT

(c) weight loss

(d) cough

(e) anaemia

37. Epididymo-orchitis:

(a) is characterised by a cough impulse

(b) is easily confirmed by fine-needle aspiration

(c) requires percussion tenderness for diagnosis

(d) in a young man may be confused with testicular torsion

(e) is relieved by vigorous exercise

38. Ruptured abdominal aortic aneurysm may cause:

(a) pain in the epigastrium

(b) pain in the back

(c) pain in the left flank

(d) pain in the right flank

(e) pain in the lower abdomen

39. Patients with ruptured aortic aneurysm:

(a) are always hypotensive

(b) may have had pain for several hours

(c) always have a pulsatile expansile mass in the abdomen

(d) rarely have femoral pulses

(e) are usually female

40. A painful tender irreducible hernia:

(a) is not strangulated

(b) is incarcerated

(c) should be repaired on the next elective list

(d) may contain non-viable bowel

(e) cannot cause intestinal obstruction

41. Small bowel obstruction:

(a) is usually due to adhesions or hernia

(b) does not cause vomiting or constipation

(c) can cause gangrenous bowel

(d) mostly resolves with nasogastric decompression and IV fluids

(e) invariably needs laparotomy

42. Large bowel obstruction:

(a) is usually due to adhesions or hernia

(b) must be distinguished from pseudo-obstruction before treatment

(c) usually requires surgery to resect the obstruction

(d) is seldom caused by colorectal cancer

(e) does not require rectal examination

43. Upper GI haemorrhage:

(a) may cause pale stool which smells of almonds

(b) typically causes raised blood urea due to partial digestion of blood

(c) is an indication for urgent upper GI endoscopy

(d) does not cause haematemesis

(e) may be caused by aspirin

44. Suspected appendicitis:

(a) is easy to distinguish from salpingitis

(b) should be treated with antibiotics if the diagnosis is unclear

(c) in females does not require a pregnancy test

(d) usually causes an elevated WBC

(e) may cause leucocytes in the urine

45. Haematuria:

(a) when painless is less likely to be due to bladder cancer

(b) requires investigation of the upper urinary tract to exclude renal carcinoma

(c) should be ignored if the patient is taking warfarin

(d) is associated with Leriche syndrome

(e) may result from a systemic rather than urological disease

46. Prostate cancer:

(a) affects women as well as men

(b) metastasises to lymph nodes and lungs but not bones

(c) is less common in men who have had more than three children

(d) can be treated with surgery, radiotherapy, hormones and chemotherapy

(e) can be screened for using serum PSA levels

47. Urethral trauma:

(a) is often present in patients with pelvic fractures

(b) is suggested by urine at the meatus and a low riding prostate on PR

(c) requires immediate catheterisation

(d) is a contraindication for retrograde urethrography

(e) should be detected in the ATLS primary survey

48. Osteoarthritis of the hip:

(a) typically causes pain in the buttock

(b) causes a raised ESR

(c) may shorten the limb

(d) affects women more than men

(e) characteristically results in loss of joint space, osteophytes and bone cysts

49. A fracture:

(a) heals more rapidly in a child than in an adult

(b) of a rib in a child is less likely to be associated with internal injury than in an adult

(c) of the pelvis causes internal blood loss of several litres

(d) should be reduced to an anatomical position before being immobilised

(e) which fails to heal should be considered for homeopathy

50. Varicose veins:

(a) are mainly a cosmetic problem and rarely cause real symptoms

(b) regress in pregnancy

(c) can cause leg ulcers

(d) should be removed if the patient has had a DVT

(e) can be treated with angioplasty

51. The causes of a mass in the right iliac fossa include:

(a) Crohn's disease

(b) ectopic pregnancy

(c) carcinoma of the caecum

(d) myelofibrosis

(e) ovarian carcinoma

52. **A young male builder falls 5 metres off scaffolding onto a paved surface. On arrival in A&E he is unconscious and hypotensive, with blood coming from his nose and left ear:**

(a) antibiotics should be given immediately to prevent meningitis

(b) skull X-rays are mandatory

(c) he should be assumed to have sustained a cervical spine injury

(d) the hypotension is a sign of serious head injury

(e) a pelvic X-ray is indicated

53. **An elderly female falls off her chair at her residential nursing home. On arrival, she smells of alcohol, and a hip flask of whisky is found in her handbag. She is drowsy, her speech is slurred and she asks to be left alone to sleep:**

(a) she should be shaken and told to wake up

(b) she might have a cervical spine injury

(c) a CT scan is indicated to look for subdural haematoma

(d) alcohol should be forbidden to all elderly nursing home residents

(e) a 12-lead ECG is indicated

54. **Two days after her hen night, a 23-year-old medical student presents to A&E with severe epigastric pain. She can remember little of the celebrations, but recalls experimenting with cocktails:**

(a) the differential diagnosis includes gastritis, pancreatitis and duodenal ulcer

(b) her serum amylase comes back at 1300. Arterial blood gases are indicated

(c) her fiancé should be advised to cancel the wedding

(d) abdominal ultrasound is indicated to look for gallstones

(e) she should be fluid restricted

55. **A 70-year-old retired stockbroker is referred by his GP with a diagnosis of intermittent calf claudication. His popliteal and pedal pulses are absent and ABPIs are 0.5 bilaterally. Duplex scanning confirms severe stenoses of both superficial femoral arteries:**

(a) he should stop smoking

(b) he should be started on a statin, even though his fasting cholesterol is low

(c) he must be advised to rest when the pain starts

(d) he is likely to go on to develop critical limb ischaemia

(e) he should undergo femoropopliteal bypass grafting as soon as possible

1. F T T F T	20. T T T T F	39. F T F F F
2. F T T F T	21. F F T F T	40. F F F T F
3. T T F T T	22. T T F T T	41. T F T T F
4. T T T F F	23. T T F T T	42. F T T F F
5. T T F T T	24. T F F F F	43. F T T F T
6. F F T T T	25. T T T T T	44. F F F T T
7. T T F F F	26. T F T T T	45. F T F F T
8. T F T T F	27. T F F T F	46. F F F T T
9. F F T T T	28. T T F T F	47. T F F F F
10. F T T T T	29. T F F F T	48. F F T T T
11. F F T T T	30. T T F F T	49. T F T T F
12. T T T F T	31. T T F F F	50. F F T F F
13. F F F T T	32. F F T F F	51. T F T F T
14. F T T T F	33. F F T T T	52. F F T F T
15. F T F T T	34. T T F F T	53. F T T F T
16. T T T F F	35. F F T T F	54. T T F T F
17. F F T T F	36. T T T T T	55. T T F F F
18. T T F F T	37. F F F T F	
19. T T T T F	38. T T T T T	

Index